Computational Vision and Medical Image Processing

Computational Methods in Applied Sciences

Volume 19

Series Editor

E. Oñate
International Center for Numerical Methods in Engineering (CIMNE)
Technical University of Catalunya (UPC)
Edificio C-1, Campus Norte UPC
Gran Capitán, s/n
08034 Barcelona, Spain
onate@cimne.upc.edu
www.cimne.com

For other titles published in this series, go to
www.springer.com/series/6899

João Manuel R. S. Tavares · R. M. Natal Jorge
Editors

Computational Vision and Medical Image Processing

Recent Trends

Springer

Editors
João Manuel R. S. Tavares
Universidade do Porto
Fac. Engenharia
Departamento de Engenharia Mecânica
Rua Dr. Roberto Frias
4200-465 Porto
Portugal
tavares@fe.up.pt

R. M. Natal Jorge
Universidade do Porto
Fac. Engenharia
Departamento de Engenharia Mecânica
Rua Dr. Roberto Frias
4200-465 Porto
Portugal
rnatal@fe.up.pt

ISSN 1871-3033
ISBN 978-94-007-3420-3 ISBN 978-94-007-0011-6 (eBook)
DOI 10.1007/978-94-007-0011-6
Springer Dordrecht Heidelberg New York London

Softcover reprint of the hardcover 1st edition 2010

Printed on acid-free paper

Springer is part of Springer Science+Business Media (www.springer.com)

Preface

Nowadays, computational methodologies of signal processing and imaging analysis for 2D, 3D and even 4D data are commonly used for various applications in society. For example, Computational Vision systems are progressively used for surveillance tasks, traffic analysis, recognition process, inspection purposes, human-machine interfaces, 3D vision and deformation analysis.

One of the main characteristics of the Computational Vision domain is its inter-multidisciplinary nature. In fact, in this domain, methodologies of several other fundamental sciences, such as Informatics, Mathematics, Statistics, Psychology, Mechanics and Physics are regularly used. Besides this inter-multidisciplinary characteristic, one of the main rationale that promotes the continuous effort being made in this area of human knowledge is the number of applications in the medical area. For instance, statistical or physical procedures on medical images can be used in order to model the represented structures. This modelling can have different goals, for example: shape reconstruction, segmentation, registration, behavioural interpretation and simulation, motion and deformation analysis, virtual reality, computer-assisted therapy or tissue characterization.

The main objective of the ECCOMAS Thematic Conferences on Computational Vision and Medical Image Processing (VIPimage) is to promote a comprehensive forum for discussion on the recent advances in the related fields and try to identify areas of potential collaboration between researchers of different sciences.

This book contains the extended versions of nineteen papers selected from works presented at the second ECCOMAS thematic conference on Computational Vision and Medical Image processing (VIPimage 2009), which was held at the Engineering Faculty of the University of Porto, Portugal. It gathers together the state-of-the-art on the subject of Computational Vision and Medical Image processing contributing to the development of these knowledge areas and showing new trends in these fields.

The Editors would like to take this opportunity to thank to the European Community on Computational Methods in Applied Sciences, the Portuguese Association of Theoretical, Applied and Computational Mechanics, the University of Porto, all sponsors, all members of the International Scientific Committee and to all Invited Lecturers and Authors.

Faculty of Engineering
University of Porto, Portugal

João Manuel R.S. Tavares
R.M. Natal Jorge

Contents

Automatic Segmentation of the Optic Radiation Using DTI in Healthy Subjects and Patients with Glaucoma

Ahmed El-Rafei, Tobias Engelhorn, Simone Waerntges, Arnd Doerfler, Joachim Hornegger, and Georg Michelson

Abstract The complexity of the diffusion tensor imaging (DTI) data and the interpersonal variability of the brain fiber structure make the identification of the fibers a difficult and time consuming task. In this work, an automated segmentation system of the optic radiation using DTI is proposed. The system is applicable to normal subjects and glaucoma patients. It is intended to aid future glaucoma studies. The automation of the system is based on utilizing physiological and anatomical information to produce robust initial estimates of the optic radiation. The estimated optic radiation initializes a statistical level set framework. The optic radiation is segmented by the surface evolution of the level set function. The system is tested using eighteen DTI-datasets of glaucoma patients and normal subjects. The segmentation results were compared to the manual segmentation performed by a physician experienced in neuroimaging and found to be in agreement with the known anatomy with 83% accuracy. The automation eliminates the necessity of medical experts' intervention and facilitates studies with large number of subjects.

Keywords Diffusion tensor imaging (DTI) · Segmentation · Optic radiation · Glaucoma

---

A. El-Rafei (✉) and J. Hornegger
Pattern Recognition Lab, Department of Computer Science and Erlangen Graduate School in Advanced Optical Technologies (SAOT), Friedrich-Alexander University Erlangen-Nuremberg, Germany
e-mail: ahmed.el-rafei@informatik.uni-erlangen.de; joachim.hornegger@informatik.uni-erlangen.de

T. Engelhorn and A. Doerfler
Department of Neuroradiology, Friedrich-Alexander University Erlangen-Nuremberg, Germany
e-mail: Tobias.Engelhorn@uk-erlangen.de; Arnd.Doerfler@uk-erlangen.de

S. Waerntges
Department of Ophthalmology, Friedrich-Alexander University Erlangen-Nuremberg, Germany
e-mail: Simone.Waerntges@uk-erlangen.de

G. Michelson
Department of Ophthalmology and Interdisciplinary Center of Ophthalmic Preventive Medicine and Imaging, Friedrich-Alexander University Erlangen-Nuremberg, Germany
e-mail: Georg.Michelson@uk-erlangen.de

J.M.R.S. Tavares and R.M.N. Jorge (eds.), *Computational Vision and Medical Image Processing: Recent Trends*, Computational Methods in Applied Sciences 19,
DOI 10.1007/978-94-007-0011-6_1, © Springer Science+Business Media B.V. 2011

1 Introduction

Glaucoma is the second leading cause of blindness in the world. The damage caused by glaucoma is irreversible. The progression of glaucoma can be delayed significantly if glaucoma is detected in early stages. Therefore, methods for screening, early diagnosis and better understanding of glaucoma and its progression are needed.

Most of the existing ophthalmic imaging modalities focus on imaging the eye in general and the retina in particular. Many studies were performed to investigate the correlation between glaucoma and retinal changes such as retinal nerve fiber atrophy, retinal vessels, and optic disk changes [16, 24, 33]. The human visual system does not only consist of the eye but it extends through the optic nerve into the brain till it reaches the visual cortex. The visual pathway consists of four neurons. The first neuron (photoreceptors) and the second neuron (amacrine and bipolar cells) lie within the retina in the eye. The third neuron (retinal ganglion cells) connects the retina with the brain. The axons of the third neuron leave the eye and end in the lateral geniculate nucleus where the fourth neuron begins. The axons of the fourth neuron neuronal cells carry the visual information and end up in the visual cortex V1. The intracerebral part of the fourth neuron is called the optic radiation. Correlation has been shown between glaucoma and neurodegeneration in parts of the visual system such as the optic nerve and the optic radiation [13, 18]. Nevertheless, the effect of glaucoma on the visual system is not yet fully addressed.

In this work we aim to provide a system for the automatic identification of the optic radiation in normal subjects and glaucoma patients. DTI is used to segment the optic radiation as it is the only imaging modality that allows for the identification of white matter fiber structure non-invasively. This is a step towards a better understanding of the changes caused by glaucoma in this part of the human visual system.

In the last two decades, diffusion tensor imaging has received a lot of attention due to its clinical applications [11,39]. Diffusion weighted imaging (DWI) is proven to be effective in the early diagnosis and investigation of cerebral diseases such as acute stroke [21, 28] and abscesses [7]. Diffusion tensor derived parameters such as the degree of anisotropy and the diffusivity parameters are used to evaluate certain neural pathologies and were found to be sensitive to white matter abnormalities. Axonal degeneration evaluated by diffusion tensor derived parameters were evident in the temporal lobe for mild cognitive impairment and Alzheimer disease patients [8, 17]. In relapsing-remitting multiple sclerosis, reduced anisotropy accompanied by increased isotropic apparent diffusion was observed correlating to the signature of Wallerian degeneration [15]. The process of normal human brain maturation and aging affecting the structure of myelin were monitored using DTI [19, 34]. Furthermore, DTI is the only imaging modality that allows tracking the white matter fibers *in vivo* and non-invasively [3,29], and it enables the construction of an atlas of white matter fibers in the human brain [27, 36].

As the basis of the DTI, diffusion weighted imaging (DWI) is based on magnetic resonance signal attenuation due to restricted diffusion of water molecules along the diffusion weighting gradient field [23,26]. The cell membranes and myelin sheaths surrounding the axons act as a guided tube for the diffusion process within the axons. Thus, they limit the diffusion in the direction perpendicular to the axons while increasing the average diffusion along the axons resulting in a highly anisotropic diffusion. The diffusion of water like molecules can be used to identify fiber orientation which coincide with the average diffusion direction and so for to depict the microstructure of the brain white matter. The diffusion tensor relies on modeling the diffusion process within a specified volume by a Gaussian process (probability density function of molecular displacement) with a zero mean. The tensor corresponds to the covariance matrix of the diffusion process and is calculated from the diffusion weighted images. Analyzing the diffusion tensor gives significant diffusion related information such as the main diffusion direction within the specified volume and the degree of anisotropy. This information is used to identify the white matter structure within the brain.

Many algorithms were proposed for the identification of white matter tracts using DTI. The dominant category is tractography which is based on following the fiber tracts using the principal diffusion direction [4,9,22,35]. Tractography suffers from accumulated tracking errors during the tracking process. Connectivity maps were suggested [20,30,38] to explore the probability of connectivity between a selected seed point and the surrounding neighborhood which can be the whole brain. Connectivity maps have the main disadvantage that they do not provide a straightforward plausible visualization of the results. The split and merge technique [6] attempts to avoid the accumulated errors of tractography by identifying short tracts. This is done by limiting the tracking process to a certain number of steps. Then it provides a degree of membership of the extracted tracts belonging to the same fiber. The practicality of the split and merge technique is limited because it does not describe the complete fiber pathway. Segmentation approaches of DTI [14,37,40] are more suitable for identifying coherent densely packed bundles of axons. The segmentation avoids the drawbacks from both connectivity maps and tractography such as tracking accumulation errors and the need to merge the individual tracts to obtain fiber bundles. Furthermore, it relies on the coherency within the fiber bundle of interest. Therefore, the segmentation approach is adopted in this work.

Most of the proposed white matter identification algorithms did not address the problem of algorithm initialization. They rely on the interaction of medical experts to select the seed points or the region of interest of the desired fiber tracts in tractography algorithms or the initialization of the segmentation engines to include the desired fiber bundle. This is a rather time consuming process and might limit the number of subjects in clinical studies that involves DTI. The proposed segmentation system utilizes the physiological properties of the optic radiation to produce a robust initialization of the proposed segmentation system in both healthy and pathological subjects with glaucoma.

The proposed segmentation system utilizes the complete tensor information in a statistical level set frame work that takes into account the Riemannian nature of the tensor space. It consists of the following steps: First the diffusion tensor and related anisotropy measures are calculated from the diffusion weighted images. The calculated diffusion tensor data is transformed into the Log-Euclidean framework and interpolated as presented in Sect. 2. In Sect. 3, DTI-data is regularized to increase the coherency of the optic radiation fiber bundle before obtaining an initial estimate of the optic radiation using thresholding and connectivity analysis. The midbrain is initially identified using a similar analysis to that of the optic radiation. The system extends the statistical level set framework for DTI segmentation developed by Lenglet et al. [25] to be used in conjunction with the Log-Euclidean dissimilarity distance as detailed in Sect. 4. The optic radiation is obtained by iteratively evolving the level set function. Finally, the output from the level set framework is adjusted based on the relative location of the optic radiation and the midbrain. Section 5 contains the results and discussion. The conclusion and future work are stated in Sect. 6.

2 Interpolation in the Space of Diffusion Tensors

The diffusion tensors are 3×3 symmetric positive definite matrices. The space of diffusion tensors is a convex subset of the vector space $\mathbb{R}^{(3)^2}$ and does not form a vector space using a Euclidean metric [12, 31]. Thus, the decomposition of the diffusion tensors could result in non-physical negative eigenvalues. Moreover, the Euclidean framework is not appropriate for dealing with tensors because the swelling effect where the average of diffusion tensors with the same determinant could result in a mean tensor with a larger determinant [10]. Thus, the Riemannian nature of the tensor space should be taken into account when handling the diffusion tensors.

Dissimilarity metrics have been proposed to overcome the limitations of the Euclidean framework. An information theoretic measure called the J-divergence is proposed [37] based on the symmetric Kullback–Leibler divergence between two Gaussian probability densities. The J-divergence distance between two diffusion tensors is given by (1) and is affine-invariant. i.e. the distance between tensors is independent from affine transformation of the coordinate system.

$$d_J\left(\mathsf{DT}_1, \mathsf{DT}_2\right) = \frac{1}{2}\sqrt{tr\left(\mathsf{DT}_1^{-1}\mathsf{DT}_2 + \mathsf{DT}_2^{-1}\mathsf{DT}_1\right) - 2n} \tag{1}$$

where $tr(.)$ is the matrix trace operator, n is the size of the diffusion tensors DT_1 and DT_2.

Fletcher and Joshi [12] deal with the space of diffusion tensors as a curved manifold called Riemannian symmetric space. They derived a Riemannian metric on the space of diffusion tensors. The proposed metric accounts for the positive definiteness constraint ensuring that the eigenvalues of the diffusion tensors are positive.

The Log-Euclidean framework proposed by Arsigny et al. [2] provides a Riemannian framework to deal with the diffusion tensors. Using this framework, the diffusion tensor space of positive semi definite matrices can be transformed into the space of symmetric matrices, i.e. a vector space. Additionally, all operations performed on vectors can be used on the vector form of the diffusion tensor in the Log-Euclidean framework. Despite the similar properties of the Log-Euclidean metric compared to other dissimilarity distances such as the J-divergence distance or the Riemannian metric by Fletcher and Joshi, the Log-Euclidean framework has a similar behavior but at a significantly lower computational cost as it involves vector operations.

The Log-Euclidean distance d_{LE} between tensors DT_1 and DT_2 is defined by

$$d_{LE}\left(\mathsf{DT}_1, \mathsf{DT}_2\right) = \parallel \log\left(\mathsf{DT}_1\right) - \log\left(\mathsf{DT}_2\right) \parallel \tag{2}$$

where log is the matrix logarithm.

The interpolation of the DTI-data is necessary in order to obtain a volumetric identification of the optic radiation. Interpolation of diffusion tensors in the Euclidean framework results in the non-physical swelling effect. This effect is also evident in interpolating two tensors, where it is possible to get an interpolated tensor that has a larger determinant than the original tensors. Interpolation in the Log-Euclidean framework avoids the swelling effect at a computationally attractive cost. The diffusion tensor DT is interpolated trilinearly at non-grid position x as the Log-Euclidean weighted sum of N tensors in a neighborhood of the non-grid position x. The weights are inversely proportional to the spatial distance between the non-grid position and the locations of the tensors in the neighborhood. The used interpolation formula is

$$\mathsf{DT}\left(x\right) = \exp\left(\frac{\sum_{i=1}^{N} w_i\left(x\right)\log\left(\mathsf{DT}\left(x_i\right)\right)}{\sum_{i=1}^{N} w_i\left(x\right)}\right) \tag{3}$$

where exp and log are the matrix exponential and logarithm respectively.

3 Initial Estimation of the Optic Radiation and the Midbrain

In this step, the optic radiation and the midbrain are initially identified. The diffusion tensor data is first regularized by applying Perona–Malik diffusion filtering [32]. Perona and Malik proposed an anisotropic diffusion filtering technique based on controlling the heat flow according to the presence of edges. The edges are estimated by the magnitude of the image gradient. The diffusivity is non-linearly inversely proportional to the magnitude of the image gradient, i.e. the diffusion is limited at large image gradients indicating the presence of an edge with high probability. Conversely, the diffusion is increased at small image gradients. The evolution of the image $f(x, y, z) : \Omega \subset \mathbb{R}_3 \rightarrow \mathbb{R}$ is governed by the following diffusion equation

$$\frac{\partial f}{\partial t} = div(\rho(\|\nabla f\|)\nabla f) \tag{4}$$

where $\rho = e^{-\frac{\|\nabla f\|^2}{k}}$ or $\rho = \frac{1}{1+\|\nabla f\|^2/k}$.

The diffusion filtering is applied to the transformed Log-Euclidean vector form of the diffusion tensors componentwise. Regularization is performed to reduce the noise and to increase the coherency inside the fiber bundles while preserving the boundaries of the fiber bundles.

The initial estimation of the optic radiation is based on the fact that the main fiber bundle of the optic radiation is dominated by diffusion in the anterior–posterior direction. Moreover, the optic radiation is a massive fiber bundle which occupies a significant part of the brain white matter. This physiological information regarding the diffusion direction and the size of the optic radiation gives a unique discrimination of the optic radiation from other fiber bundles.

The diffusion tensor is analyzed using eigen-decomposition as given by (5) to determine the principal diffusion direction (PDD) which is the eigenvector of the tensor corresponding to the largest eigenvalue. The degree of anisotropy is determined by the fractional anisotropy (FA) [5] and is calculated from the diffusion tensor eigenvalues using (6).

$$\mathsf{DT} = \begin{bmatrix} \mathbf{e_1} \; \mathbf{e_2} \; \mathbf{e_3} \end{bmatrix} \cdot \begin{pmatrix} \lambda_1 & 0 & 0 \\ 0 & \lambda_2 & 0 \\ 0 & 0 & \lambda_3 \end{pmatrix} \cdot \begin{bmatrix} \mathbf{e_1} \; \mathbf{e_2} \; \mathbf{e_3} \end{bmatrix}^T \tag{5}$$

where $\mathbf{e_1}$, $\mathbf{e_2}$ and $\mathbf{e_3}$ are the diffusion tensor eigenvectors corresponding to λ_1, λ_2 and λ_3 which are the diffusion tensor eigenvalues in a descending order.

$$FA = \sqrt{\frac{3}{2}} \frac{\sqrt{(\lambda_1 - \lambda)^2 + (\lambda_2 - \lambda)^2 + (\lambda_3 - \lambda)^2}}{\sqrt{\lambda_1^2 + \lambda_2^2 + \lambda_3^2}} \tag{6}$$

where $\lambda = \frac{(\lambda_1+\lambda_2+\lambda_3)}{3}$.

The image is analyzed on a voxel by voxel basis to create a binary mask representing the initial optic radiation. The vector corresponding to principal diffusion direction has three components: the anterior–posterior component (AP), the left-right component (LR), and the superior–inferior (SI) component. The three components at each voxel are compared and the foreground voxels of the binary mask are selected to have a dominant AP component. The foreground voxels satisfies the inequalities given by (7) that is the AP-component is greater than a user specified factor (AP_{thres}) of the sum of the other two components and a fractional anisotropy value greater than 0.2. The fractional anisotropy threshold is used to ensure the coherency of the fiber bundle and that the partial volume effects [1] are avoided. In DTI the partial volume effects are the result of the limitation of the tensor model to describe complex fiber situations such as fiber crossing or branching situations within a voxel. This results in a reduced fractional anisotropy and a misleading principal diffusion direction. The remaining voxels that do not satisfy the selection criteria are set as the background of the binary image.

$$AP > AP_{thres} \times (LR + SI) \quad \text{and} \quad FA > 0.2 \tag{7}$$

A three dimensional six-neighborhood connectivity analysis is performed on the binarized image. Connected objects are determined and the optic radiation is initially identified as the largest object dominated by diffusion in the anterior–posterior direction. This estimation will be used in the segmentation step as an initialization of the level set.

The analysis applied to estimate the optic radiation is similarly applied to identify the midbrain. The analysis takes into account that the midbrain is characterized by diffusion in the superior–inferior direction and is located in the neighborhood of the centers of the axial brain slices. The relative position of the estimated midbrain to the optic radiation will be used in a later step to refine the segmentation of the optic radiation.

4 Segmentation Using a Statistical Level Set Framework

The segmentation is performed in two steps. First, the DTI is segmented using a statistical level set framework. The initially estimated optic radiation as described in Sect. 3 is used as the initial surface. Second, the results from the level set framework are adjusted based on anatomical information between the midbrain and the optic radiation.

We extend the surface evolution framework developed by Lenglet et al. [25] to work with the Log-Euclidean dissimilarity measure given in (2). In the following we present briefly the mathematical formulation of the level set framework in the case of the Log-Euclidean framework. For further details see [2,25]. The diffusion tensor $\mathsf{DT}(x)$ at voxel x is mapped to the space of symmetric matrices and transformed into a vector form $\beta(x)$ using the following mapping:

$$\beta(x) = vec\,(\log(\mathsf{DT}(x))) \tag{8}$$

where *vec* is the mapping of the 3×3 symmetric matrices to the corresponding six dimensional vectors with adjusted relative weights of the matrix coefficients according to the similarity distance used.

Using the notation in (8), the mean, covariance matrix and Gaussian distribution of diffusion tensors can be defined as:

$$\mu_{LE} = \frac{1}{N}\sum_{i=1}^{N} \beta(x_i) \tag{9}$$

$$Cov_{LE} = \frac{1}{N-1}\sum_{i=1}^{N} (\beta(x_i) - \mu_{LE})(\beta(x_i) - \mu_{LE})^T \tag{10}$$

$$P_{LE}(\beta(x_i)) = \frac{1}{\sqrt{(2\pi)^6 |Cov_{LE}|}} \times \exp\left(-\frac{(\beta(x_i) - \mu_{LE})^T \, Cov_{LE}^{-1} (\beta(x_i) - \mu_{LE})}{2}\right) \quad (11)$$

The spatial gradient of the diffusion tensor in the vector space is given by

$$|\nabla\beta(x)|^2 = \frac{1}{2}\sum_{k=1}^{3}\sum_{s=\pm 1} tr\Big((\beta(x) - \beta(x + s \times i_k)) \times (\beta(x) - \beta(x + s \times i_k))^T \Big) \quad (12)$$

where i_k, k =1, 2, 3 denotes the canonical basis of $\mathbb{R}_3$. $s \in \{1, -1\}$ denotes the forward and backward approximations of the gradient, tr is the trace of a matrix.

The idea of the statistical surface evolution is to seek the optimal partitioning of the tensor image (β in the Log-Euclidean case) by maximizing a posteriori frame partition probability for the diffusion tensor image with image domain Γ. This is done in a level set framework, where the image is partitioned into three regions based on a level set function ϕ: inside Γ_{in}, outside Γ_{out} or on the boundary Γ_B. The boundary is defined as the zero-crossing of ϕ. The probability distributions of the tensors inside (p_{in}) and outside (p_{out}) regions are modeled by Gaussian distributions on tensors using (11). The partition probability is given by

$$P(\beta|\phi) = \prod_{x\in\Gamma_{in}} p_{in}(\beta(x)) \prod_{x\in\Gamma_{out}} p_{out}(\beta(x)) \prod_{x\in\Gamma_B} p_b(\beta(x)) \quad (13)$$

The boundary probability distribution p_b is selected to have a value of approximately one for high gradients of the diffusion tensors (using (12) for gradient calculations) and a value of approximately zero for low gradients as the following relation indicates:

$$p_b(\beta(x)) \propto \exp(-g(|\nabla\beta(x)|)) \quad (14)$$

where $g(u) = 1/(1 + u^2)$.

This leads to the energy minimization formulation:

$$E(\phi, \mu_{LE_{in/out}}, Cov_{LE_{in/out}}) = \nu \int_{\Gamma} \delta(\phi)|\nabla\phi| dx + \int_{\Gamma} \delta(\phi)|\nabla\phi| g(|\nabla\beta(x)|) dx - \int_{\Gamma_{in}} \log(p_{in}(x)) dx - \int_{\Gamma_{out}} \log(p_{out}(x)) dx \quad (15)$$

where δ is the Dirac delta function.

The following Euler–Lagrange equation is used to evolve the level set function

$$\frac{\partial \phi}{\partial t} = \delta(\phi)\left((\nu + g(|\nabla \beta(x)|))\, div\left(\frac{\nabla \phi}{|\nabla \phi|}\right) + \frac{\nabla \phi}{|\nabla \phi|} \cdot \nabla g(|\nabla \beta(x)|) + \log\left(\frac{p_{in}}{p_{out}}\right)\right) \tag{16}$$

The level set function in (16) is evolved iteratively to obtain the desired segmentation and the statistics are updated after each iteration.

The output from the level set framework contains the fiber bundle of the optic radiation and additional bundles connected to it such as traces of the optic tract. The reason for this is that the optic tract is connected to the optic radiation and the diffusion direction is also anterior–posterior in the connection area so traces of the optic tract are segmented as well. The lateral geniculate nucleus (LGN) connects the optic radiation to the optic tract and is located laterally to the midbrain. Therefore, the LGN position can be used to separate the optic tract from the optic radiation. Based on this anatomical information, the segmented region is automatically adjusted in order to confine the segmentation results to the part representing the optic radiation. The relative position of the segmented optic radiation to the midbrain is used instead of the relative position to the LGN because the midbrain is larger, more reliable to identify and in turn more robust. The midbrain is previously identified in the initialization step. The plane corresponding to the anterior boundary of the segmented midbrain is selected as the separation level between the optic radiation and the optic tract. The segmentation results anterior to the selected plane are eliminated leaving the optic radiation and approximately eliminating the part corresponding to the optic tract.

5 Results and Discussion

Eighteen subjects were examined by ophthalmologists and categorized into two age matched groups. The first group represents the subjects that were diagnosed with primary open angle glaucoma and the other group represents the normal subjects. The glaucoma group contains nine subjects with a mean $\pm$ standard deviation age of 66 $\pm$ 11.8 years with seven females and two males, while the normal group contains nine subjects with a mean$\pm$standard deviation age of 67.1 $\pm$ 8.1 years with six females and three males. Further ophthalmological and neuroradiological examinations were performed and did not provide indications of microangiopathy or irregularly developed optic radiation.

The subjects were scanned using a 3T-MRI scanner. The diffusion weighted images were acquired using a single-shot, spin echo, echo planar imaging (EPI) as an imaging sequence with repetition time (TR) 3400 ms, echo time (TE) 93 ms, field of view (FoV) $230 \times 230\,\text{mm}^2$, acquisition matrix size of 128×128 reconstructed to

256×256, seven signal averages, and partial Fourier acquisition of 60%. The axial slices have a thickness of 5 mm and 1 mm interslice spacing. Diffusion weighting were applied with a maximal b-factor of 1000 s/mm^2 along 15 icosahedral directions complemented by one scan with b = 0. The diffusion tensors were calculated from the measured diffusion weighted images along with fractional anisotropy, eigenvectors and eigenvalues on a voxel by voxel basis.

The segmentation system is applied to the DTI-datasets and the optic radiation in the two groups is identified. The left side of Fig. 1 shows the final segmented optic radiation on non-diffusion weighted axial slices with b = 0 from two sample subjects. The color coded fractional anisotropy representation of the DTI-data is demonstrated on the right side of the figure.

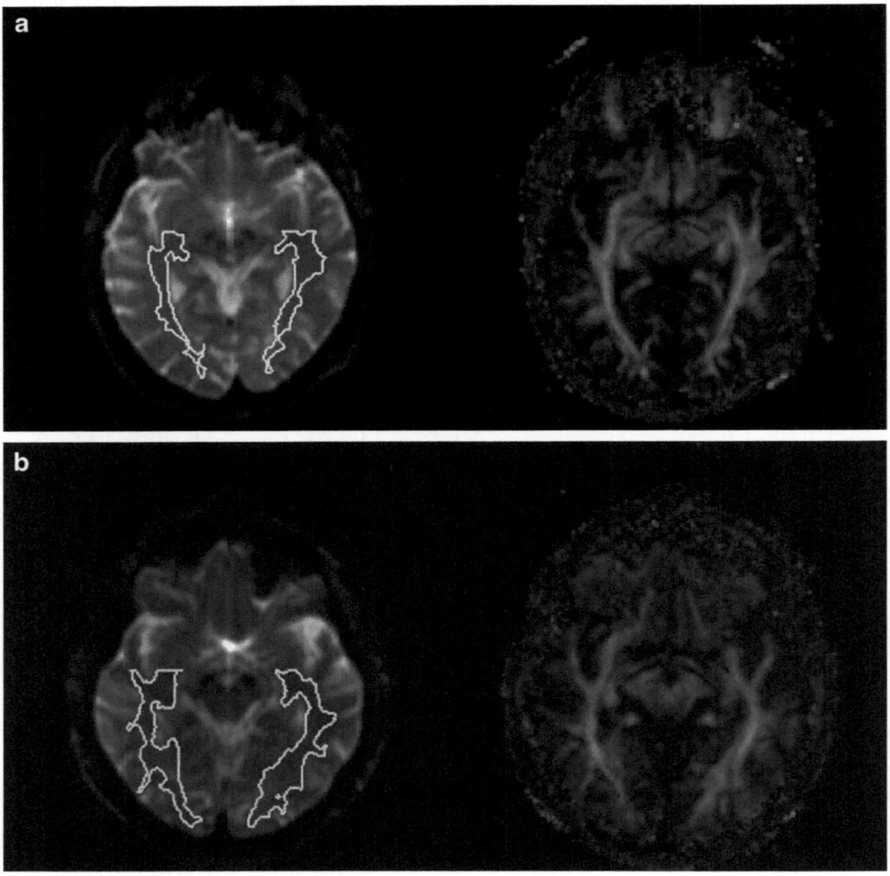

Fig. 1 Segmentation of the optic radiation in two sample subjects shown on a non-diffusion weighted image (b = 0) on the *left* side. (**a**) Segmented optic radiation on a sample subject. (**b**) Segmented optic radiation on a second sample subject. The color coded fractional anisotropy image is shown on the *right* side. The main fiber bundle of the optic radiation and the lateral geniculate nucleus (LGN) of the visual pathway are clearly identified. The examples indicate the fiber structure variability of the optic radiation among different subjects

The segmentation results were evaluated by comparing them with a manual segmentation of the optic radiation main fiber bundle performed by a physician experienced in neuroimaging. The accuracy of the segmentation system is calculated as the percentage of the overlap volume between the automatic segmentation results and the manual segmentation to the total volume of the manually segmented optic radiation. The segmentation accuracy is summarized in Table 1. The accuracy of the segmentation results is 82.71% for the normal subjects and 82.76% for the glaucoma group.

The analysis of the segmentation errors showed that the errors typically occur in the region where the optic radiation branches in the proximity of the visual cortex. Due to the branching of the optic radiation in this region, the incoherency increases and the anterior–posterior direction is no longer the dominating diffusion direction which is the principal segmentation assumption for the proposed algorithm. Another source of errors is the relatively small coherent fiber bundles intersecting the optic radiation and sharing the anterior–posterior diffusion direction near the intersection location. Figure 2 shows the mentioned classes of errors on a sample subject as indicated by arrows.

The effect of glaucoma on the visual system specifically the optic nerve and the optic radiation was investigated in [13]. The correlation between glaucoma and diffusion tensor derived parameters such as fractional anisotropy and mean diffusivity was studied. The fractional anisotropy was found to be significantly lower in the

Table 1 The segmentation accuracy of the normal subjects and glaucoma patients

Subjects' class	Number of subjects	Segmentation accuracy
Normal subjects	9	82.71%
Glaucoma patients	9	82.76%

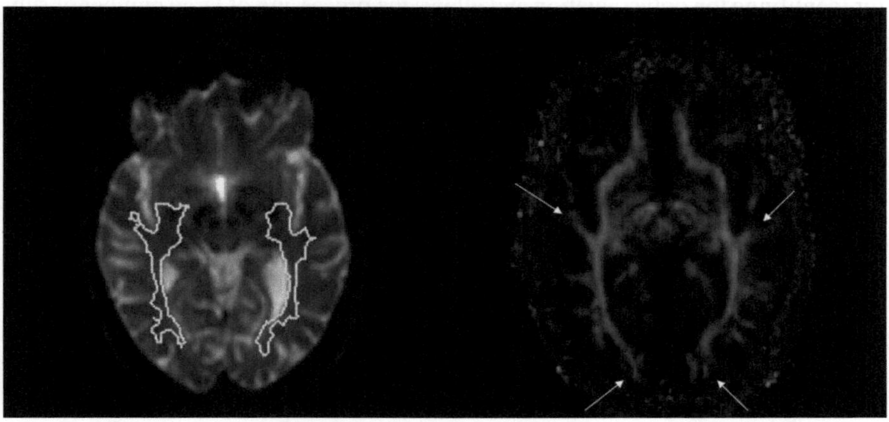

Fig. 2 The errors of segmentation of the optic radiation demonstrated on a sample subject as indicated by arrows

glaucoma group when compared to the normal subjects. On the other hand, the mean diffusivity was significantly higher in glaucoma patients than in the normal subjects. This yields that the diffusion tensors within the optic radiation are generally affected by the presence of the neurologic pathology of glaucoma. Despite these findings, the proposed automated segmentation algorithm has approximately the same accuracy for normal subjects and glaucoma patients. This robustness is due to the dependence of the system on the physiological and anatomical properties which are slightly affected by glaucoma.

The high individual variability of the brain fiber structure and the special nature of DTI-data require great attention when dealing with the segmentation of major fiber bundles. The diffusion tensor contains information about the diffusion direction and the degree of diffusion anisotropy. So, the segmentation based on anisotropy measures or diffusion directions only results in a loss of information and inaccuracy in segmentation. Employing a Euclidean metric for measuring the similarity between diffusion tensors ignores the Riemannian nature of the tensor space and does not represent adequately the dissimilarity between tensors. Most of the proposed segmentation algorithms do not address the problem of system initialization which is usually done by a medical expert or roughly. This leads to an increased number of system iterations and the necessity for an experienced medical user. The proposed segmentation system overcomes the mentioned problems and eliminates the variations due to human intervention.

6 Conclusion and Future Work

A system has been proposed for the automatic segmentation of the optic radiation using DTI based on dissimilarity measure and the coherency property within the optic radiation fiber bundles. The automation eliminates medical-experts' intervention for identifying the optic radiation and allows the processing of large number of subjects. The system initialization problem is addressed by utilizing prior knowledge about the physiological and anatomical properties of the optic radiation to automatically provide robust estimation of the optic radiation. The incorporation of the Log-Euclidean framework in the statistical level set framework is suitable and efficient for DTI segmentation because it accounts for the Riemannian nature of the tensor space and incorporates the whole tensor information in a probabilistic framework. The system is implemented and tested using real DTI-data. The experimental results indicate that the system shows high efficiency in determining the main fiber bundle of the optic radiation for normal subjects as well as pathological subjects with glaucoma.

The automated identification of the optic radiation will be utilized in a following study to investigate the correlation between glaucoma and the quantification of the changes occurred in the optic radiation. This aims to give further insight into the glaucoma disease and its effect on the various parts of the human visual system. The identification of the optic radiation connectivity on the visual cortex is another future goal. This requires the development of a robust tractography algorithm to be able to accurately identify the highly variable branches of the optic radiation while taking into consideration the complex fiber situations (e.g. crossing, branching, etc. . .) and the uncertainties in the diffusion tensor data.

Acknowledgements The authors would like to thank Dr. B. Acar from Bogazici University (www.vavlab.ee.boun.edu.tr) for the valuable discussion of the segmentation system. The authors gratefully acknowledge funding of German academic exchange service (DAAD) and the Erlangen Graduate School in Advanced Optical Technologies (SAOT) by the German National Science Foundation (DFG) in the framework of the excellence initiative.

References

1. Alexander, A.L., Hasan, K.M., Lazar, M., Tsuruda, J.S., Parker, D.L.: Analysis of partial volume effects in diffusion-tensor MRI. Magn. Reson. Med. **45**(5), 770–780 (2001)
2. Arsigny, V., Fillard, P., Pennec, X., Ayache, N.: Log-Euclidean metrics for fast and simple calculus on diffusion tensors. Magn. Reson. Med. **56**(2), 411–421 (2006)
3. Basser, P.J., Jones, D.K.: Diffusion-tensor MRI: theory, experimental design and data analysis – a technical review. NMR Biomed **15**(7-8), 456–467 (2002)
4. Basser, P.J., Pajevic, S., Pierpaoli, C., Duda, J., Aldroubi, A.: *In vivo* fiber tractography using DT-MRI data. Magn. Reson. Med. **44**(4), 625–632 (2000)
5. Basser, P.J., Pierpaoli, C.: Microstructural and physiological features of tissues elucidated by quantitative-diffusion-tensor MRI. J. Magn. Reson. B **111**(3), 209–219 (1996)
6. Bozkaya, U., Acar, B.: SMT: Split and merge tractography for DT-MRI. In: MICCAI, Brisbane, Australia. Lecture Notes in Computer Science, vol. 4792, pp. 153–160. Springer (2007)
7. Cartes-Zumelzu, F.W., Stavrou, I., Castillo, M., Eisenhuber, E., Knosp, E., Thurnher, M.M.: Diffusion-weighted imaging in the assessment of brain abscesses therapy. Am. J. Neuroradiol. **25**(8), 1310–1317 (2004)
8. Chen, T.F., Lin, C.C., Chen, Y.F., Liu, H.M., Hua, M.S., Huang, Y.C., Chiu, M.J.: Diffusion tensor changes in patients with amnesic mild cognitive impairment and various dementias. Psychiatr. Res. Neuroimaging **173**(1), 15–21 (2009)
9. Conturo, T.E., Lori, N.F., Cull, T.S., Akbudak, E., Snyder, A.Z., Shimony, J.S., Mckinstry, R.C., Burton, H., Raichle, M.E.: Tracking neuronal fiber pathways in the living human brain. Proc. Natl. Acad. Sci. USA **96**(18), 10422–10427 (1999)
10. Corouge, I., Fletcher, P., Joshi, S., Gouttard, S., Gerig, G.: Fiber tract-oriented statistics for quantitative diffusion tensor MRI analysis. Med. Image Anal. **10**(5), 786–798 (2006)
11. Dong, Q., Welsh, R.C., Chenevert, T.L., Carlos, R.C., Maly-Sundgren, P., Gomez-Hassan, D.M., Mukherji, S.K.: Clinical applications of diffusion tensor imaging. J. Magn. Reson. Imag. **19**, 6–18 (2004)
12. Fletcher, P.T., Joshi, S.C.: Riemannian geometry for the statistical analysis of diffusion tensor data. Signal Process. **87**(2), 250–262 (2007)
13. Garaci, F.G., Bolacchi, F., Cerulli, A., Melis, M., Span, A., Cedrone, C., Floris, R., Simonetti, G., Nucci, C.: Optic nerve and optic radiation neurodegeneration in patients with glaucoma: In: Vivo Analysis with 3-T Diffusion-Tensor MR Imaging. Radiology **252**(2), 496–501 (2009)
14. Hamarneh, G., Hradsky, J.: DTMRI segmentation using DT-snakes and DT-livewire. In: IEEE International Symposium on Signal Processing and Information Technology, pp. 513–518 (2006)
15. Henry, R.G., Oh, J., Nelson, S.J., Pelletier, D.: Directional diffusion in relapsing-remitting multiple sclerosis: A possible in vivo signature of Wallerian degeneration. J. Magn. Reson. Imag. **18**(4), 420–426 (2003)

16. Hoffmann, E., Zangwill, L., Crowston, J., Weinreb, R.: Optic disk size and glaucoma. Surv. Ophthalmol. **52**(5), 32–49 (2007)
17. Huang, J., Friedland, R., Auchus, A.: Diffusion tensor imaging of normal-appearing white matter in mild cognitive impairment and early alzheimer disease: Preliminary evidence of axonal degeneration in the temporal lobe. Am. J. Neuroradiol. **28**(10), 1943–1948 (2007)
18. Hui, E., Fu, Q., So, K., Wu, E.: Diffusion tensor MR study of optic nerve degeneration in glaucoma. In: Engineering in Medicine and Biology Society, 2007. EMBS 2007. 29th Annual International Conference of the IEEE, pp. 4312–4315 (2007)
19. Huppi, P.S., Murphy, B., Maier, S.E., Zientara, G.P., Inder, T.E., Barnes, P.D., Kikinis, R., Jolesz, F.A., Volpe, J.J.: Microstructural brain development after perinatal cerebral white matter injury assessed by diffusion tensor magnetic resonance imaging. Pediatrics **107**(3), 455–460 (2001)
20. Jones, D.: Tractography gone wild: Probabilistic fibre tracking using the wild bootstrap with diffusion tensor MRI. IEEE Trans. Med. Imag. **27**(9), 1268–1274 (2008)
21. Lansberg, M.G., Norbash, A.M., Marks, M.P., Tong, D.C., Moseley, M.E., Albers, G.W.: Advantages of adding diffusion-weighted magnetic resonance imaging to conventional magnetic resonance imaging for evaluating acute stroke. Arch. Neurol. **57**(9), 1311–1316 (2000)
22. Lazar, M., Weinstein, D.M., Tsuruda, J.S., Hasan, K.M., Arfanakis, K., Meyerand, M.E., Badie, B., Rowley, H.A., Haughton, V., Field, A., Alexander, A.L.: White matter tractography using diffusion tensor deflection. Hum. Brain. Mapp. **18**(4), 306–321 (2003)
23. Le Bihan, D., Mangin, J., Poupon, C., Clark, C., Pappata, S., Molko, N., Chabriat, H.: Diffusion tensor imaging: concepts and applications. J. Magn. Reson. Imag. **13**(4), 534–546 (2001)
24. Lee, S., Uhm, K., Hong, C.: Retinal vessel diameter in normal and primary open-angle glaucoma. Kor. J. Ophthalmol. **12**(1), 51–59 (1998)
25. Lenglet, C., Rousson, M., Deriche, R.: DTI segmentation by statistical surface evolution. IEEE Trans. Med. Imag. **25**(6), 685–700 (2006)
26. Mori, S., Barker, P.B.: Diffusion magnetic resonance imaging: Its principle and applications. Anat. Rec. **257**(3), 102–109 (1999)
27. Mori, S., Oishi, K., Jiang, H., Jiang, L., Li, X., Akhter, K., Hua, K., Faria, A.V., Mahmood, A., Woods, R., Toga, A.W., Pike, G.B., Neto, P.R., Evans, A., Zhang, J., Huang, H., Miller, M.I., van Zijl, P., Mazziotta, J.: Stereotaxic white matter atlas based on diffusion tensor imaging in an ICBM template. Neuroimage **40**(2), 570–582 (2008)
28. Moseley, M.E., Cohen, Y., Mintorovitch, J., Chileuitt, L., Shimizu, H., Kucharczyk, J., Wendland, M.F., Weinstein, P.R.: Early detection of regional cerebral ischemia in cats: Comparison of diffusion- and T2-weighted MRI and spectroscopy. Magn. Reson. Med. **14**(2), 330–346 (1990)
29. Nucifora, P., Verma, R., Lee, S., Melhem, E.: Diffusion-tensor MR imaging and tractography: exploring brain microstructure and connectivity. Radiology **245**(2), 367–384 (2007)
30. Parker, G.J., Haroon, H.A., Wheeler-Kingshott, C.A.: A framework for a streamline-based probabilistic index of connectivity (PICo) using a structural interpretation of MRI diffusion measurements. J. Magn. Reson. Imag. **18**(2), 242–254 (2003)
31. Pennec, X., Fillard, P., Ayache, N.: A riemannian framework for tensor computing. Int. J. Comput. Vision **66**(1), 41–66 (2006)
32. Perona, P., Malik, J.: Scale-space and edge detection using anisotropic diffusion. IEEE Trans. Pattern. Anal. Mach. Intell. **12**(7), 629–639 (1990)
33. Polo, V., Larrosa, J., Ferreras, A., Mayoral, F., Pueyo, V., Honrubia, F.: Retinal nerve fiber layer evaluation in open-angle glaucoma. Ophthalmologica **223**(1), 2–6 (2009)
34. Salat, D., Tuch, D., Greve, D., van der Kouwe, A., Hevelone, N., Zaleta, A., Rosen, B., Fischl, B., Corkin, S., Rosas, H.D., Dale, A.: Age-related alterations in white matter microstructure measured by diffusion tensor imaging. Neurobiol. Aging **26**(8), 1215–1227 (2005)
35. Staempfli, P., Jaermann, T., Crelier, G., Kollias, S., Valavanis, A., Boesiger, P.: Resolving fiber crossing using advanced fast marching tractography based on diffusion tensor imaging. NeuroImage **30**(1), 110–120 (2006)
36. Wakana, S., Jiang, H., Nagae-Poetscher, L., van Zijl, P., Mori, S.: Fiber tract-based atlas of human white matter anatomy. Radiology **230**(1), 77–87 (2004)

37. Wang, Z., Vemuri, B.: DTI segmentation using an information theoretic tensor dissimilarity measure. IEEE Trans. Med. Imag. **24**(10), 1267–1277 (2005)
38. Yörük, E., Acar, B., Bammer, R.: A physical model for MR-DTI based connectivity map computation. In: MICCAI, Palm Springs, CA. Lecture Notes in Computer Science, vol. 3749, pp. 213–220. Springer (2005)
39. Zhou, X.: Diffusion tensor imaging: techniques and clinical applications. Engineering in Medicine and Biology Society, 2004. IEMBS '04. 26th Annual International Conference of the IEEE **2**, 5223–5225. San Francisco, CA, USA (2004)
40. Zhukov, L., Museth, K., Breen, D., Whitaker, R., Barr, A.: Level set modeling and segmentation of DT-MRI brain data. J. Electronic Imag. **12**(1), 125–133 (2003)

Real Time Colour Based Player Tracking in Indoor Sports

Catarina B. Santiago, Armando Sousa, Luís Paulo Reis, and Maria Luísa Estriga

Abstract In recent years there has been a growing interest by the sport's experts (teachers and coaches) in developing automatic systems for detecting, tracking and identifying player's movements with the purpose of improving the players' performance and accomplishing a consistent and standard analysis of the game metrics. A challenge like this requires sophisticated techniques from the areas of image processing and artificial intelligence. The objective of our work is to study and develop hardware and software techniques in order to build an automatic visual system for detecting and tracking players in indoor sports games that can aid coaches to analyse and improve the players' performance. Our methodology is based on colour features and therefore several colour image processing techniques such as background subtraction, blob colour definition (RGB and HSL colour spaces) and colour blob manipulation are employed in order to detect the players. Past information

C.B. Santiago (✉) and A. Sousa
FEUP – Faculty of Engineering of the University of Porto, Rua Dr. Roberto Frias, s/n 4200-465, Porto, Portugal
and
INESC – Institute for Systems and Computer Engineering of Porto, Campus da FEUP, Rua Dr. Roberto Frias, 378, 4200-465, Porto, Portugal
e-mail: catarina.santiago@fe.up.pt; asousa@fe.up.pt

L.P. Reis
FEUP – Faculty of Engineering of the University of Porto, Rua Dr. Roberto Frias, s/n 4200-465, Porto, Portugal
and
LIACC – Artificial Intelligence and Computer Science Lab, University of Porto, Portugal, Rua Dr. Roberto Frias, s/n 4200-465, Porto, Portugal
e-mail: lpreis@fe.up.pt

M.L. Estriga
FADEUP – Faculty of Sports of the University of Porto, Rua Dr. Plácido Costa, 91, 4200-450, Porto, Portugal
and
CIFI2D – Centre of Research, Education, Innovation and Intervention in Sport, Sports Faculty, University of Porto, Rua Dr. Plácido Costa, 91, 4200-450, Porto, Portugal
e-mail: lestriga@fade.up.pt

J.M.R.S. Tavares and R.M.N. Jorge (eds.), *Computational Vision and Medical Image Processing: Recent Trends*, Computational Methods in Applied Sciences 19,
DOI 10.1007/978-94-007-0011-6_2,

and players' velocity allow the tracking algorithm to define probable areas. Tests conducted with a single IP surveillance camera on the sports hall of the Faculty of Sports from the University of Porto showed detection rates from 72.2% to 93.3%.

Keywords Colour image processing · Object tracking · Game analysis

1 Introduction

In sports, especially at high level competition a small advantage of one team regarding another can be of great importance and decisive for a match or even a complete championship.

Therefore, teams are always trying to improve their performance and tactics in order to gain this advantage. So, it could be of greater help to record the game sequence from strategic points where the field can be completely surveyed and where the movements of all players may be recorded with precision. This way, after the game, the team's coach can identify their weak points and define measures to improve the team global behaviour.

Besides acquiring high quality images it would also be interesting to track the players and analyze their behaviour during the game: covered area, number of shoots and goals, number of passes, interaction between players, etc.

An automatic system such as this would bring many advantages, namely it would be able to handle a huge amount of data and perform a systematic evaluation, that is a very time consuming task and not always systematic when performed by a human being.

In this chapter we present the approach used for developing an automatic and intelligent visual system for detecting and tracking players in indoor sports games.

The main objectives are to design a vision system that is able to cover the entire field, detect each player individually and track his/her movements. One of the requirements for this system is that it must not cause any interference in the game, no special tags or colours should be placed neither in the area of action nor on the players, since most of the championships do not allow it.

A system like this is highly complex since it involves objects that are all very similar, constantly moving, changing of shape and getting together which makes an hard task to individualize and consistently identify and track each player. In fact, occlusion and player merging make the task of player identification very difficult.

This chapter is divided into eight sections. The initial sections introduce the topic under analysis including some background information, motivation and related work. The two subsequent sections (3 and 4) provide a description of the projected and implemented architectures and give a detailed explanation of the image processing system which includes the players' detection and tracking. Section 5 shows the results achieved so far and the last section refers to the conclusions and some future work.

2 Related Work

In recent years there has been a growing interest in developing automatic systems for detecting, tracking and identifying player's movements. Some works on the specific area of player tracking have been developed but the majority is intended to outdoor sports namely soccer. In outdoor sports it is very hard to mount a camera system and therefore most of the systems are developed upon images provided by broadcast TV cameras, either single camera or multiple camera systems.

Liu, Jiu et al. [1] use an approach based on a single moving broadcast camera system. Their system doesn't need to be manually initialized since it is able to learn the models of both the background and the players. The background is modelled using a dominant colour learning algorithm and a Haar feature based boosting cascade algorithm is able to represent the players. After this initial learning phase to model the players and the background, the detection and tracking are built upon a Markov Chain Monte Carlo data association method.

FIFA World Cup 2006 was their test platform and from the results their method seems to have high detection and labelling precision, around 90%.

On the opposite side Iwase and Saito [2] propose a dedicated eight camera system which is able to minimize the effects of occlusion. Each camera is treated as an independent system called inner-camera and is responsible for detecting and tracking the players based on very simple features such as colour, area and distance a player has moved. Whenever the inner-camera system is not able to detect the player due to occlusions, not detections or by the players being outside the angle of view an inter-camera process is, in most of the cases, able to identify the players. The geometrical relationships between the cameras is calculated based on planar homography in projective geometry. Their system only covers the penalty area and therefore they are not able to give a good insight of the entire game.

One of the most interesting systems, Aspogamo, is presented by Beetz, Michael et al. [3,4]. This system is able to analyze sports games using an ontology of models of the game that has as primitives the players' positions, motion trajectories and ball actions. The player detection is performed using first an intensity variance detection to isolate areas of interest and afterwards the players are identified using a combination of three colour templates: one for the shirt, another for the shorts and the last one for the socks of the players. Occlusions are identified using geometric constraints of shape and size. The multiple target tracking is done with a Rao-Blackwellized Resampling Particle Filter with fixed lag. This system is also able to track the ball using a particle filter algorithm.

Regarding indoor sports one of the most promising, mature and relevant work is Sagit developed by Pers et al. [5,6]. They use a two fixed camera system placed in the ceiling of the sports hall that provides a bird's eye view.

A detailed explanation for camera temporal and spatial calibration and error analysis is given and the main objective of their work was to follow trajectories. Three different algorithms are compared and described, one based on motion detection, another on RGB (colour) tracking and a last one on a colour and template tracking. They apply their method to several sports such as handball, basketball and squash. However their system is much operator dependent and is used offline.

Several authors apply Kalman filter techniques to address some of these problems, for example Liu et al. [7] give a detailed explanation on their efforts to track skaters in a skating competition. They use a hierarchical model of two components: helmet – identified by a template matching approach and body – detected by a colour histogram matching method combined with an unscented Kalman filter.

Chris and Boyle [8] use a single camera system and apply a multiple object condensation scheme to a five player soccer game. Initially a sample (that corresponds to a bounding box) of each player is detected, then through a propagation algorithm the fitness of each bounding box is evaluated and adjusted. They also include an improved predictive stage that incorporates estimates of positions from a Kalman filter.

The significance of such systems to the area of knowledge of sports can be assessed by the work of Marko Sibila et al. [9] as they evaluate the importance of cyclic movements on handball. With the Sagit platform they were able to perform a study about identifying the differences of volume and intensity in large-scale cyclic movement activities performed by handball players.

In latter years there has also been a great development in robotics soccer and numerous papers were published [10–14] describing several features developed for image processing and tracking algorithms tested with success. Some of these features due to the similarity between indoor sports can also be explored.

3 Architecture

There are several types of cameras available in the market. Mainly for convenience reasons this work was based on a Sony SNCDM110 IP security camera. Recently, colour cameras based on GigEthernet interface have been introduced in the market therefore some considerations on a system based on these cameras are also drawn.

With this kind of technology it is possible to place the cameras far away from the processing system and it is quite easy to mount a multi-camera system using a standard, low cost Ethernet switch.

Due to the dynamics of indoor sports games, where players are constantly moving the best spot to place the camera is in the ceiling of the sports hall which gives a birds-eye perspective [5]. This way there will be no obstacles between the camera and each player and there will be a clear view of the ball, except when occlusion occurs due to a player.

The indoor sport that uses the biggest field area is handball. A handball field has 20×40 m which represents a very large area to be covered and also a very large amount of information to be processed and taken care of. Therefore special attention must be paid when choosing the cameras resolution and frame rates.

Using a system based on a moving camera would not be cheaper and would not prevent dark areas in the game that could eventually be of interest to a coach. The system would also be prone to aging and mechanical problems. Due to these limitations a fixed system seems to be the best choice.

3.1 Projected Solution

The vast area to be covered makes it impossible to use a single camera; therefore a four GigEthernet fixed camera system was projected. The camera placement as well as the system architecture is shown in Fig. 1.

The cameras chosen have resolutions of 640 × 480 pixels and maximum frame rates of 60fps. This implies a high quantity of data delivered by each camera and therefore the architecture is based on a two processor system.

3.2 Tested Solution

Due to some constraints it was not possible to implement the full system. Therefore, all the results presented in this paper were achieved using a single Sony SNCDM110 camera fixed above the 6 m handball line (Fig. 2).

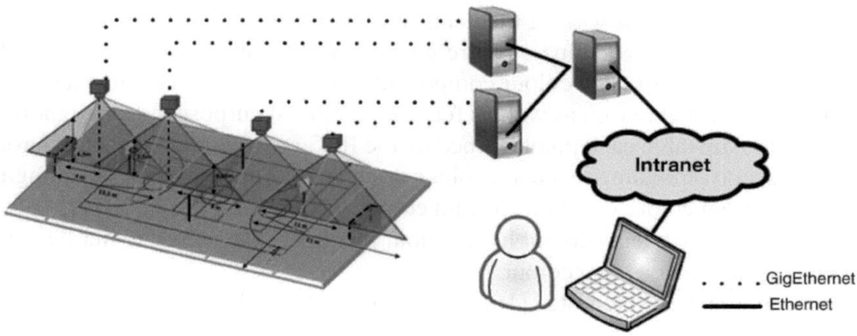

Fig. 1 System architecture

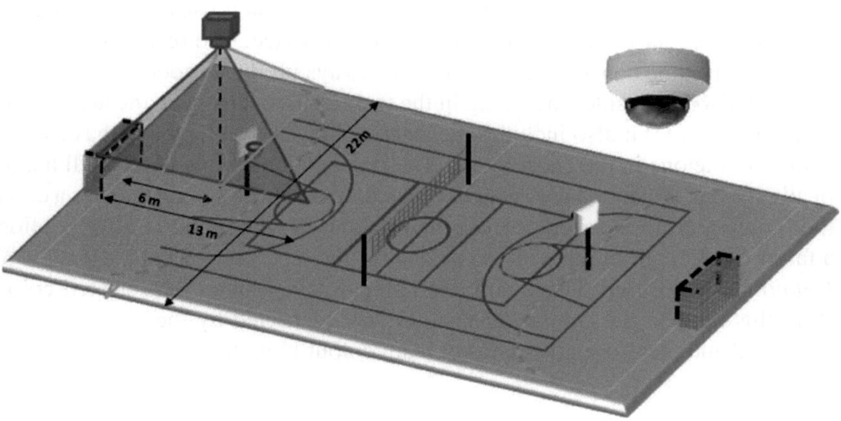

Fig. 2 Camera placement for the tested solution

4 Image Processing

One of the most important systems in this kind of application is the image processing. It must be robust enough so that the tracking algorithm can have solid bases to work with.

In this case the image processing system is based on blob definition and each player is seen as a colour blob. In order to have a clean interface with the images received from the camera we used the OpenCV library [15].

The following subsections describe the steps towards the players' detection.

4.1 Team Definition

The first step consists on defining the colour blobs for each team that correspond to sub-spaces of the entire colour space. This is a very important task since a good colour calibration will influence the success of the subsequent steps.

These colour sub-spaces are stored in a special lookup table that corresponds to a three dimensional vector with 32 elements in each dimension, this way each colour component (red, green and blue) is represented by the five most significant bits. The least significant bits of each colour component represent very slight changes in the colour itself, for that reason as well as for computational purpose they are ignored.

In this lookup table each point defined by the R, G and B components can have a few values, corresponding to a team colour or no team. The set of points belonging to the same team colour constitute a team colour sub-space.

Besides this, each team colour has a colour identifier that is used to mark a pixel that belongs to a given team colour.

Three approaches were tested [16], the first using the Red, Green and Blue (RGB) colour space and the other two using the Hue, Saturation and Luminance (HSL) colour space (which allow minimizing the shadow and light variations effects):

- *Physical range* – This is the simplest method tested and uses only the area selected by the user to define the team colour sub-space. The results showed that this is a very time consuming task that not always produces good results.
- *Physical flood* – Besides including in the team colour sub-space the area defined by the user (seed) it also includes the surrounding area as long as it has a colour similar to the one in the chosen area. The propagation among pixels will happen in all physical directions in a recursive way until reaching a pixel that has a colour too far away from the seed or from the previous neighbour. This novelty allows a faster colour calibration with very good results.
- *Colour grow* – Based on growing the colour space around the selected colour. With this method the colour expansion is not restricted by the physical neighbourhood and therefore gives a faster team colour blob definition.

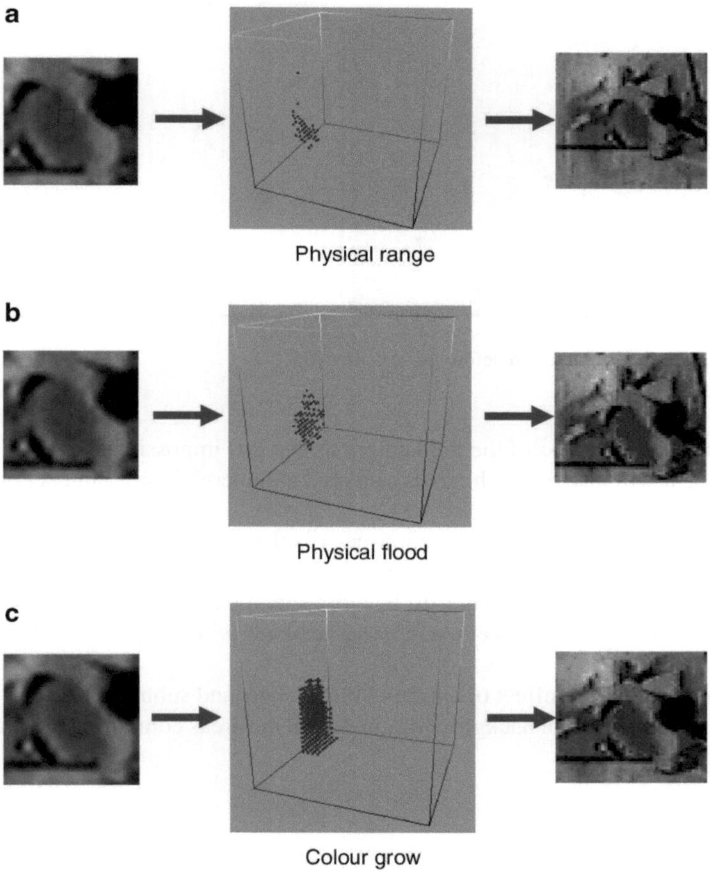

Fig. 3 Team colour sub-spaces resulting from different colour calibration techniques: (**a**) Physical Range, (**b**) Physical Flood, (**c**) Colour Grow

The colour team sub-spaces resulting from applying these three different techniques can be seen on Fig. 3. In this figure the team colour sub-space is identified with the green colour.

4.2 Background Subtraction

Most of the image area has non-useful information. In fact the regions of interest are the ones that include a player so it makes sense to perform a background subtraction in order to highlight the zones where the players are. To perform this subtraction an empty image of the field is collected a priori.

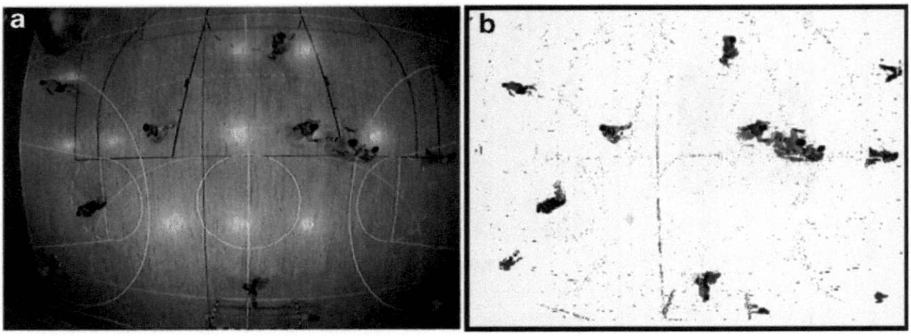

Fig. 4 Background subtraction before (**a**) and after (**b**)

Due to the brightness of the field empty image it is impossible to simple subtract it, because it will also have a huge impact on the players' figures almost eliminating them from the image.

Therefore a conditional subtraction per pixel is performed [16], which means that the subtraction occurs only if the pixel under analysis has a colour similar to the one of the background image. To be more specific the two pixels are not exactly subtracted but the pixel in the image under analysis will be updated with the white colour.

Figure 4 shows the effect of applying the background subtraction.

With this conditional background subtraction the areas containing the players are clearly highlighted.

4.3 Colour Detection

The first action towards the players' localization is to detect the colours of their uniforms. Since the colour sub-spaces for each team have already been calibrated and stored in the colour lookup up table it is necessary to scan the entire image to detect and mark pixels that belong to either one of those colour sub-spaces.

During this scan each pixel colour is tested to see if it has an entry on the colour lookup table. If it corresponds to a team colour then the colour of the pixel is replaced with the team colour identifier.

4.4 Blob Aggregation and Characterization

At this point there is only information if a pixel belongs to a given colour team or no team, it is still necessary to establish a relationship between pixels belonging to the same colour blob. A colour blob corresponds to a region, in the image, where pixels of the same colour team sub-space are concentrated.

The algorithm responsible for establishing this relationship comprises two steps. The first one is based on a per line scan detection and the information is stored in a way similar to that of a run-length encoding using three parameters: y, x_{min} and x_{max}. Whenever a pixel belonging to a team colour is reached the subsequent pixels of the same line are checked to see if they belong to the same team colour. An outline of the algorithm is presented next.

```
for y:=0 to imageMaxY
  for x:=0 to imageMaxX
    curColour:=getColourFromImage(x,y)
    if curColour<>-1 then
      Segment(SgmCount++).Colour:=curColour
      Segment(SgmCount).Start:=x
Segment(SgmCount).End:=findEndSegment(curColour,x,y)
      if Segment(SgmCount).End <>-1
        SgmCount++
      end if
    end if
  end for
end for
```

Where the findEndSegment function is described by:

```
findEndSegment(curColour,xStart,y)
  for x:=xStart to endOfLine
    while getColourFromImage(x,y)=curColour
      x++
    end while
    xEnd:=x
    while getColourFromImage(x,y)<>curColour
      x++
    end while
    if xEnd-x>BLOBDISTANCE
      break
    end if
  end for
  if xEnd-x>BLOBSIZE
    return xEnd
  else
    return -1
    end if
  end findEndSegment
```

As a result from the previous procedure a series of single lines are identified as belonging to a specific colour team and they still need to be joined to form a single blob, which represents the second step.

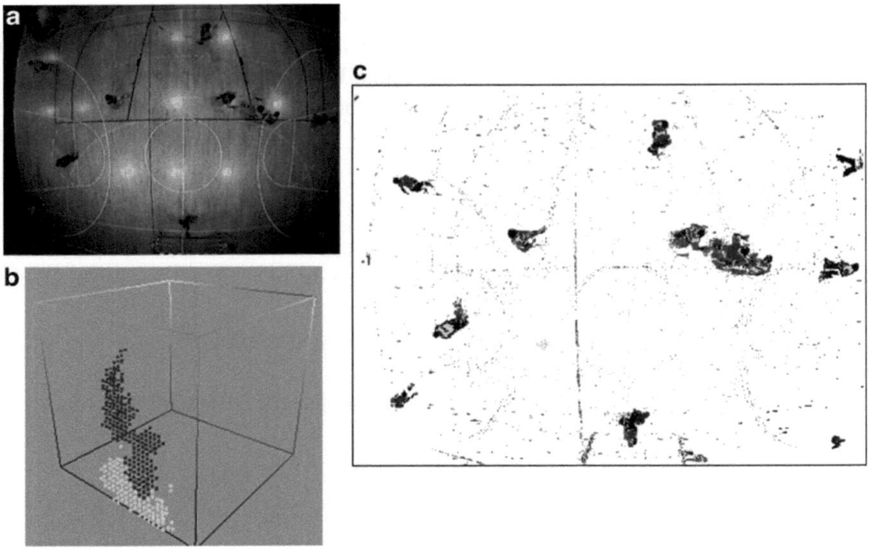

Fig. 5 Colour detection and blob aggregation. Original image (**a**), teams colour subspaces (**b**) and image after processing (**c**)

If the distance between two of these lines is small and they belong to the same colour team they are considered as being part of the same blob and are connected together.

Once the blob aggregation is performed it is possible to characterize each blob, namely determine its maximum and minimum x and y positions, the area it occupies, the rectangle that best fits the blob and its centre of mass.

Figure 5 shows the result of these processing techniques including the colour regions of each team.

Despite the two team colour sub-spaces being too near the players from each team can be properly identified as demonstrated by the bottom image of the above image.

Two features are used in order to determine if a colour blob can represent a player: the area of the colour blob and the colour density inside the rectangle that best fits it.

4.5 Real World Transformation

Once the players are completely identified and the blobs characterization is performed it is still necessary to perform the conversion into the real world coordinates.

This real world transformation comprises two parameters one, as seen from the previous images is the barrel distortion, that in this case is quite severe and the other corresponds to a scaling factor between the coordinates of the image (that are in pixels) into the coordinates of the real world (in centimetres).

In order to compensate for these two factors Eq. 1 was considered [16]:

$$\begin{bmatrix} x_R \\ y_R \end{bmatrix} = \left(1 + kr^2\right) \begin{bmatrix} S_x \times x_D \\ S_y \times y_D \end{bmatrix} \tag{1}$$

$(1 + kr^2)$ term denotes the barrel effect distortion, being k the barrel distortion coefficient. (S_x,S_y) represents the scale factor, (x_R,y_R) are the real world coordinates and (x_D,y_D) are the distorted coordinates that correspond to the image coordinates.

In this equation the parameters that need to be found are the k and the (S_x,S_y), so that the real world coordinates for any given pixel can be determined.

The (S_x,S_y) can be easily calculated aided by the lines of the field and using the ratio between the real world distance and the pixels distance. For example, measuring the pixels used to define the inner area of the 6 m line.

Using this method both on the x axis as well as on the y results in: S = (2.94 cm, 2.80 cm).

For determining the k factor an approach based on the least square method was used. Let's ignore for now the scale factor and using the y component of Eq. 1 an expression like the one in Eq. 2 would be obtained:

$$\begin{aligned} &y_D = -y_D r^2 k + y_R \Leftrightarrow y = mx + b, \\ &where \quad y = y_D,\ x = -y_D r^2,\ m = k\ and\ b = y_R \end{aligned} \tag{2}$$

Applying the least squares method results in:

$$\begin{aligned} m &= \frac{n\sum_{i=1}^{n}\left(-y_D r^2 \times y_D\right) - \left(\sum_{i=1}^{n} -y_D r^2\right) \times \left(\sum_{i=1}^{n} y_D\right)}{n\sum_{i=1}^{n}\left(-y_D r^2\right)^2 - \left(\sum_{i=1}^{n} -y_D r^2\right)^2} = k \\ b &= \frac{\left(\sum_{i=1}^{n} y_D\right) \times \left(\sum_{i=1}^{n}\left(-y_D r^2\right)^2\right) - \left(\sum_{i=1}^{n} -y_D r^2\right) \times \left(\sum_{i=1}^{n} -y_D r^2 \times y_D\right)}{n\sum_{i=1}^{n}\left(-y_D r^2\right)^2 - \left(\sum_{i=1}^{n} -y_D r^2\right)^2} = y_R \end{aligned} \tag{3}$$

To accomplish a good calculation of the k coefficient is good practice to choose a line that covers the entire field. Figure 6 depicts the outcome of applying the barrel "undistortion" equation.

After the coordinates are transformed into the real world it is possible to determine the exact amount a player has run and if during a move is in a good position.

4.6 Player Tracking

Once the players are detected it is possible to perform their tracking. As stated before the main parameters that characterize each player are the area and the centre of mass.

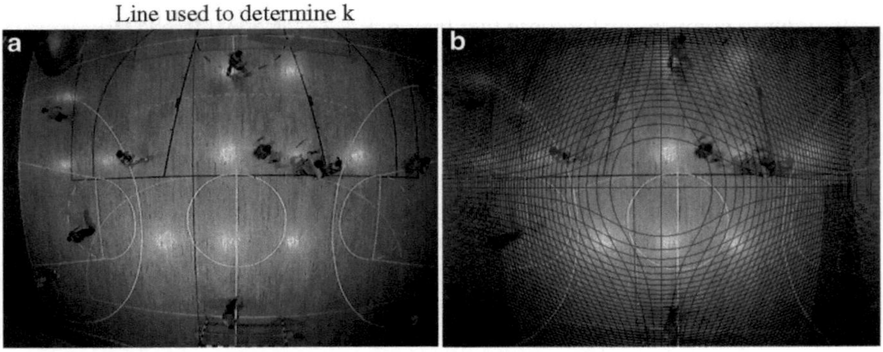

Fig. 6 Image before (**a**) and after applying the barrel "undistortion" expression (**b**)

The method adopted is based on the past information and on defining a probable area around each player that defines his/her next position. This probable area takes into account the position and the velocity of the player.

Once a new frame is picked, the processing system starts by identifying all the colour blobs and those that are identified as being a player are characterized.

The characterization parameters will be compared with the ones from the previously identified blobs and if they fit inside the probable area of one of those blobs then the new blob is assumed as being the sequence.

5 Results

This section presents the results achieved so far and gives a description of the test platform used.

Tests were conducted at the FADEUP's sports hall during handball training sessions of the Futebol Clube do Porto junior teams with training vests. Due to the short period the camera was available (the camera was lent by Sony Portugal) it was only possible to capture a few videos and not always under the best conditions.

5.1 Overview

Figure 7 demonstrates the final result after applying the image processing and the tracking techniques.

Merging between players of the same team seems to be the strongest factor to loose player identification.

Experiments also evidenced that the colour calibration of each team is a key factor to have a good player detection, and a combination of the physical flood and colour grow techniques produced the best results.

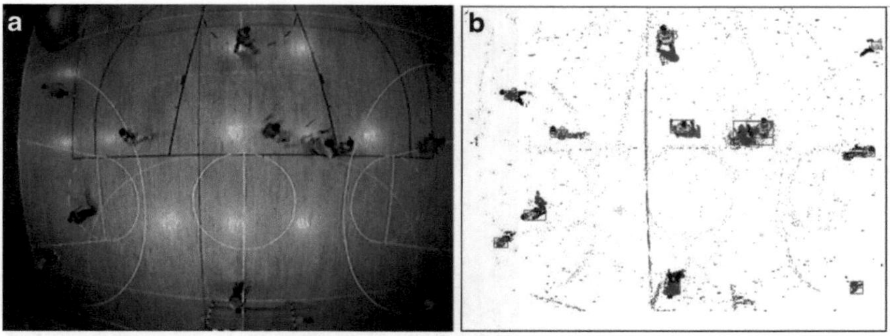

Fig. 7 Image before (**a**) and after (**b**) processing

Regarding the tracking algorithm the results are still scarce, mainly because we were only able to cover a small portion of the field and therefore when a player leaves this area the tracking algorithm is not able to follow him.

However when the player stays in the visible region the tracking behaviour is satisfactory and even when a player is not detected in one frame it is able to recover the track in the subsequent frames.

5.2 *Sample Footage*

The following results were obtained using a 60 s' portion (which corresponds to 900 frames) of a video recorded at a handball training session of the Futebol Clube do Porto junior team, filmed with permission at the Faculty of Sports of the University of Porto on the 25 April 2009.

The video was filmed in MJPEG with resolution of 640 × 480 pixels, 15 fps and compression ratio of 1/6.

The sample footage used has a particularity that is common on training sessions but not on real game situations, both teams have very similar equipments only differing in a dark blue vest the dark blue team wears above the same equipment of the light blue team.

5.3 *Player Detection*

Robust player detection plays a very important role since it establishes solid foundations where the tracking algorithm can build upon. Therefore the first tests were oriented to determine the player detection robustness.

The left side of Fig. 8 shows the team colour definition used in this batch of tests (green colour identifies the light blue team and yellow colour the dark blue team)

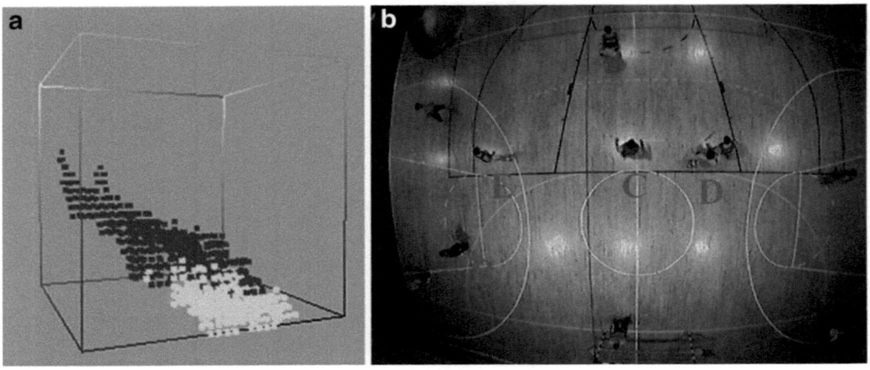

Fig. 8 Team colour definition (*left*) and players under detection (*right*)

Table 1 Player detection rate

Player	Detection rate (%)
A (goalkeeper)	76.2
B (dark blue team)	72.2
C (dark blue team)	88.0
D (light blue team)	93.3
E (dark blue team)	75.2

where it is possible to see that due to the equipment similarity the two team colours have an interlaced region which makes it even harder to identify players whose equipment colour is on this frontier.

On the right side of the same figure players used to evaluate the detection rate are highlighted and identified with letters

Table 1 provides the detection rates for each highlighted player.

From these results it is possible to see that players' detection rates ranged from 72.2% (player D) until 93.3% (player D). It is also noticed that the detection algorithm had better performance at the centre of the image because this area had a better illumination (there were some missing light bulbs on the sides of the field mainly near the goal) and also corresponded to the area seen by the centre of the lenses where the image is better.

Player B had the lowest detection rate (72.2%) followed by player E (75.2%). The first case is explained by the fact that, during the sample footage, the player stayed most of the time in the extremity of the image where the two above mentioned conditions were not gathered. On the second case the player was from the dark blue team but stayed the majority of time with his flank towards the camera where the most visible area of the equipment was the sleeve (of light blue colour) and therefore the player was miss classified as belonging to the wrong team.

Player C was also from the dark blue team but had a satisfactory detection rate because he consistently stayed on the centre of the image with his backs towards the camera.

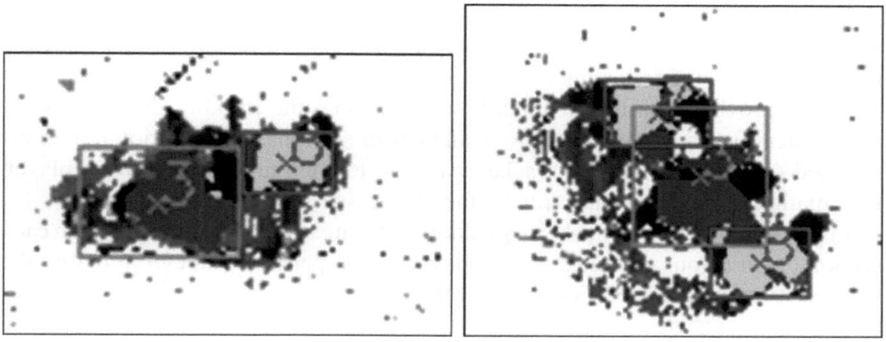

Fig. 9 Correct player identification during a merge situation

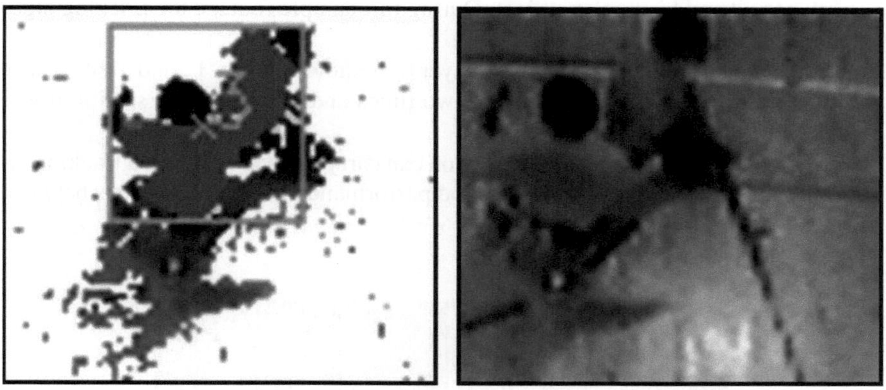

Fig. 10 Merging between players of the same team

It was also possible to verify that a player belonging to the light blue team (player D) had better chances of being well detected

Further tests showed that during merge situations with players from different teams the detection was able to perform correctly as can be seen on Fig. 9.

Nevertheless when two players of the same team got close enough to occur merging (Fig. 10) the detection algorithm considered them as being a single individual.

The image on the right side shows clearly that the camera "saw" the sleeves from both players touching.

5.4 Player Tracking

The performance of the tracking algorithm was evaluated by the time it continuously managed to track a player.

As stated before a good tracking algorithm is based on solid player detection, therefore a lower detection rate will imply a worse player tracking which is proved by the results on the following figures and tables.

Tables provide information about how many times the tracking algorithm lost a player identified by a higher or lower number of sections. Each section represents a period of time in which the tracker was able to continuously follow the player. Information about the distance run by the player is also given.

Figures provide a graphical visualization of the area covered by the player in each section (each colour identifies a section tracked properly). Although in reality the set of sections belong to the same player the tracking algorithm sees each portion as belonging to a different player.

We present the results achieved for player B and C (recall 5.3).

Figure 11 and Table 2 represent the data for player B. Initially the player was tracked in section dark grey, but 14.2 s later the player was not detected for a long enough period and his track was lost. During this sample footage the tracking algorithm lost the player three times.

We could achieve better results on player C as shown on Fig. 12 and Table 3. The tracking algorithm only lost the player two times and on the second section it was able to follow the player during 30 s.

As stated before, merging and occlusion can carry many troubles in a tracking algorithm, nevertheless tests showed a good performance when this happens between players from opposite teams.

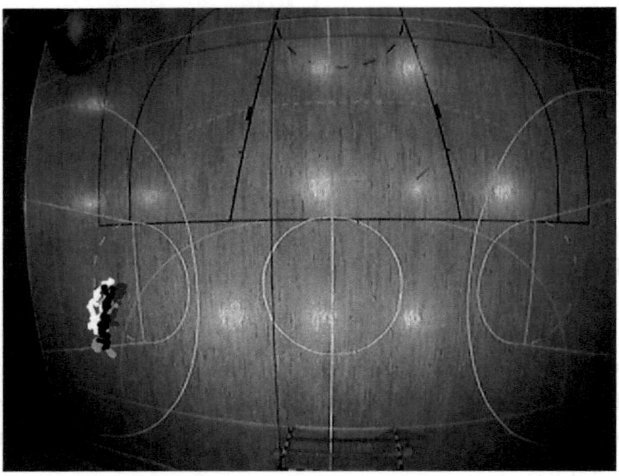

Fig. 11 Spatial occupation of player B

Table 2 Player B sections during tracking

Section	Duration (s)	Distance (cm)
Dark grey	14.2	12.3
Light grey	14.4	8.1
White	16.2	9.7
Black	12.2	8.3

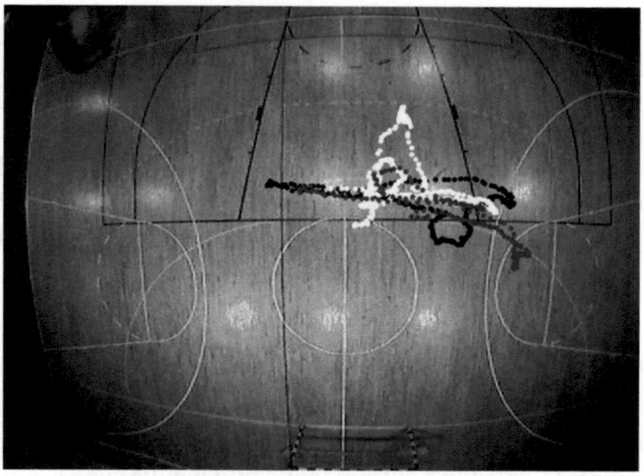

Fig. 12 Spatial occupation of player C

Table 3 Player C sections during tracking

Section	Duration (s)	Distance (cm)
Black	16.6	23.2
White	30.0	31.3
Grey	13.1	21.8

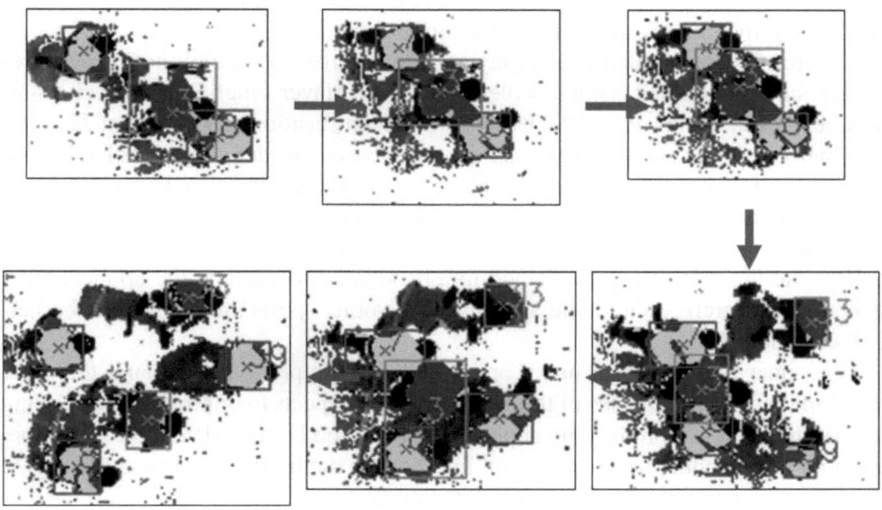

Fig. 13 Tracking during a merging situation

Figure 13 shows the result of the tracking algorithm during the right side merging of Fig. 9. This sequence of screenshots evidences that, despite occurring a merging between several players, the algorithm was capable of identifying correctly the players during and after the merging period.

Of course that during the merging some players were seen much bigger (example of player three), but in the general sense it is able to detect all the players and position their centre of mass (cross inside the rectangle) in more or less the correct position.

These tests were performed in a laptop computer with 1MB L2 cache and powered by an Intel T2130 processor running at 1.86 GHz, under Windows Vista operative system and, in average, each frames takes around 65 ms to be processed.

6 Conclusions and Future Work

This chapter presented a system for tracking players in indoor sports games. The main objectives were to develop a system that could handle such a complex problem, recognize each team player and follow their movement all over the field.

The system is composed of two main blocks, one concerned with image processing where several colour techniques are applied in order to identify the players and the other responsible for tracking the players throughout the field.

Tests conducted using an IP surveillance camera and a sample footage of 60 s showed that most of the time players are correctly identified has being part of either team. This is a good result taking into consideration the several artefacts the camera produces and the many light effects present on this scenario (mirror of the lights, shadows of the players, and barrel effect among others).

The results also evidence that players detection based on blob notion achieves good results, although it is not completely robust to player's merging and occlusions. The best result achieved was 93.3% of correct identification and the worst 72.2%.

Finally the last step, player tracking, was based on defining a probable area around the previous position of the player using the centre of mass position and the maximum theoretical player velocity. The minimalistic presented tracking algorithm was able to correctly and continuously follow a player during 30 s.

Despite the tests being conducted in a handball environment the application is generic and therefore should be able to analyse other sports images such as basketball or volleyball.

It is clear that there are many opportunities to improve and expand the work developed so far. Maybe one of the most important aspects to improve is the tracking algorithm in order to reduce its dependency on a good player detection. Therefore Kalman filter techniques and artificial intelligence methodologies may be explored in order to improve the algorithm's performance.

It would also be interesting to implement the complete engineering solution and test it in a real game situation where the players have very distinct equipments (with official team colours).

Acknowledgments The authors would like to thank Sony Portugal for the cost free usage of the camera used for the tests. The presented work was also partially funded by Fundação Gulbenkian through a PhD scholarship and by Portuguese FCT, under project PTDC/EIA/70695/2006 – ACORD – Adaptative Coordination of Robotic Teams.

References

1. Liu, J., Tong, X., Li, W., Wang, T., Zhang, Y., Wang, H., Yang, B., Sun, L., Yang, S.: Automatic player detection, labeling and tracking in broadcast soccer video. Pattern Recognit. Lett. **30**(2), 103–113 (2009)
2. Iwase, S., Saito, H.: Tracking soccer players based on homography among multiple views. In: Proceedings of SPIE – The International Society for Optical Engineering, Lugano, Italy **5150**(3), 283–292 (2003)
3. Beetz, M., Gedikli, S., Bandouch, J., Kirchlechner, B., von Hoyningen-Huene, N., Perzylo, A.: Visually tracking football games based on TV broadcasts. In: Proceedings of the 20th International Joint Conference on Artifical intelligence, pp. 2066–2071. Morgan Kaufmann Publishers Inc., San Francisco, CA (2007)
4. Beetz, M., von Hoyningen-Huene, N., Kirchlechner, B., Gedikli, S., Siles, F., Durus, M., Lames, M.: ASPOGAMO: Automated sports games analysis models. Int. J. Comput. Sci. Sport **8**(1), 4–12 (2009)
5. Pers, J., Kovacic, S.: Computer vision system for tracking players in sports games. In: Proceedings of the First International Workshop on Image and Signal Processing and Analysis, 2000, pp. 81–86. Pula, Croatia (2000)
6. Pers, J., Bon, M., Kovacic, S., Sibila, M., Dezman, B.: Observation and analysis of large-scale human motion. Hum. Mov. Sci. **21**(2), 295–311 (2002)
7. Lui, G., Tang, X., Huang, J., Liu, F., Sun, D.: Hierarchical model-based human motion tracking via unscented Kalman Filter. In: Proceedings of the 11th International Conference on Computer Vision, pp. 1–8. IEEE Computer Society Press, Washington, DC (2007)
8. Needham, C.J., Boyle, R.D.: Tracking multiple sports players through occlusion, congestion and scale. In: Proceedings of the British Machine Vision Conference 2001, vol. 1, pp. 93–102. Manchester, UK (2001)
9. Šibila, M., Vuleta, D., Pori, P.: Position related differences in volume and intensity of large scale cyclic movements of male players in handball. Kinesiology **36**(1), 58–68 (2004)
10. Sousa, A: Arquitecturas de Sistemas Robóticos e Localização em Tempo Real Através de Visão. Feup Edições, Porto, Portugal (2003)
11. Moreira, A., Sousa, A., Costa, P.: Vision based real-time localization of multiple mobile robots. In: 3rd International Conference on Field and Service Robotics, pp. 103–106. Helsinki, Finland (2001)
12. D'Andrea, R., Lee, J.W., Hoffman, A., Yahaya, A.S., Cremean, L.B., Karpati, T.: Big Red: The Cornell small league robot. Lecture Notes in Computer Science 1856: 89–98 (2000)
13. Reis, L.P., et al.: Robust vision algorithms for quadruped soccer robots. In: Proceedings of CompImage 2006 – Computational Modelling of Objects Represented in Images: Fundamentals Methods and Applications, pp. 367–372. Coimbra, Portugal (2007)
14. Reis, L.P., Neves, A., Sousa, A.: Real-Time Vision in the RoboCup – Robotic Soccer International Competitions, Computer Vision in Robotics – VipIMAGE 2009 – II ECCOMAS Thematic Conference on Computational Vision and Medical Image Processing, pp. 319–324. Porto, Portugal (2009)
15. Bradski, G., Kaehler, A.: Learning OpenCV. O'Reilly Media, USA (2008)
16. Sousa, A., Santiago, C., Reis, L.P., Estriga, M.L.: Automatic detection and tracking of handball players. In: Proceedings of the VipIMAGE 2009 – II ECCOMAS Thematic Conference on Computational Vision and Medical Image Processing, pp. 213–219. Porto, Portugal (2009)

Visualization of the Dynamics of the Female Pelvic Floor Reflex and Steady State Function

Christos E. Constantinou, Qiyu Peng, and Sadao Omata

Abstract Female urinary incontinence has been recently termed a "silent epidemic", requiring systematic attention and a multidisciplinary approach towards economically ameliorating its impact. In this paper we examine the role of the pelvic floor (PF) in maintaining urinary continence by evaluating the dynamics produced during its voluntary and reflex activation. Analytical methods for the acquisition and subsequent ultrasound analysis of movement of PF structures during maneuvers that are associated with exercises are presented to enable the development of criteria and unique new parameters that define the kinematics of PF function. Principal among these parameters, are displacement, velocity, acceleration and the trajectory of pelvic floor landmarks facilitating functional and anatomical visualization. Different methods of movement detection, including motion tracking algorithms and segmentation algorithms were developed to acquire new dynamic parameters of Pelvic structures during different maneuvers. 2D animation was applied to enhance the ultrasound imaging and highlight the timing of the movement and deformation to fast and stressful maneuvers, which are important for understanding the neuromuscular control mechanisms in urinary continence. Parameters were derived using image processing of non-invasive trans-perineal scanning and probe measurements from asymptomatic volunteers as well as patients presenting with relevant pathology. In each case the results are visualized using a graphic interface deigned to illustrate the significant factors separating the continent from the incontinent subjects.

Keywords Ultrasound · Biomechanics · Segmentation · Biomechanics

---

C.E. Constantinou (✉), Q. Peng, and S. Omata
Stanford University School of Medicine (Urology), Stanford, CA 94395-5118, USA
e-mail: ceconst@stanford.edu; qpeng@lbl.gov; omalab3@ee.ce.nihon-u.ac.jp

J.M.R.S. Tavares and R.M.N. Jorge (eds.), *Computational Vision and Medical Image Processing: Recent Trends*, Computational Methods in Applied Sciences 19,
DOI 10.1007/978-94-007-0011-6_3,

1 Introduction

1.1 Clinical Problem

Functionally the role of the Pelvic Floor (PF) is multiple, ranging from control of urinary and fecal continence to orgasm, conception and birth and in the containment intra abdominal organs such as the uterus, vagina, bladder and rectum. Principal among PF disorders, is urinary incontinence and prolapse, accounting for over 400,000 operations in the USA in 1987 [25], and nearly a third of these were re-operations. It is estimated that 30 ∼ 50% of women in Europe and the USA are affected by Urinary incontinence [10]. Stress Urinary Incontinence (SUI), the involuntary leakage of urine on coughing, sneezing, exertion or effort, is the most common form of urinary incontinence in women. The scientific understanding of normal PF function is limited and consequently treatment of these prevalent, disabling conditions is, at best, inefficient. As a consequence SUI has been termed a "hidden epidemic", affects a large percentage of the population, particularly at the later stages of life. In our long-term studies of the mechanism of urinary continence, we realized it is important to develop a method to visualize, measure and model the dynamic responses of the pelvic floor, including the timing of the movement of pelvic structures, consequent trajectories and the dynamic parameters of movement in order to understand the mechanism of urinary continence and establish a more objective basis for the clinical diagnoses and the evaluation of the treatments of SUI patients in clinics.

In the present communication the functional characteristics of the female pelvic floor are considered using two distinct approaches, ultrasound imaging [48,50], and direct measures of contractility using a vaginal probe [15]. These two measurement methodologies were used using the same population of subjects and consequently provide a comparable means of visualizing the results in each case.

1.2 Anatomical Considerations

Due to the location of the PF defining its normal function is challenging. The PF is under neural control and is a complex 3D arrangement of muscle and connective tissue, attached to the bony pelvis and sacrum. The PFM is a collective name for the levator ani and ischiococcygeus. The levator ani muscle consists of the pubococcygeus, the puborectalis, and the iliococcygeus muscles. The pubococcygeus and the puborectalis muscles form a U-shape as they originate from the pubic bone on either side of the midline and pass behind the rectum to form a sling. The iliococcygeus muscle arises laterally from the arcus tendineus levator ani and forms a horizontal sheet that spans the opening in the posterior region of the pelvis, thereby providing a "shelf" upon which the pelvic organs rest [26]. The muscles and fascias of the pelvic diaphragm are inserted on the ischial spines either directly or indirectly through the sacrospinous ligament and the tendinous arch of the pelvic fascia. The result of a PFM contraction can be thought to be a medial pull on the ischial spines to produce a more rigid and narrower PF [1].

1.3 Functional Considerations

Many measurement tools for PFM function quantify the strength of contraction but PFM strengthening is not the only intervention used clinically in rehabilitation of patients with PFM disorders. Indeed there are many methods of measuring PFM activity such as palpation, visual observation, electromyography, dynamometers, ultrasound, and magnetic resonance imaging (MRI). Each tool has its own qualities and limitations [9]. Most recently, using a reliable instrumented speculum, incontinent women demonstrated lower values in passive force, endurance and speed of contraction than continent women, however, differences between the two groups for maximal force reached the statistically significant level only in the endurance parameter [44]. PFM strengthening exercises do diminish the symptoms of SUI [6,46] yet a number of studies have demonstrated that strength of PFM contraction does not always correlate to continence state or action on the urethra [39, 44, 60], so what is it about PFM rehabilitation that helps? Little research has focused upon the mechanisms of therapeutic change to help identify the specific critical muscle components of training [47] so it is unknown whether PFM training mimics the normal physiological behavior of the PFM or is an compensation strategy, nor whether a strengthening program is indeed the most efficient method of conservative rehabilitation. It seems appropriate to determine whether other properties of muscle function are also important in defining PFM function and dysfunction, as well as gaining a greater understanding of why PFM rehabilitation in women with SUI is effective.

1.4 Contribution of Imaging

Previous visualization studies using ultrasound or MRI show that a voluntary contraction of the Pelvic Floor Muscles (PFM) changes the ano-rectal angle (ARA) [22] and can displace the urethra in a direction towards the pubic symphysis [19,27,43]. Yet why does a correct PFM contraction in some women increase the intra urethral pressure, but in others it does not? [11] It is known that in continent women there is recruitment of PFM motor units [23] and an increase in intra-urethral pressure [18] prior to an increase in intra-abdominal pressure (IAP) during a cough. Is the increase in intra-urethral pressure caused by an automatic, pre programmed activation of the PFM? If so, is this pre-activation lost or delayed in SUI? Certainly there are altered PFM activation patterns during a cough, measured by EMG in women with SUI compared to healthy volunteers [24], with shorter activation periods, lack of response or paradoxical inhibition, so how does this alteration affect the trajectory of urogenital structures?

Visualization studies have described the displacement of the urethra or bladder neck that occurs from the start to finishing point of a cough, a PFM contraction and Valsalva maneuver, yet none so far have either mapped the trajectory throughout the maneuver, or defined the automatic function of the PFM, especially in response to sudden rises in intra-abdominal pressure (IAP) during a cough. Are the differences in women with PF disorders just a difference of amplitude of displacement, or are the specifics of the journey important too?

The PFM, along with the diaphragm and abdominal muscles are also thought to contribute in generating intra-abdominal pressure (IAP). Disorders of breathing and incontinence have a strong association with low back pain (LBP) [58] and subjects with LBP generate more IAP during low load tasks and have alterations in the timing of trunk muscle activity [30, 35] than those without LBP. Small studies of continent women have shown that the Abdominal muscles and PFM co-activate [45, 55], is this true for a larger group size, and are there any differences in women with SUI or other PF disorders? To answer those important clinical questions, it is essential to establish reliable methods for the evaluation of the PF function. The reliable methods to evaluate the changes of the PF functions will be helpful for the physicians or clinicians to identify those patients who are likely to be rehabilitated by PF exercises instead of by surgery.

MRI imaging was introduced to study the anatomical components of the PF and thereby contribute to better understand mechanism of continence [12, 40, 59, 61]. Different methods have been applied to process and analyze the MRI image to acquire the 2D anatomy of the PF with higher spatial resolution and speed of image acquisition [13, 32, 33]. MRI imaging in 3D, reported in the recent research literature, was achieved by reconstructing sequential 2D images acquired in the axial and sagittal plane [4, 31]. While 3D MRI imaging provides very useful insight into the anatomical configuration, the amount of time required to acquire 3D volume data is too long to record any dynamic information of the PF activities. Therefore, current 3D MRI studies are limited to analyze the passive response of the PF under a certain loading or straining [51]. MRI imaging is also too expensive to be used in regular clinical examination.

1.5 Diagnostic Methods

In current clinical practice, manual muscle testing per vagina is the technique used by most clinicians to evaluate a PFM contraction using a five point modified Oxford Grading ordinal scale [41]. It can measure whether or not there is a correct contraction and the strength of it. The main limitation of this method is the length of time the assessment takes and the ease with which most clinicians, other than physiotherapists, could incorporate it into their clinical practice. Vaginal palpation has also been criticized for its lack of reliability and sensitivity in the measurement of pelvic floor muscles strength for scientific purposes [8]. Because of the inherent limitations of vaginal palpation, other methods such as vaginal cones, hydrostatic pressure, surface, needle and wire EMG are currently tested to assess PF function and the improvement of PF function in conservative treatment. The clinical applications of those methods are limited because they are invasive and inconvenient to be applied in regular clinical examination.

2D ultrasound imaging can acquire dynamic information on the morphology of the urogenital organs. In particular, perineal, introital and trans-vaginal ultrasound has become an imaging platform for the evaluation of the PF and for the treatment planning of many uro-gynecological conditions [8]. By its nature, 2D ultrasound imaging provides a very large amount of dynamic data that cannot be visually assimilated by the observer in its totality, particularly during fast occurring events. Such dynamic events contain information relating the integrity of the supporting structures of the bladder neck, the role of the PF, and the compliance of pelvic floor structures [5]. Furthermore, because the urogenital structures are anatomically interconnected, ultrasound-based dynamic imaging can substantiate urodynamic observations of the effective distribution of pressure transmission to the urethra. State-of-the-art 3D ultrasound imaging techniques provide 3D visualization of the pelvic floor structures with higher resolution. However, current 3D ultrasound machines are not fast enough for the purpose of visualization the movement of tissues in fast and stressful maneuvers like coughing, which may provoke urinary incontinence. Besides, as 3D imaging is cost prohibitive for the majority of clinicians it is anticipated that 2D ultrasound will be, for the foreseeable future, the measuring and feedback tool of clinical choice.

1.6 Evaluation of the Dynamic Function of the PF Using 2D Ultrasound Imaging

In real time ultrasound imaging, the diagnostically important information of the dynamic response of the PF cannot be assimilated and quantified by the observer during the scanning process. The trajectories and the timings of the movement of the PF tissues, which may be more important than the amplitudes in the mechanism of female urinary continence, are usually ignored. Current quantitative measurements of 2D ultrasound images can only tell us about the resting position of the urethra and the displacement at the end of events such as Valsalva, voluntary PFM contraction and coughing. The difficulties with accurately determining the finishing point of any maneuver, are numerous and are a potential source of error. The operator has either had to make multiple on-screen measurements, or determine the exact peak moment, or end position of the maneuver, freeze it, and then measure the change in position manually on screen or within in built electronic calipers. Without correcting for probe movement relative to the pubis symphysis the percentage errors range from 18–87%. In addition measuring only the re-positioning of urogenital structures is of limited value because intermediary anatomical changes are not registered.

In order to develop more sensitive measures to define normal PF function pilot studies were performed to capture and visualize the sequence of dynamic changes the PFM produced on the urethra, vagina and rectum using digital image-processing methods. The approach taken is to use an edge extraction algorithm to outline the coordinates of the symphysis, urethra and rectum interfaces on a frame-by-frame basis for sequences of stress inducing events such a cough, Valsalva and voluntarily induced PF contractions. During each event, the trajectory of the boundary of each structure was identified to characterize the sequential history of the ensuing movement. The resulting image analysis focused to reveal the anatomical displacement of the urogenital structures and to enable the evaluation of their biomechanical parameters in terms of displacement, velocity and acceleration. On the basis of these observations, we expect that the urogenital response to PF contractions can be quantified and the mechanism of UI, including the trajectories and timing of the PF activities, can be elucidated. Given that ultrasound imaging contains a considerable amount of useful data which can be obtained with the minimum of invasion to the patient, it is appropriate to find a way that this information be revealed, displayed quantitatively and quantitatively measure, analyze and describe the whole of the movement during a particular maneuver. We have accounted for movement of the probe, relative to the structures being examined and do not rely upon the operator to capture the precise moment at the end of the maneuver. Confidence is required none the less to validate the ultrasound approach with subjects of a broad age group and disposition. The visualization of the PF activities using 2D ultrasound imaging is likely to develop new measures of the PF functions that are more sensitive and specific than current methods. Those measures are useful for categorizing different sub groups of patients within a particular pathology and determining the most appropriate treatment intervention.

2 Methods

2.1 Coordinate System of the Anatomic Structures

Visual examination of the ultrasound images suggested that the displacement of the PF tissues during maneuvers contains components that can best be defined as a ventral (anterior) component towards or dorsal (posterior) component away from the symphysis pubis and a cephalad (superior) component upwards or caudad (inferior) component downwards. This is supported by other studies that suggest that in a functional PFM contraction, the bladder neck has been shown to move in a ventrocephlad direction increasing the closure pressure within the urethra as it is displaced towards the symphysis pubis and during valsalva, as the intra-abdominal pressure (IAP) increases, the bladder neck moves in an dorsal-caudad direction.

Therefore, an orthogonal coordinate system fixed on the bony landmark, the symphysis pubis, was established (Fig. 1). The two axes of the coordinate system are parallel and vertical to the urethra at rest respectively. The coordinate system is fixed during the maneuver, so when the subject deforms the bladder (State 2 in Fig. 1), the coordinate system will maintain its original position and the ensuing trajectory of urogenic structures can be measured relative to this fixed axis.

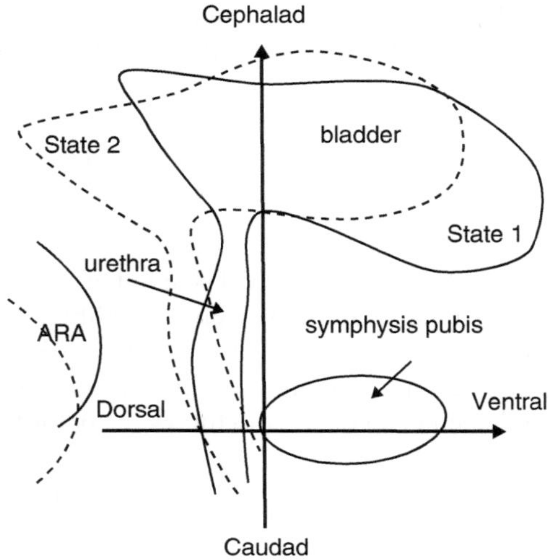

Fig. 1 The orthogonal coordinate system fixed on the symphysis pubis. The two orthogonal components (ventral-dorsal and cephalad-caudad components) of the tissues displacements reflect PF functions of squeezing the urethra and supporting the bladder respectively (Reprinted from Peng et al. 2006)

2.2 Motion Tracking Algorithms

A readily visible, clearly resolved anatomical structure in perineal ultrasound imaging is the angle the rectal ampulla forms with the anal canal, the ano-rectal angle (ARA). The movement of ARA can be used to analyze the PFM function because the sling of the PFM or Levator Ani muscles wrap around the anorectal junction, and its displacement is closely associated with a PFM contraction

In order to accurately map the trajectory of the ARA in response to a cough it is necessary to maintain each frame indexed to the symphysis pubis, which is a stationary, rigid, non deforming structure. However, the movement of the ultrasound probe in experiments could cause a motion artifact in the image of the symphysis pubis. Therefore, the motion artifact of the symphysis pubis needs to be tracked and subtracted from the motion of the ARA. To accomplish the task of indexing, we developed an adaptive motion tracking algorithm based on matching template to measure the movement of the symphysis pubis.

Initially, a template of the symphysis pubis is manually defined in the first frame of the ultrasound video. The template is then compared with the second image frame with different offsets in both x and y direction. The matched position in the second image frame is defined as the position where the difference function $D(k,l)$, given by Eq. (1), has the minimum value.

$$D(k,l) = \sum_{i=0}^{M-1} \sum_{j=0}^{N-1} \left| T_{i,j} - P_{i+k,j+l} \right| \tag{1}$$

where, $T_{i,j}$ $P_{i+k,j+l}$ and are the template and the image to be matched respectively. M and N is the size of the template. k and l are offsets for matching at different position.

The template for the matching the following image frames is then updated according to Eq. (2) and the matching procedure is repeated until the last image frame.

$$T(n) = \frac{1}{n}\sum_{i=0}^{n-1} S(i) = \frac{n-1}{n}T(n-1) + \frac{1}{n}S(n-1) \qquad n \geq 2 \tag{2}$$

where, $S(i)$ is the matched position of the symphysis pubis in image frame i.

A similar adaptive matching algorithm is used to track the motion of ARA. However, ARA is a soft tissue structure which deforms, particularly in fast maneuvers like coughing. Therefore, a weight coefficient is introduced to speed up the updating of the template in order to follow the deformations:

$$T(n) = w \cdot T(n-1) + (1-w) \cdot S(n-1) \qquad n \geq 2 \tag{3}$$

where, w is the weight coefficient, $w \in [0, 1]$. In practice, w is set to a value between 0.7 and 0.8 according to the extent of the ARA deformation.

To decrease the effect of the size and position of the initial template, manually defined in the first image frame, the tracking procedure is performed four times with different initial templates and the results are averaged. The relative movement of ARA to the symphysis pubis is then derived by subtracting the motion of symphysis pubis from that of ARA.

Figure 2 illustrates the results of the motion tracking of a healthy subject's symphysis pubis and ARA in supine. Figure 2a shows the ultrasound image at rest and the ventral-cephalad coordinate system. The motion tacking of the symphysis pubis and ARA are shown in Fig. 2b and c respectively. The relative movement of ARA shown in Fig. 2d, is derived by subtracting the motion of symphysis pubis from that of ARA and then transforming the image coordinate system to the ventral-cephalad coordinate system.

2.3 Image Segmentation Algorithms

Because the urogenital structures are anatomically interconnected, ultrasound based dynamic imaging can substantiate urodynamic observations of the effective distribution of pressure transmission to the urethra closure mechanism. However, urethra and bladder, which are the container or path of the urine, may have huge deformation in maneuvers. The above-mentioned motion tracking algorithms based on matching are not applicable in the movement analysis of the urethra and bladder.

Therefore, an image segmentation algorithm needs to be designed to segment the boundaries of the urethra and bladder. The movement analysis of the urethra and bladder can then be based on the tracking of the typical anatomic position, such as Urethro-Vesical Junction (UVJ), on the boundaries of the urethra and bladder.

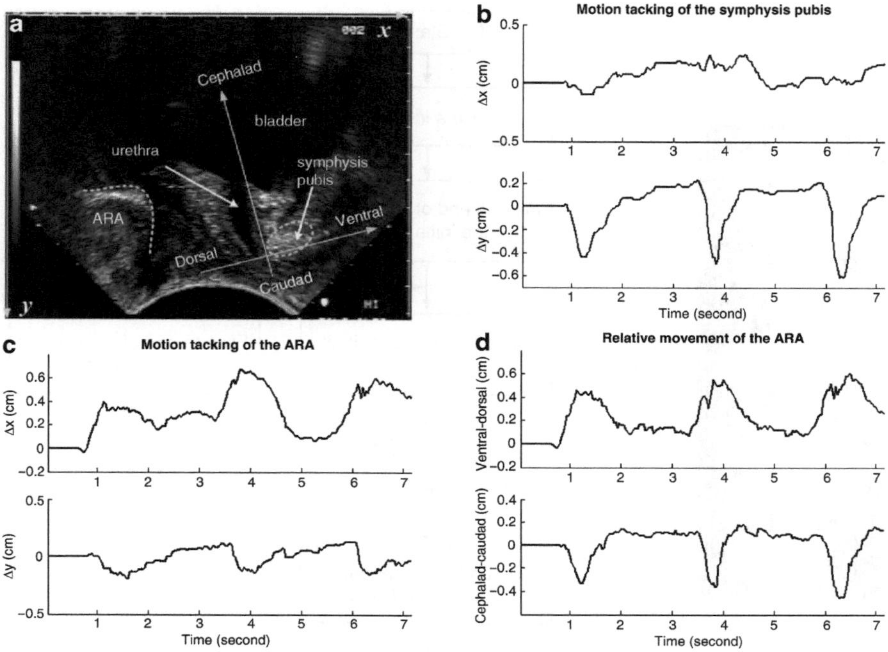

Fig. 2 The motion tracking of a healthy subject's symphysis pubis and ARA in supine. (**a**) The ultrasound image and the coordinate system. (**b**) The motion tracking of the symphysis pubis and the ARA (**c**). (**d**) The ventral-dorsal and cephalad-caudad components of the displacement of the ARA (Reprinted from Peng et al. 2007)

Test results show that the segmentation algorithms usually do not work well because of the speckle noise in the ultrasound images, the movement and out-of-plane rotation of the ultrasound probe, and especially the huge deformations of the urethra and bladder during fast, stressful maneuvers like coughing. Therefore, a simple and effective segmentation algorithm based on "virtual ruler" was developed for the segmentation of the urethra and bladder.

To begin, the original ultrasound images with integer values were converted to binary images with logical value of 0s (black) and 1s (white). Otsu's method, which minimizes the intra-class variance of the black and white pixels, was used to determine the threshold for the conversion. All pixels in the intensity image with value less than the threshold have value 0 (black) in the binary image. And all other pixels have value 1 (white) in the binary image. Then, the isolated pixels (individual 1s that are surrounded by 0s) were removed from the binary images by combining morphological operations of dilation and erosion.

The boundaries of anterior and posterior edges of urethra and bladder were then segmented in the binary images using the automatic segmentation algorithm shown in Fig. 3. An initial point on the edge to be segmented was chosen, and one end of a virtual ruler was fixed on the initial point. The virtual ruler was then rotated around the initial point until it hit a non-zero point on the edge. The fixed end of the virtual

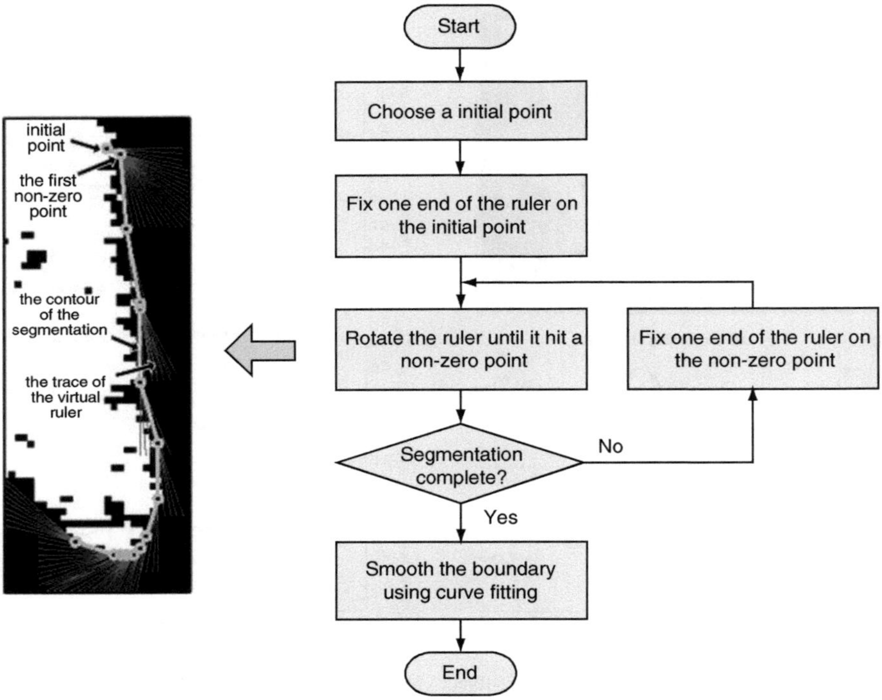

Fig. 3 Flow chart of automatic image segmentation. (Modified and reprinted in part from Peng et al. 2007)

ruler was then moved to the non-zero point. The virtual ruler was rotated around the fixed point again until it hit a new non-zero point on the edge. The procedure of moving and rotating the virtual ruler was repeated until the contour of the whole boundary was acquired. The length of the virtual ruler is an adjustable parameter to obtain different resolution of the segmentation. The shorter the virtual ruler, the more detailed information will be elucidated in the segmentation. However, the results of the segmentation will be affected by the noise in the ultrasound images if the virtual ruler is too short. Therefore, the length of the virtual ruler was set from 4 to 16 pixels. After the segmentation, smoothing spline, a nonparametric fitting method available in MATLAB® curve-fitting toolbox, was applied to smooth the segmented boundaries of tissues. The smoothing parameter was set to $p = 0.8$ to obtain the most reasonable results.

3 Results

We analyzed perineal ultrasonography of 22 asymptomatic females and nine Stress Urinary Incontinent (SUI) patients with a broad age distribution and parity. Figure 4 illustrates the differences between continent and SUI women in the magnitude and

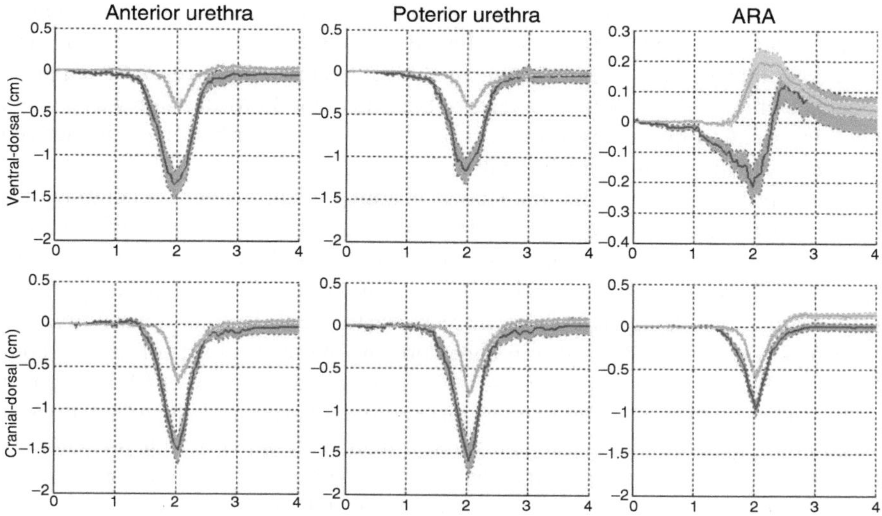

Fig. 4 Ventral-dorsal and cranio-caudal displacements of the anterior UVJ, posterior UVJ and ARA during a cough in supine. The Standard Error (SE) of the displacements is marked by the thickness of the colored areas. The continent and the SUI women are shown in green and red respectively

ventral-dorsal and cranio-caudal displacement during a cough. As clearly indicated by Fig. 4, both the direction and temporal sequence of the ARA movement are distinctly different between the continent and SUI women. During a cough, in continent women the ARA moves ventrally towards the SP. In SUI women the ARA moves dorsally away from the SP. Furthermore, the amplitude of the maximum caudal movement of the SUI women' ARA and UVJ are larger than those of the continent women. T-tests were performed to compare the continent and SUI women. The results indicate that the ARA and UVJ displacements of the continent and SUI women are significantly different ($P < 0.0001$) in both the ventral-dorsal and cranio-caudal direction.

Results given by Fig. 4 imply that the PFM of the continent women function vary differently from those volunteers with SUI. It appears that the functional PFM in continent women, provide support to the urogenital structures prior to and during a cough, acting like a brake, to resist or limit the dorsal-caudal movement that occurs as IAP inevitably rises during a cough. In women with SUI, this PFM "brake" appears to have been applied late, or is diminished, demonstrated by the increased displacement of the ARA and the increased velocity and acceleration. The pilot results quantitatively demonstrated the characteristic mechanical response of the ARA to the cough reflex of asymptomatic women. Evidence was provided to show that continent and asymptomatic women can clearly and significantly be identified from those with SUI on the basis of a number of parameters such as the displacement, velocity and acceleration of the ARA movement. Furthermore these studies were obtained using the non-invasive nature of transperineal ultrasound, the significance of the results are of current practical clinical value in evaluating women with SUI. As a consequence of the degree of the analytical treatment applied to the temporal sequence of the data, important aspects of the role of the PFM function was gained. Such information may prove critical in identifying the contribution of the derived parameters to the mechanisms of continence.

Our approach is one of the first studies enabling quantification, generating new dynamic parameters of PFM function. It incorporates original software, which is not operator dependent, thereby improving the reliability of the measurement tool. Our approach of processed Ultrasound imaging of the pelvic floor provides significant new information relating to its dynamic response to stress. This non-invasive type of information is potentially of use in understanding the mechanisms of urinary continence, which is a silent epidemic severely affecting the quality of life of women with Urinary Incontinence. Potentially, this approach can help lay the foundations of determining a more reliable pragmatic assessment of PFM function and eventually improve the rehabilitation of women with SUI and other pelvic floor disorders. Furthermore these studies suggest that the anatomical and physiological changes of the PF in women with SUI can be highlighted by analyzing the activities of an anatomical triangle comprising of the Urethra-Vesical Junction (UVJ), Ano-Rectal Angle (ARA) and Symphysis Pubis (SP). On this basis we developed a software package of 2-D ultrasound image processing for the analysis and visualization of the static and dynamic responses of the UVJ-ARA-SP triangle to provide a sensitive and reliable tool for the clinical diagnoses.

3.1 Quantitative Analysis of the Static Characters of the UVJ-ARA-SP Triangle

The UVJ-ARA-SP triangle is an anatomical triangle comprising of the Urethra-Vesical Junction (UVJ), Ano-Rectal Angle (ARA) and Symphysis Pubis (SP). The reasons we introduce the concept of the UVJ-ARA-SP triangle into the evaluation of the PF functions are:

1. The PF is a complex 3D arrangement of muscle and connective tissue, attached to the bony pelvis. The SP is the best stationary, rigid and bony landmark in 2D perineal ultrasound imaging for the measurement of the relative movement of the other PF tissues including PFM, vaginal, urethra and bladder.
2. The activities of the ARA are closely associated with the activities of PFM which is under the neural control, because the sling of the PFM wraps around the ARA.
3. The activities of the UVJ are important in the UI mechanisms. UVJ are closely associated with the changes of the abdominal pressures which may lead to UI when PFM cannot response appropriately.

The UVJ, ARA and SP are the most readily visible, clearly resolved anatomical structure in perineal ultrasound imaging. The concept of UVJ-ARA-SP triangle enables the systematic evaluation of the overall PF responses to incontinence stimulus like cough. We manually derived the UVJ-ARA-SP triangles of 17 asymptomatic females and five SUI patients in supine and in standing. Figure 5 shows the UVJ-ARA-SP triangles of asymptomatic females and SUI patients are distinct in both supine and standing.

The UVJ-ARA-SP triangle has 11 geometric parameters including dorsal-ventral and cranial-caudal coordinates of ARA and UVJ (four parameters), length of three sides (three parameters), three internal angles (three parameters) and the area (one parameter). Those parameters are of important anatomic and physiological information related to the PF functions.

Table 1 compares the mean of the seven parameters of the UVJ-ARA-SP triangles of 17 healthy subjects and five SUI patients in supine and standing. The healthy

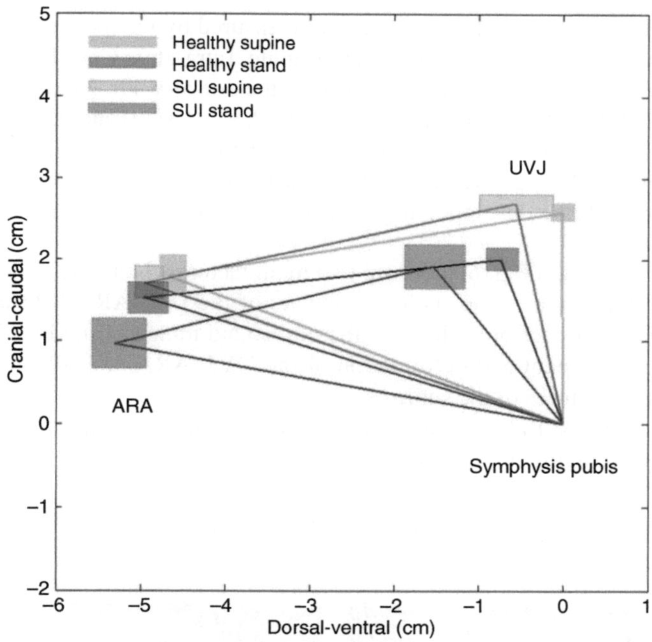

Fig. 5 The UVJ-Pubis-ARA triangles of 17 asymptomatic females and five SUI patients. Healthy supine: green; Healthy stand: blue; SUI supine: magenta; SUI stand: red. The Standard Error (SE) is shown by the transparent bars in different colors

Table 1 Parameters of the UVJ-ARA-SP triangles (Healthy subjects: 17, SUI patients: 5)

			Angle (degree)			Length of sides (cm)		
		Area (cm^2)	UVJ	ARA	SP	UVJ-SP	ARA-SP	ARA-UVJ
Healthy subjects	Supine	6.00	80.87	30.65	68.48	2.58	4.99	4.71
	Stand	4.39	103.89	23.55	52.55	2.13	5.19	4.24
SUI patients	Supine	6.19	89.09	31.70	59.21	2.75	5.24	4.50
	Stand	4.32	114.74	24.49	40.77	2.46	5.39	3.87

subjects and SUI patients has similar changes in those seven parameters (Area: ↓, UVJ angle: ↑, ARA angle ↓, SP angle: ↓, UVJ-SP side: ↓, ARA-SP side: ↑, ARA-UVJ side: ↓) when they stood up. Those changes of those parameters reflect the descent of the PF tissues and the responses of the PFM in stand. Table 1 also shows the differences between the healthy subjects and SUI patients. For example, the SUI patients have larger UVJ angle and longer ARA-SP side. Those parameters reflect the fact that the SUI patients have descended PF because of the pathological changes of the mechanical properties of their connective tissues and the dysfunctions of their PFM.

3.2 *Automatic Detection of the UVJ-ARA-SP Triangle*

Manual analysis of the same pilot data were measured by independent observers to test the reliability of the UVJ-Pubis-ARA triangle. Intra-class Correlations (ICC) of the single measures are calculated. The ICC in the dorsal-ventral and cranial-caudal directions are 0.696 (95% Confidence Interval: [0.506 0.822]) and 0.720 (95% Confidence Interval: [0.540 0.837]) respectively indicating satisfactory the reliability of the measurement. To improve the reliability further, algorithms of ultrasound image processing need to be developed to characterize the static parameters of the UVJ-ARA-SP triangle.

As demonstrated in Fig. 6, there are two main factors which affect the reliability of the characterization of the static parameters of the UVJ-ARA-SP triangle. The first factor is the higher noise level in the ultrasound image of the PF. The second factor is the movement and deformation of the UVJ, ARA and SP caused by the changes of the postures of the subjects.

The Signal-Noise-Ratio (SNR) of the ultrasound image of the static PF can be improved by averaging multi-images:

$$SNR_{average} = \sqrt{N} \cdot SNR_{machine} \tag{4}$$

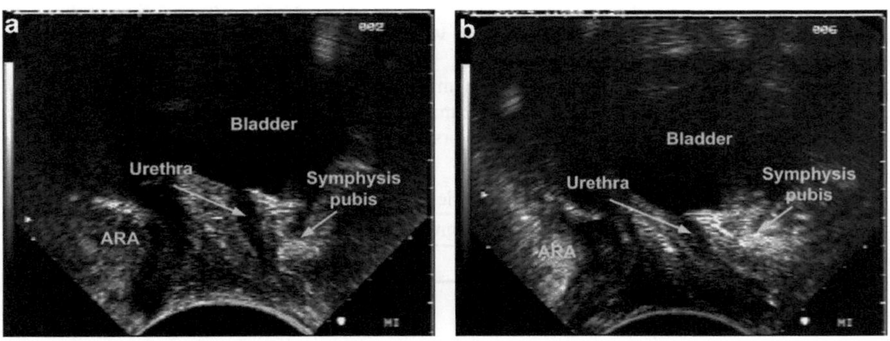

Fig. 6 The effects of the subject's postures on the geometry of the pelvic tissues

where, $SNR_{machine}$ is the SNR of the ultrasound machine. N is the number of ultrasound images been averaged. $SNR_{average}$ is the SNR of the averaged image.

However, the subjects and ultrasongraphers may not be able to keep absolutely stationary when the images for averaging are acquired. If that occurs, the movement artifacts will be produced when the images are averaged directly. Therefore, the algorithm to track the movement of the rigid body in our preliminary studies can be applied on the SP. Then, all the frames can be matched and averaged to produce a single image with higher SNR. The UVJ in the enhanced static ultrasound image can be detected automatically by the image segmentation algorithms. The movement and deformation of the SP and ARA caused by the changes of the postures of the subjects can also be registered and detected by the motion tracking algorithms.

3.3 *Quantitative Analysis of the Dynamic Characters of the UVJ-ARA-SP Triangle*

The activities of the UVJ-ARA-SP triangles in different maneuvers are of important information about the physiological mechanisms of the PF. That information cannot be assimilated and quantified by the observer in regular ultrasound imaging. The techniques of the digital ultrasound image processing and animation will highlight that information and enable the quantitative measurement and analysis of that information.

Based on the motion tracking and segmentation algorithms we developed in the pilot study, the trajectories of the UVJ-ARA-SP triangles in different maneuvers can be visualized using the techniques of animation. A method of the visualization is demonstrated in Fig. 7a. The trajectories of the UVJ and ARA are overlapped with the real ultrasound image and displayed in the polar coordinate systems to visualize the directions and routes of the UVJ and ARA in three maneuvers including PFM contraction, cough and Valsalva.

Figure 7a clearly visualized the typical responses of the healthy subject's PF in different maneuvers:

1. In PFM contraction, PFM pushed urethra and bladder towards the ventral and cranial direction. The movement of the UVJ was smaller than that of the ARA, because UVJ was moved passively.
2. In Valsalva, the increased abdominal pressures pushed UVJ and ARA towards the dorsal and caudal direction. The movement of the ARA was smaller than that of the UVJ. The possible reason is that the increased abdominal pressures passed UVJ before they reached the ARA.
3. In cough, the trajectories of the ARA and UVJ are distinct because PFM activated in response to the increased abdominal pressures in cough. The ventral movement of the ARA may lead to the increases of the abdominal pressures in the urethra to prevent UI. The dorsal-caudal movement of the UVJ in cough was smaller than that in Valsalva because of the responses of the PFM in cough.

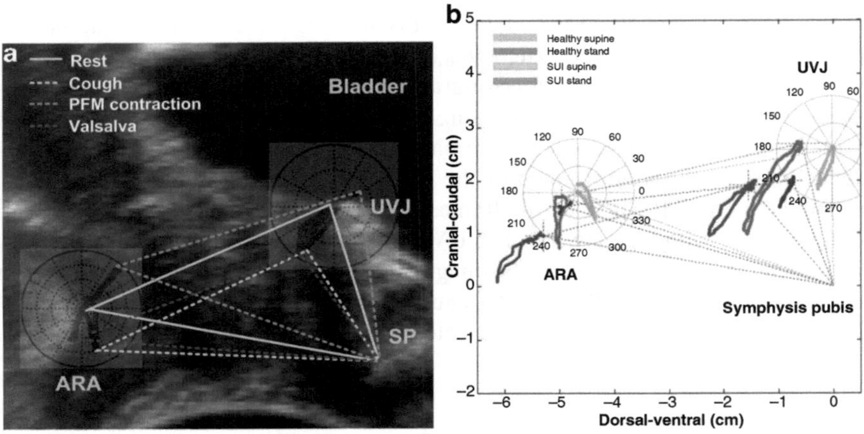

Fig. 7 (**a**) The trajectories of the UVJ-ARA-SP triangles of a healthy subject in supine. The UVJ-ARA-SP triangles at rest, in cough, in PFM contraction and in Valsalva are shown by the yellow solid lines, yellow dotted lines, green dotted lines and magenta lines respectively. (**b**) The average trajectories of the UVJ-ARA-SP triangles of 17 healthy subjects and five SUI patients in cough. The healthy subjects in supine, the healthy subjects in stand, the SUI patients in supine and the SUI patients in stand are shown in green, blue, magenta and red respectively

Figure 7a is the first visualization of the overall responses of the healthy subject's PF. Figure 7b shows there are significant differences between the trajectories of the UVJ-ARA-SP triangles of healthy subjects and SUI patients in cough. Therefore, such kind of visualization is highly likely to develop into a sensitive and reliable method for the clinical evaluation of the PF functions.

3.4 Quantitative Measurement of Dynamic Parameters of the UVJ-ARA-SP Triangle

As indicated, the UVJ-ARA-SP triangle has 11 geometric parameters which are of important anatomic and physiological information related to the PF functions. The changes of those parameters in different maneuvers can be derived from the above-mentioned analysis of the trajectories (D.2.1). Figure 8 shows the changes of the seven parameters of the UVJ-ARA-SP triangles of 17 healthy subjects and five SUI patients in cough. Figure 8 is of some very interesting information need to be studied further: (1) For the SUI patients, the three internal angles of the UVJ-ARA-SP triangles at the center of the cough (2 s in Fig. 8a) were the same in supine and in stand. The same phenomenon is found in Valsalva. (2) In stand, the length of the ARA-SP side of the triangle increased at the center of the cough. That may explain why the possibility of UI increases when the SUI patients cough in stand.

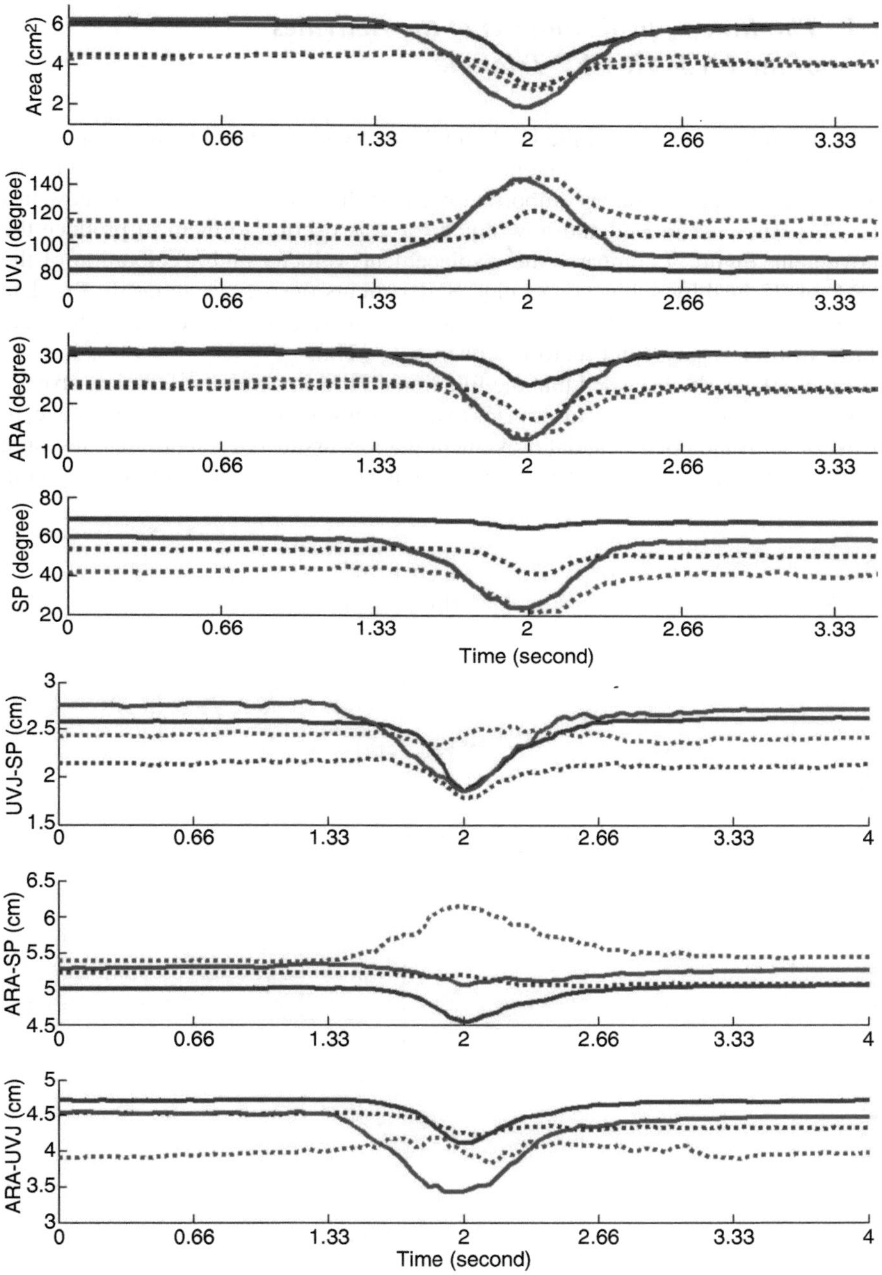

Fig. 8 (**a**) Area, UVJ angle, ARA angle, SP angle, (**b**) UVJ-SP side, ARA-SP side and ARA-UVJ side of the UVJ-Pubis-ARA triangle in cough. Blue solid: healthy subjects in supine; blue dotted: healthy subjects in stand; Red solid: SUI patients in supine; Red dotted: SUI patients in stand

3.5 The Kinematical Analysis of the Activities of the UVJ-ARA-SP Triangle

Velocity and acceleration of the UVJ and ARA, two important kinematics parameters, can be derived from the first and second derivative of their displacement. The velocity and acceleration are important because they are associated with how fast the PF tissues are moved and how much force is exerted to them to produce the movement. Figure 9 compares the displacement, velocity and acceleration of the ARA of 22 healthy subjects and nine SUI patients during coughing. In the data pre-processing, the velocity and acceleration were smoothed using an eight-order Butterworth low-pass filter (cutoff frequency = 3 Hz).

Figure 9 clearly disclosed that the functional PFM in continent females, provide support to the urogenic structures prior to and during a cough, acting like a brake, to resist or limit the dorsal-caudal movement that occurs as intra-abdominal pressure (IAP) rises during a cough. This hypothesis is supported both by comparing both

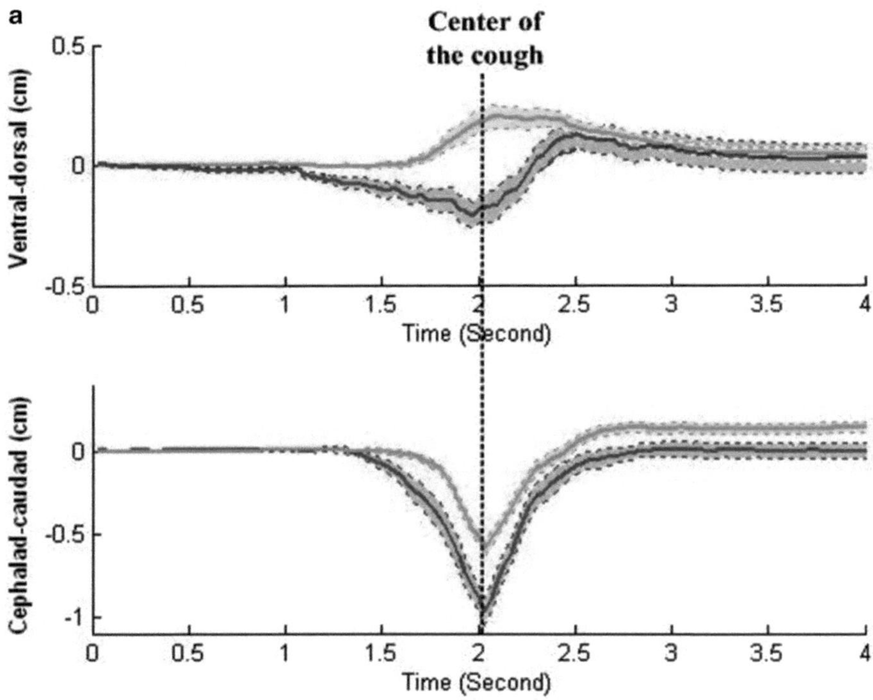

Fig. 9 Mean and SE of the ventral (positive)-dorsal (negative) and cephalad (positive)-caudad (negative) components of the (**a**) displacement, (**b**) velocity and (**c**) acceleration of the ARA in supine during coughing. The healthy subjects and the SUI patients are shown in green and red respectively. The SE of the signals is marked by the colored areas

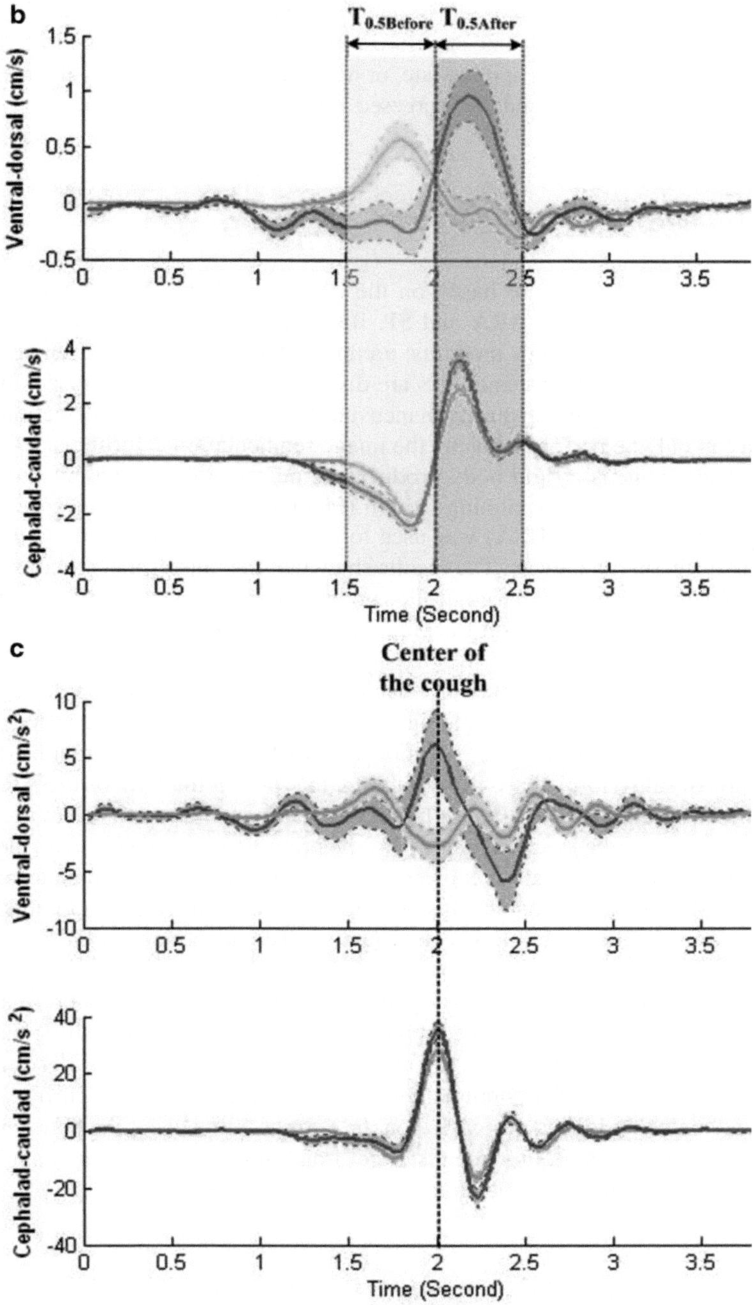

Fig. 9 (continued)

the overall direction and magnitude of displacement as well as the reduced velocity and acceleration of the urogenic structures. In women with SUI, this PFM "brake" appears either to have been applied late, or not at all, demonstrated by the increased displacement of the ARA and the increased velocity and acceleration.

3.6 Motion Tracking Algorithms

All quantitative analysis are based on the detection of the three main anatomic structures including UVJ, ARA and SP. Because of the differences in their mechanical properties (Young's modulus: urethra < ARA < SP), the movement of the UVJ, ARA and the SP in maneuvers are distinct. The urethra is very flexible and may have huge deformation during maneuvers. The reliable motion detection of the urethra can only be performed using the image segmentation algorithms.

The pubic bone is a rigid body produces no deformation during maneuvers. In our pilot studies, a 3D positioning system (Flock of Birds, FOB, Ascension technology Corporation VA, USA) was used to trace the movement of the ultrasound probe in different maneuvers. The results show that the out-of-plane rotation of the ultrasound probe can easily be controlled under a certain range ($< \pm 5°$). Therefore, as shown in Fig. 9, the motion tracking algorithm works very well in the motion detection of the SP (Fig. 10).

The ARA is flexible and may produce non-negligible deformation during some maneuvers. In the pilot study, a weight coefficient is introduced to speed up the updating of the template in order to follow the ARA deformations (demonstrated in Fig. 11a). Besides, to increase the reliability, the motion tracking of the ARA was performed four times with different initial templates and the results were averaged. Those methods worked well in majority of the preliminary data. However, the ARA deformations in some coughs went so fast that the updating of the template couldn't follow it. Therefore, new algorithms need to be developed for the motion tracking of the ARA with faster and larger deformation. The adaptive matching algorithm with two matching templates demonstrated in Fig. 11b is one of the algorithms we are developing for that purpose. Firstly, the new algorithm performs a pre-matching using a pre-template, which is the weighted average of the last matching template and the matched zone of the last frame. Secondly, a new template is derived from the weighted average of pre-template and the matched zone of the current frame. A second matching is then performed on the current frame using the new template. The new algorithm can follow the faster deformations and is potentially applicable to improve the reliability of the motion tracking of the ARA in cough.

3.7 Visualization of the Dynamic Profiles of the Urethra

Urethra is the path of urine and it works as a "valve" in the mechanism of urinary continence during maneuvers. The opening and closure mechanism of the urethra

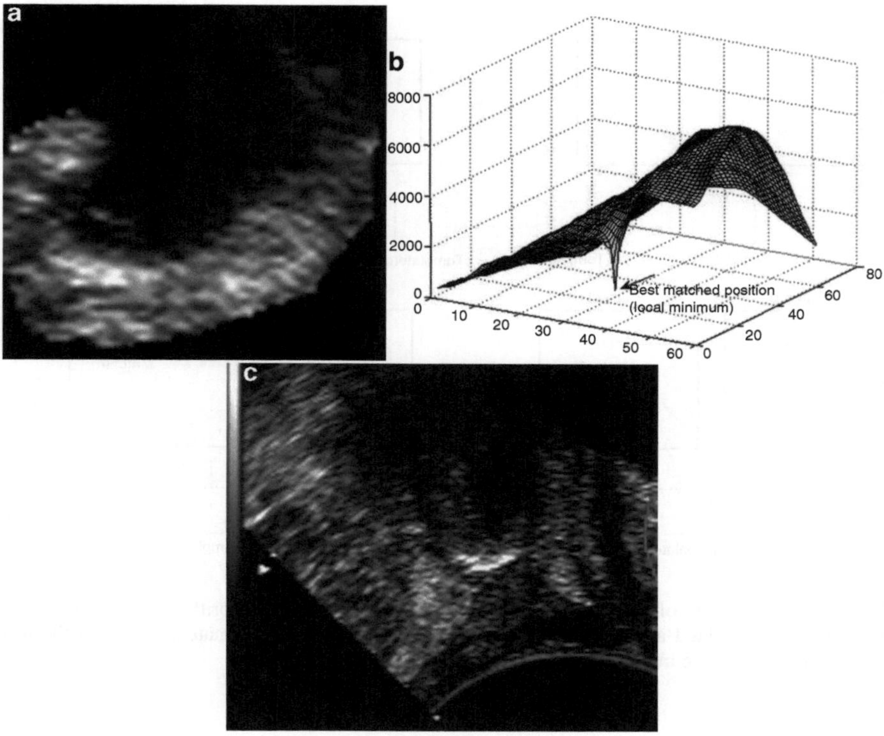

Fig. 10 (**a**) The matching template of the SP. (**b**) Difference function of the matching template and an ultrasound frame. (**c**) Matched SP in the ultrasound frame is marked by the red boundary

in fast and stressful maneuvers can be highlighted by visualization of the movement profile of the urethra. The segmentation algorithms enabled the visualization of the dynamic profiles of the urethra. As shown in Fig. 12a, the anterior and posterior edges of the urethra was segmented and divided into eight evenly-spaced segmentations. The movements of the eight segments during coughs, contractions and valsalvas were then tracked. Figure 12b–d show the typical ventral-dorsal movement profiles of a healthy subject's anterior edge of the urethra during coughs, contractions and valsalvas respectively.

Figure 12 discloses that the further the distance between the position on the anterior edge of urethra and the posterior inferior margin of the SP, the bigger the absolute value of the displacement of the position during maneuvers. There is more displacement at the proximal end compared to the distal end of the urethra.

The displacement of the (ARA) is closely associated with a PFM contraction. Motion tracking algorithms quantitatively evaluate the movement of the ARA in different maneuvers. However, the deformation of the ARA also contains important physiological information and is mainly determined by the dimension and location of the PFM as well as the strength of the PFM contraction (Fig. 13).

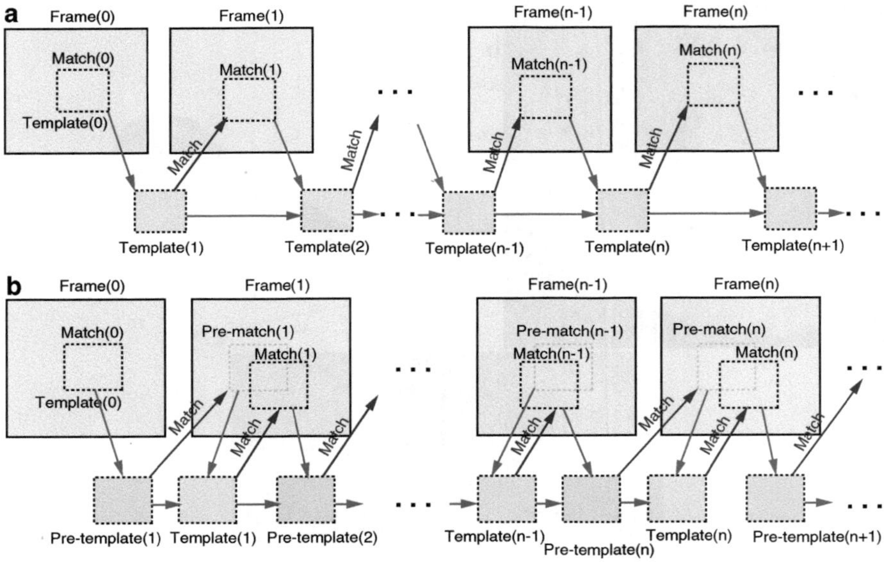

Fig. 11 The updating of the matching template in the motion track algorithms (**a**) the matching template n is weighted average of the matching template n-1 and the matched zone in the last frame. (**b**) An adaptive matching algorithm with two matching templates

3.8 Visualization of the Timing of the Dynamic Profiles

Clinical studies imply that the PFM of the normal subjects have two mechanisms to prevent the urine from incontinence in maneuvers like coughing. (1) The well-functional PFM contractions give the bladder and the posterior edge of the urethra more support in the cephalad direction, when the abdominal pressure increases and pushes the bladder towards the caudad direction. (2) The well-functional PFM contraction pushes the urethra against the symphysis pubis in ventral direction and therefore increases the closure pressure in urethra, when the increased abdominal pressure pushes the urethra towards the dorsal direction.

Appropriate timing control of the PFM contraction may be more important than the amplitude of the pressures produced by the PFM contraction in preventing UI. The normal subjects' PFM contraction pushed the ano-rectal junction to the ventral direction (towards the urethra) before the increased abdominal pressures was able to push the ano-rectal junction and urethra to the dorsal direction. By contrast, the SUI patients' PFM contractions were behind the increased abdominal pressures in timing. As a result, the ARA and urethra were pushed dorsally at first and then rebounded back to the ventral direction with higher velocity. Those movements are likely to reduce the closure pressures in the urethra.

Therefore, visualization methods, which can highlight the timing of the movement of pelvic tissues in fast, stressful maneuvers, will facilitate the understanding

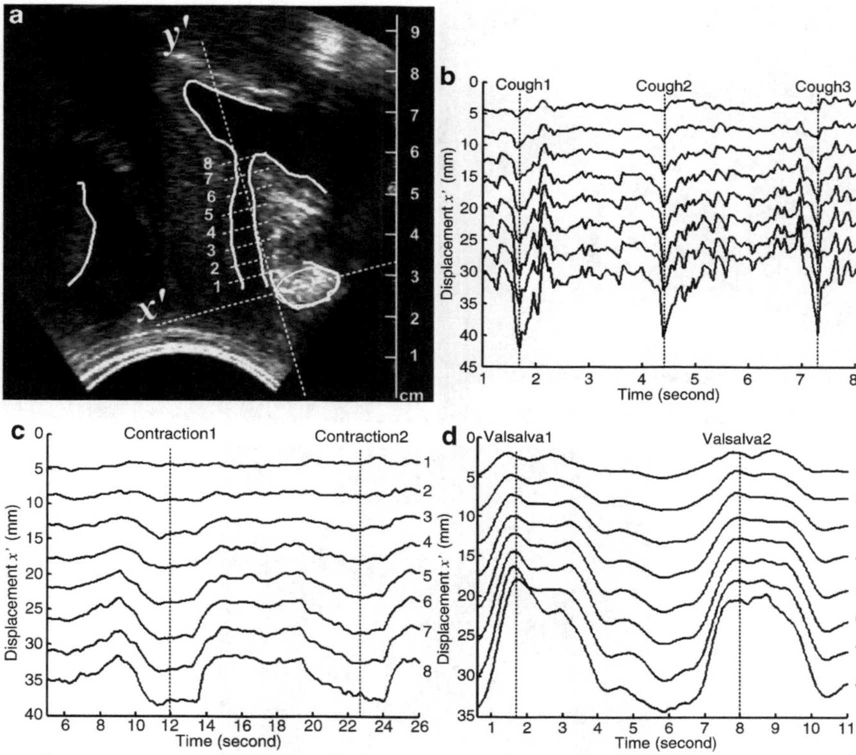

Fig. 12 Displacement of eight evenly-spaced positions (**a**) on the anterior edge of the urethra during (**b**) coughs, (**c**) contractions and (**d**) Valsalvas. Y axis is the displacement in ventral-dorsal direction

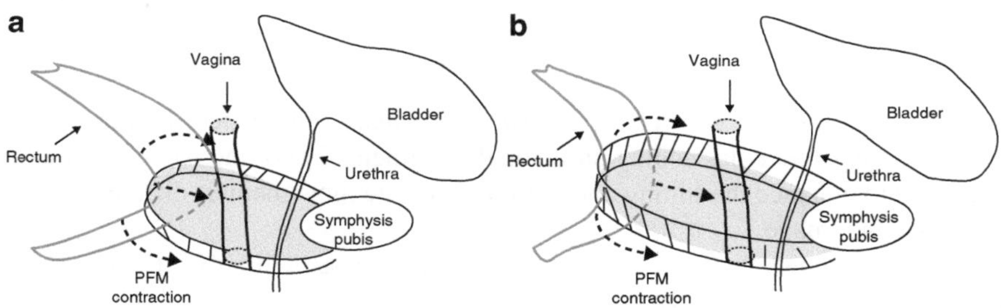

Fig. 13 The deformations of the rectum under different PFM pressures. (**a**) The ARA is acute when the PFM is narrow and the strength of the PFM contraction is strong. (**b**) The ARA is round when the PFM is wide and the strength of the PFM contraction is not very strong. The deformation is also affected by the stiffness of the rectum and the contents within it

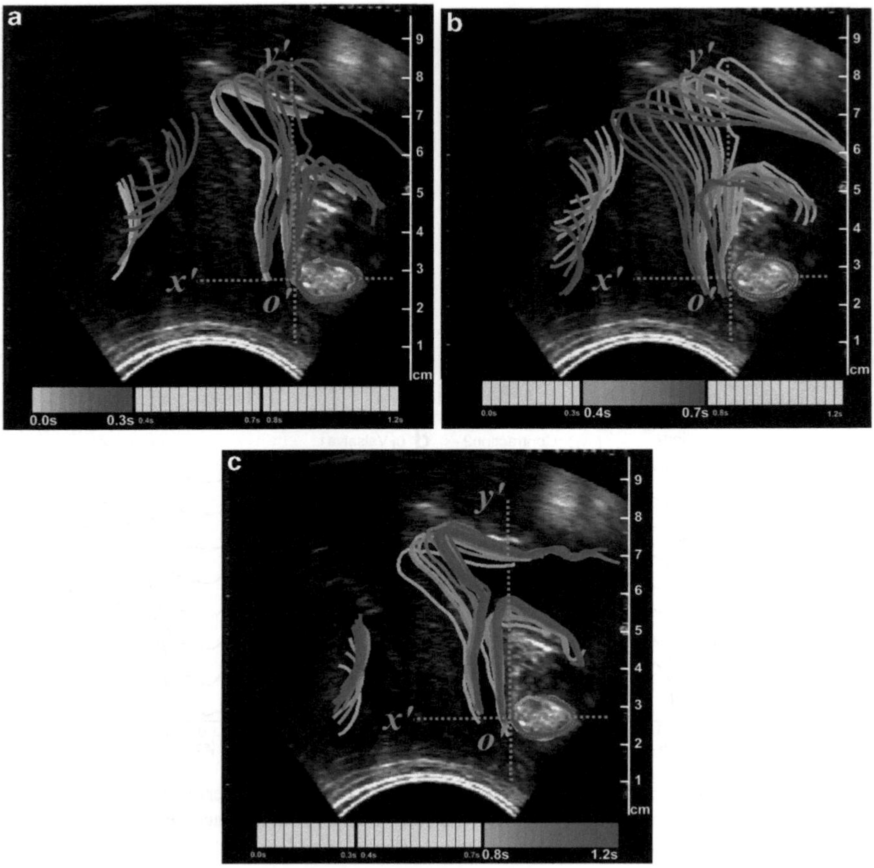

Fig. 14 The timing of the movement of tissues in pelvic floor during a typical cough in a healthy volunteer

of the neuromuscular control mechanisms in urinary continence. In Fig. 14, 14 and 15, transparent color coding based on the segmentation of the ARA and urethra was used to enhance the timing and amplitude of the movement of different tissues in ultrasound image.

Figure 14 shows the timing of the movement of tissues in pelvic floor during a typical cough in a healthy volunteer. There are three typical phases to the displacement of the urogenic structures. During the first 0.3 s they move in a ventral-cephlad (forward and up) direction (Fig. 14a) before moving in a dorsal-caudal (back and down) direction (Fig. 14b), over passing the initial resting position (0.4–0.7 s) before moving from the rightmost position back to the initial resting position (Fig. 14c) as the volunteer finishes the cough (0.8–1.2 s).

Figure 15 shows the timing of the movement of tissues in pelvic floor during a typical PFM contraction in the same volunteer. As the volunteer contracts her PFM,

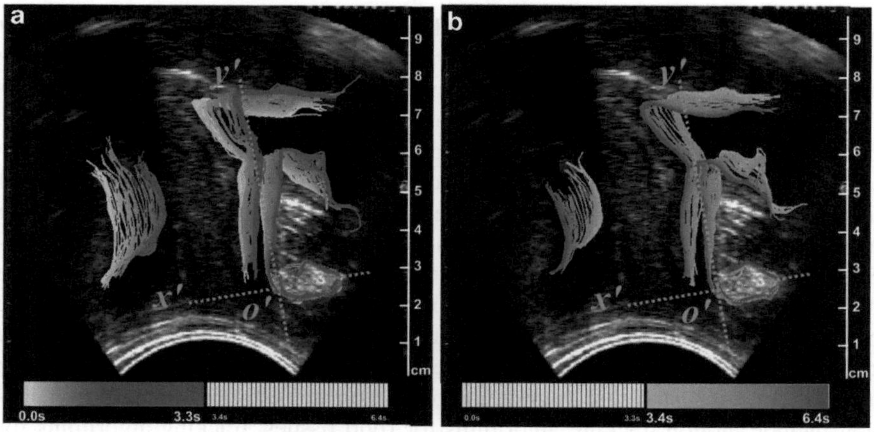

Fig. 15 The timing of the movement of tissues in pelvic floor during a typical PFM contraction

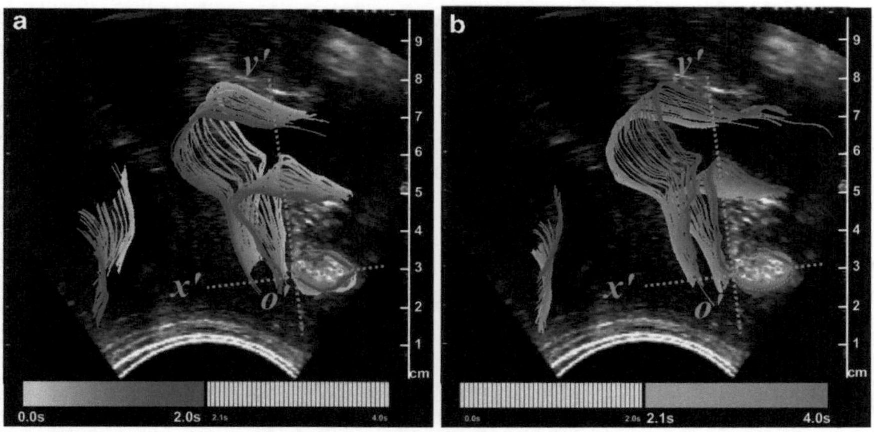

Fig. 16 Timing of the movement of tissues in pelvic floor during a typical Valsalva

(Fig. 15a) the urogenic structures move in a ventral-cephlad direction (forward and up). As she releases the contraction, or relaxes the PFM (Fig. 15b) the tissues return to the original resting position.

Figure 16 shows the timing of the movement of tissues in pelvic floor during a typical Valsalva. As the volunteer performs this forced expiration technique, the urogenic structures move from their resting position in a dorsal-caudal direction (down and back) (Fig. 16a) before returning to their resting position as the volunteer completes the maneuver (Fig. 16b).

Differences in the mechanical properties and function of the complicated anatomic structures in PF can be divided into three types. The first type includes the rigid tissues such as SP, which produce no deformation during maneuvers. The second type includes the soft tissues such as ARA, which deform slightly in fast maneuvers like coughing. The third type includes the soft tissues such as urethra and bladder, which are the container or path of the urine and may have huge deformation in maneuvers. Therefore, different algorithms for movement detection, including motion tracking algorithms and segmentation algorithm need to be developed and integrated for the analysis of different types of tissues. Because of these considerations it is essential to develop 2-D ultrasound image processing approaches to analyze both the static and dynamic responses of the UVJ-ARA-SP triangle and to further reveal its physiological and clinical significance in the mechanism of urinary continence. It is expected that upon completion of this the project, the mechanism of PF function can be better identified and more sensitive clinical diagnoses and treatment outcome measures for SUI can be developed. To do this it is suggested that Algorithms of motion tracking and image segmentation include motion tracking algorithms for rigid tissues, tracking algorithms for tissues which deform slightly in different maneuvers (ARA), automatic or manual (for images with bad quality) segmentation algorithms for soft tissues which may have large deformation in different maneuvers. Furthermore, static and dynamic measurement of the UVJ-ARA-SP triangle should include the establishment of the clinical meaningful coordinate system.

It is also desirable to enhance the 2D ultrasound images to incorporate the overlap of the UVJ-ARA-SP triangle on the 2D dynamic ultrasound images using animation techniques to highlight the timing and trajectories of the movement and deformation of the UVJ-ARA-SP triangle. Finally it would be of practical utility to be able to overlap the profiles of the urethra and ARA on the 2D dynamic ultrasound images using animation techniques to highlight the timing of the opening and closure mechanisms of the urethra and deformations of ARA.

4 Bio Mechanical Properties of Pelvic Floor Function Using the Vaginal Probe

The contribution of forces facilitating continence were evaluated using a probe [15] specifically fabricated for vaginal insertion and considered analogous imaging results. Measurements were taken in the region of deep, middle and superficial vaginal levels and processed to generate the spatial distribution function of activity as stimulated by stimuli. Eight closure forces were evaluated at each level and a graphical visualization produced to illustrate the temporal and spatial distribution produced by active and passive stimuli. The convergence of multiple neuromuscular inputs to the pelvic floor muscles (PFM) contributes to the pro-continence guarding reflexes. Clinically it was established that voluntary pre-contraction of the PFM produces a dramatic reduction of stress urinary incontinence (SUI). The effect of pre-contraction (knack) is interpreted as a consequence of the mechanical stabilization of the vesical neck resulting in reduced mobility. Transmission studies suggest that the pro-continence biomechanical forces involved are applied by the supporting structures of the-urethra and indicate a considerable PFM contribution. Practically, localization of the region of action of the PFM can be made directly using vaginal palpation and more recently using probes. Vaginal probes currently in use are spatially limited in localizing the region over which forces from PFM are applied. Consequently neither the strength nor distribution of the forces involved has been recognized. Using a novel directional vaginal probe, we demonstrate in this paper the distribution of forces applied to the vaginal wall. The spatial and temporal distribution of PFM activation was mapped along the proximal, mid and distal vaginal wall. We repeatedly used the knack to activate a voluntary pre-contraction followed by the cough reflex as a test stimulus employing asymptomatic volunteers. Using the technology afforded by the vaginal probe, we identified and visualized the temporal and spatial distribution bio mechanical forces produced by PFM. The probe consisted of four force transducers mounted circumferentially at 90° on a 23 mm shaft. Transducers were covered with a lubricated female condom. Upon insertion into the vagina, with patient supine, sensors made contact with the vaginal wall and contact pressures in the different four directions were measured (Fig. 23).

In cough and knack experiments, the subjects were tested with two postures (supine and standing) on the different position of the vaginal walls (superficial, middle and deep). To measure the pressure in more directions, the probe was rotated 30° $\sim$ 45° in some experiments (Fig. 1).

Figure 3 typically shows the pattern of a cough and knack pressures recorded from the posterior aspect of the vagina (Figs. 17 and 18).

Values shown are defined as follows: Peak value of pressures in cough; Peak value of pressures in knack; Mean value of pressures in the PFM contraction stage of the precontraction (Figs. 19 and 20).

These figures show the peak pressures distribution of normal subjects during the cough and pre-contraction compared the distribution of the peak pressures during cough and knack (Fig. 21).

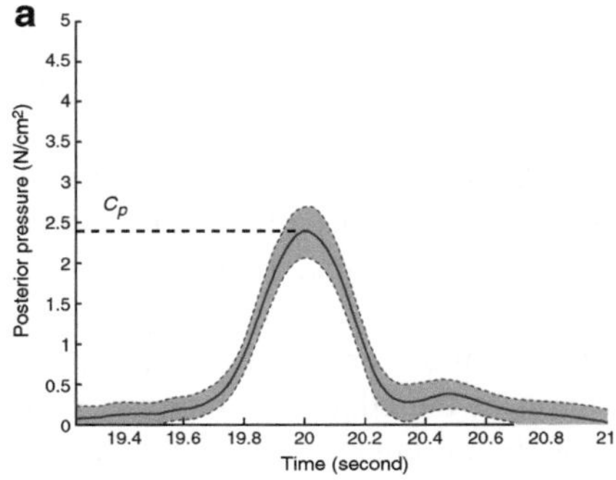

Fig. 17 Curve showing force generated by a cough

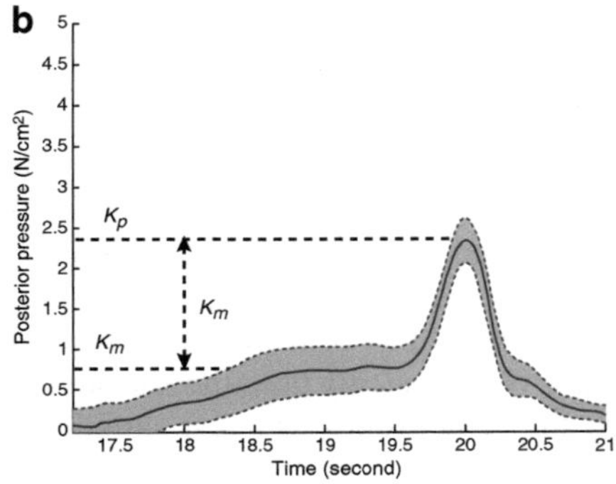

Fig. 18 Curve showing force generated by a precontraction

4.1 *Temporal/Spatial Visualization*

Considering the temporal response at each location, it is possible to represent the waveform as well as the distribution of pressures as illustrated by Fig. 22 showing the onset of closure pressures consequent to a cough stimulus of a healthy subject.

4.2 *Resting Closure Profiles*

Dynamic probe measurements shown are superimposed over the resting pressures generated by the pelvic floor muscles. Such static pressures are therefore additional to the dynamic effects of the various stimuli. The distribution of closure forces of each of the four directions can be assessed in both the supine and standing position. To do that the probe after insertion can be pulled-through the vagina at an approximate speed of 2 cm/sec manually while recording was done. Measurements were performed both at rest and during a PFM contraction for each subject. In order to prevent the inevitable fatigue of the subjects in maintaining PFM at maximum contraction, subjects were advised to moderate contraction intensity to half strength.

The static distribution of forces obtained was evaluated was averaged and a 2D image was constructed is shown by Fig. 24 (Fig. 25).

Maximum closure forces were on a position 1.98 ± 0.34 cm proximal from the introitus. Positions of the max anterior pressures at rest in continent and SUI groups were similar, 1.52 ± 0.09 cm and 1.69 ± 0.13 cm proximal from the introitus, respectively. In each group, this position was not changed by PFM contraction. Maximum closure forces were recorded on a position that is the closest to the location of the edge of symphysis pubis which is estimated to be at a distance of 1.98 ± 0.34 cm proximal from the introitus of vagina.

The positions of the maximum anterior pressures at rest in continent and SUI groups were similar, 1.52 ± 0.09 cm and 1.69 ± 0.13 cm proximal from the introitus of vagina, respectively. In each group, this position was not changed by PFM contraction.

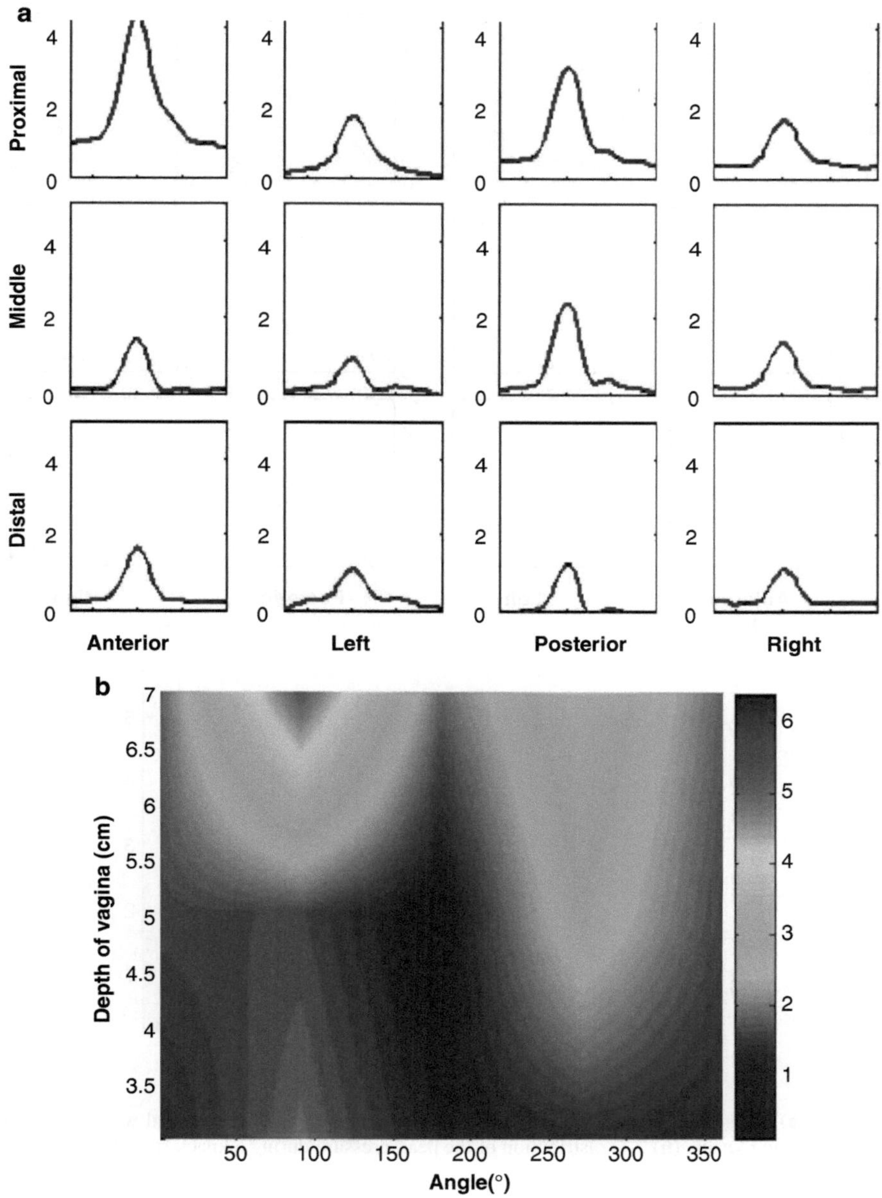

Fig. 19 (**a**) The instantaneous waveform of a cough reflex at different location with respect to time, while (**b**) the spatial distribution at the maxima

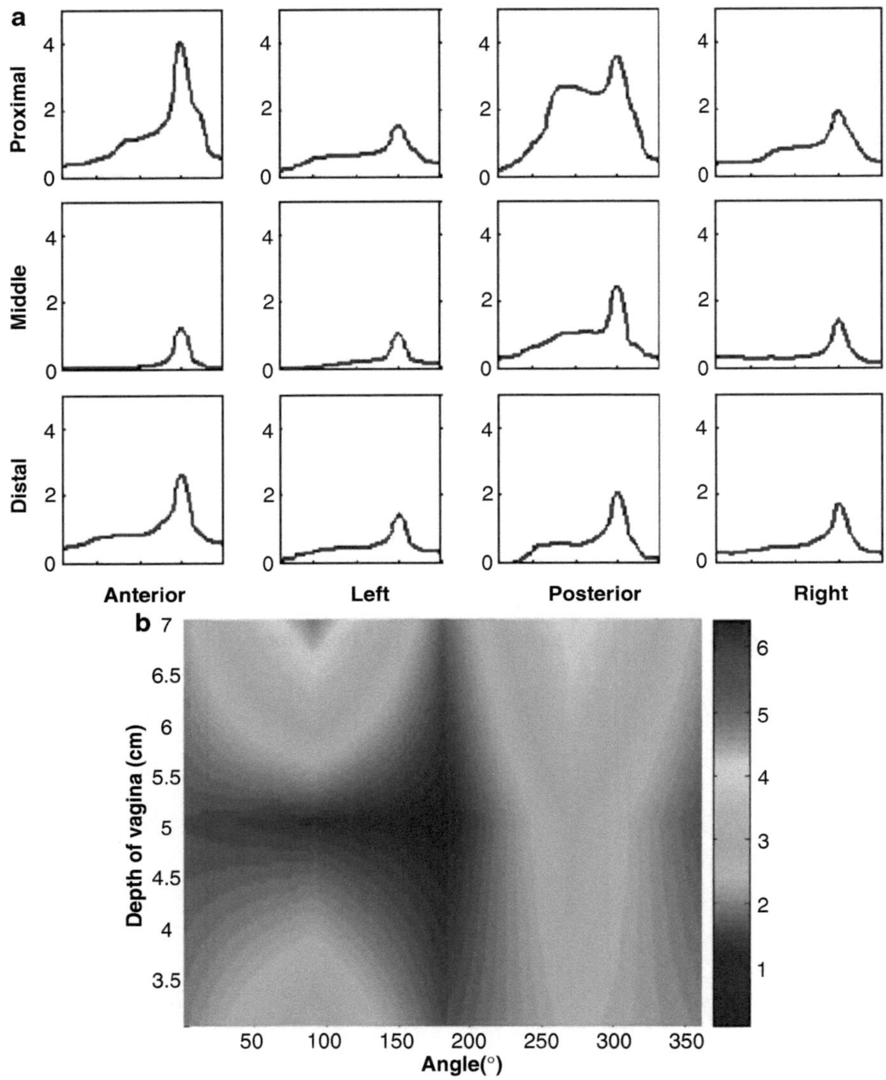

Fig. 20 (**a**) Pressure in four directions on three different positions of the vaginal wall of normal subjects during knack. (**b**) 2-D distribution of the peak pressure during a knack stimulus

5 Discussion

Analysis derived from segmented video clips show, in time resolved increments shown are given by www.urltobedefined.com and demonstrates that the activation of the PFM in continence displaces the urethra towards the pubis while in SUI there

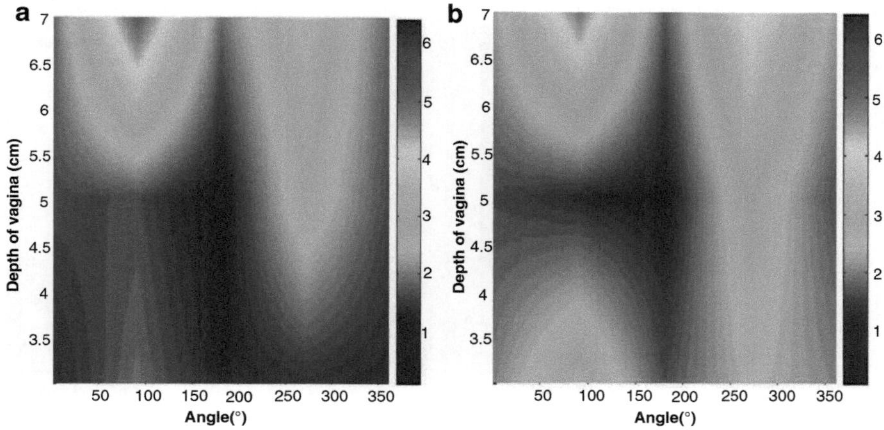

Fig. 21 2-D distribution of the peak pressure on the vaginal wall during (**a**) cough and (**b**) knack

was an absence of ventral displacement. In the SUI group displacement was over a significantly greater distance, with also a significantly different trajectory rebounding with an increased velocity. Max acceleration forces were applied for a longer time before the restoring forces were sufficient to re-establish equilibrium suggesting that in SUI the urethra was exposed to uncontrolled transverse acceleration, and was displaced over twice as far at almost twice the velocity of the continent. The distribution and visualization of closure forces along the vagina of continent and SUI women using a novel vaginal probe device was evaluated. The principle of the experimental design is to simulate the force distribution around the vagina as modified by PFM contraction that is analogous to a digital vaginal examination.

In undertaking PFM strength measurements its important to keep in mind that it is appropriate to incorporate the influence of insertion of pressure/force measuring device to the vagina. Consequently the incremental pressures most directly reflect the strength of PFM accurately suggesting that difference between the posterior and anterior are a consequence of vaginal deformation due to the forces around the vagina generated by the probe. When the mechanical measurements of PFM strength are considered in terms of continence, it is worth considering that the time constants inherent to the vaginal probe are comparatively low and provide only one dimension of the mechanism of continence. In a complimentary study where visualization studies were done using ultrasound imaging it was showed that a voluntary contraction of the PFM displaces the urethra in a direction towards the pubic symphysis and compress the urethra. Urethral closure pressure measurement studies demonstrated a significant increase of the maximum urethral closure pressure with voluntary PFM contraction. In conclusion we present a medical device to facilitate our approach of measuring vaginal pressure that can be used to differentiate SUI from control and provide new parameters defining PFM contraction. It is expected that the information revealed by the use of this probe ca provide a tool to quantitatively evaluate patients and lead to an understanding of the mechanisms through which the PF maintains continence.

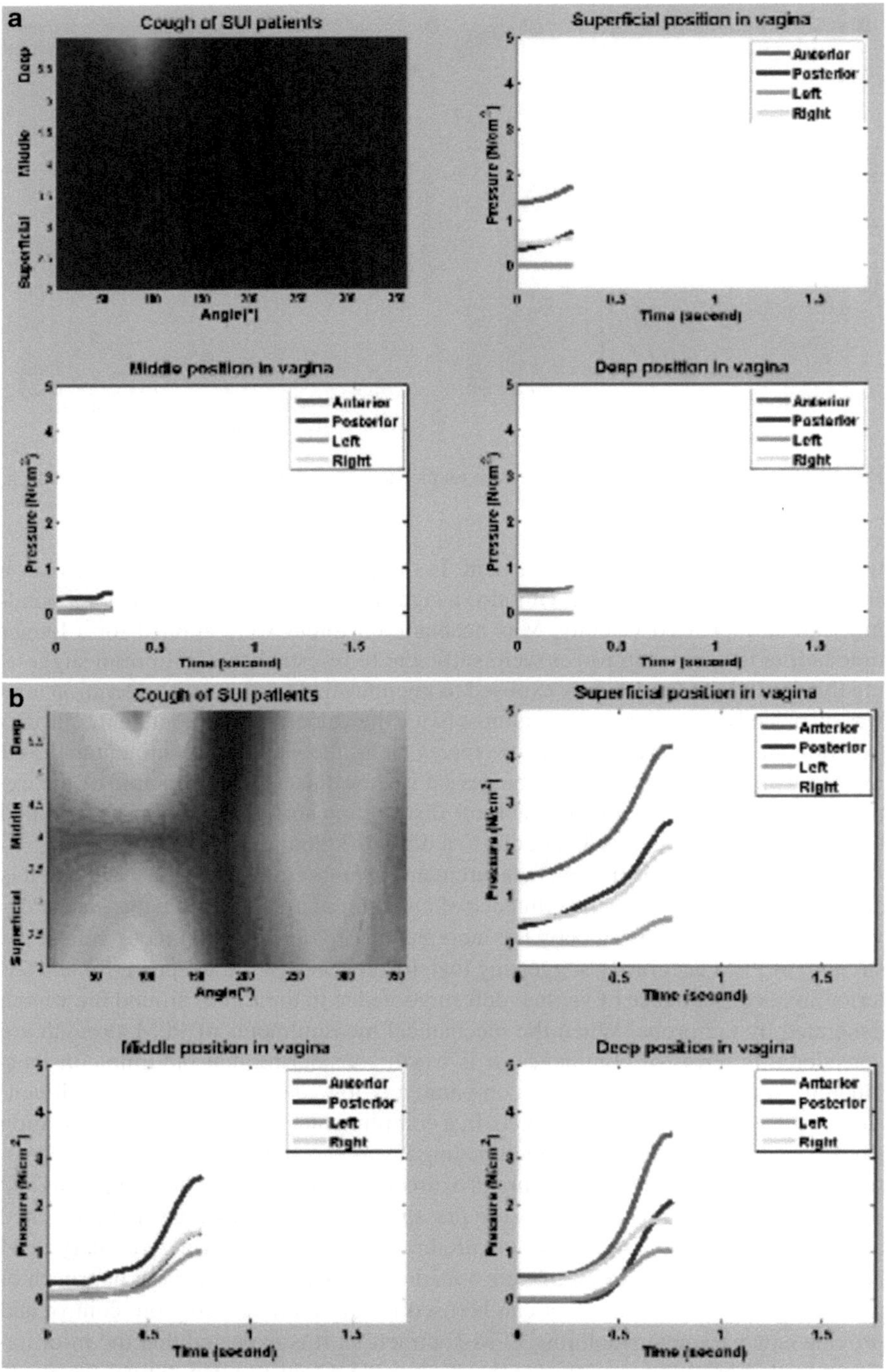

Fig. 22 Onset of closure pressures and their distribution during (**a**) caught and (**b**) a knack

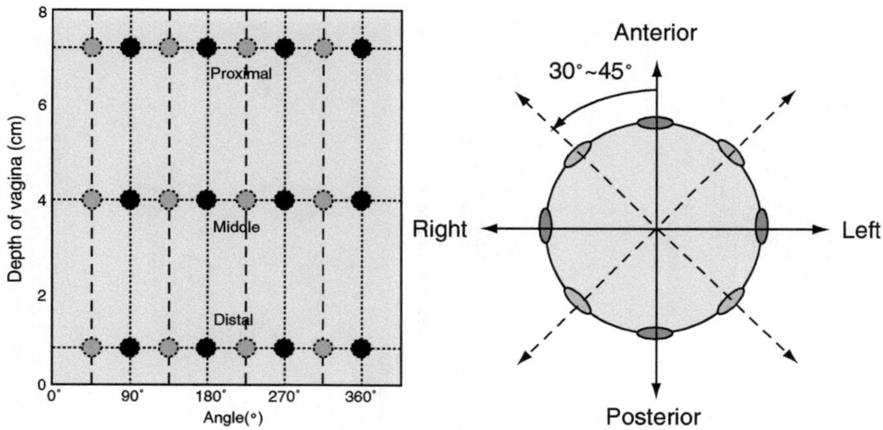

Fig. 23 Positions measured by the probe pressure sensors. The gray points are measured by rotating the probe 30° ~ 45°

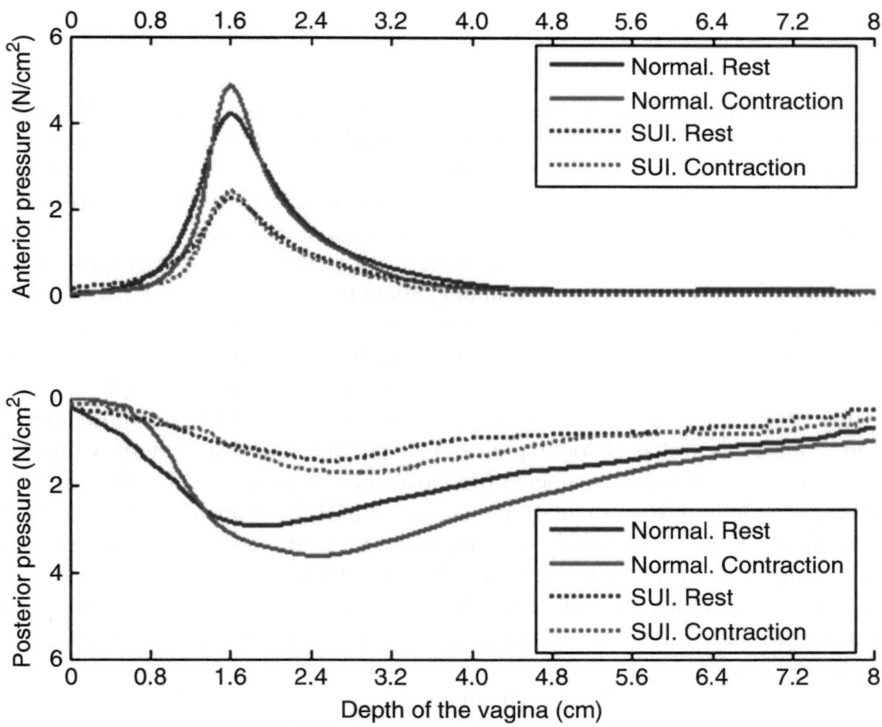

Fig. 24 Profile of vaginal closure pressures in healthy and incontinent women

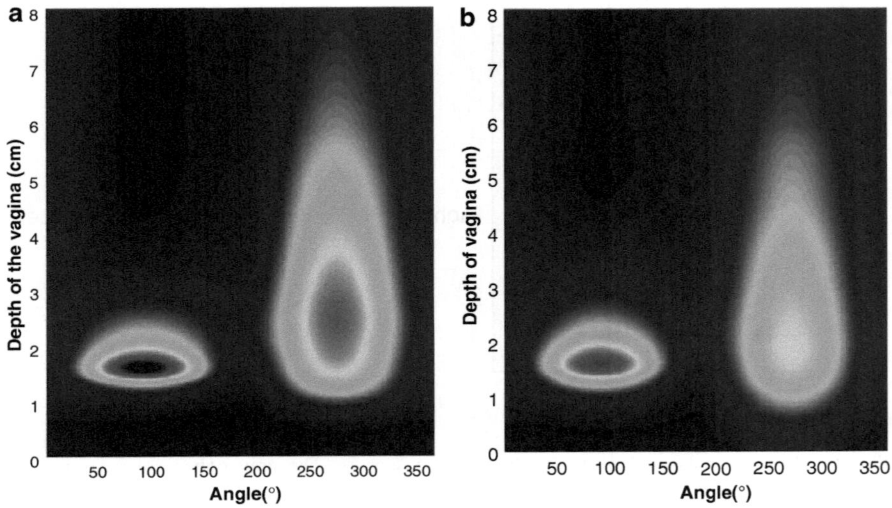

Fig. 25 Visualization of the closure pressures of healthy subjects corresponding to profile measurements of Fig. 23

In evaluating continence using ultrasound we employed principles of image analysis and visualization to demonstrate a mechanism that can best define the lower urinary tract as a highly controlled dynamic system. This analysis enabled for the first time the characterization of new parameters that proved useful in the identification of some of the mechanisms involved in maintaining continence. In view of the fact that current clinical assessment schemes are at best qualitative, translational research requiring minimum patient invasion, can potentially enable a better diagnosis of the functional machinery involved in maintaining continence.

Approach presented demonstrates a novel application of imaging that has the potential to bring new insights in our ability to track the timing of complex motion of the pelvic floor during the rapid events, not possible with casual observation. Furthermore, the value of looking at a more complex assessment tool, with new biomechanical parameters extracted from available visualizations, has the potential of distinguishing different underlying causes of SUI, be it anatomical, poor PFM strength due to neuronal damage in comparison to good muscle function with poor underlying urethral function and trauma. Developing a tool that enables simultaneous and reproducible, operator-independent, information about anatomy and PFM function will allow inroads for a great deal of subsequent research into the continence mechanisms.

In conclusion the challenge remains to develop options to derive the important parameters, with reduced invasion, exposure and cost. In this context it is appropriate to confront the challenge of urodynamics by considering the value of information that can be obtained from imaging. Thus while pressure measurements using a probe can be confounded by many variables, imaging provides data on the relationship of spatial/temporal parameters. Current imaging and computational technology enables the acquisition of unprecedented amounts quantitative information and data reduction. Furthermore imaging provides spatially accurate and unambiguous representation of the forces acting upon the urethra, vagina, bladder, and other abdominal structures that is difficult to measure using pressure sensors.

What is important is that the reflex actions recruited to respond to incontinence occur over short periods of time, seconds, and attention is necessary to resolve the mechanisms involved during these critical moments. With these concepts in mind, application of ultrasound imaging provides a challenging opportunity for the diagnosis and more importantly the cause of incontinence. The principles on which such a claim can be made are based on the fact that imaging examines the unrestrained response of the critical anatomical structures to incontinence producing events as well as the contribution of the PFM. More specifically, application of imaging enables the concurrent visualization and response of the bladder, urethral and pelvic anatomy to abdominal pressure changes likely to create incontinence. To benefit from the large amount of information available from ultrasound imaging, the application of complex motion analysis of the bladder, urethra and the PFM, can be used to provide valuable dynamic data to determine the mechanism of continence. Furthermore as a translational research priority, it is highly constructive to apply visualization technologies that would extract and parameterize the dynamics of PFM function to the fullest extent possible. Finally we demonstrated, using video computer graphic overlays, which movements are characteristic of normal function in continent subjects as distinct from those with SUI. Visualizations of ultrasound imaging, using motion tracking, contouring and segmentation of the dynamics of the bladder urethra and PFM can therefore be very critical.

Acknowledgements This work was funded in part by NIH, grant 1R21 EB 001654 and R01 EB006170. We like to acknowledge the contributions of R. Jones and V. Wolfe for assistance in data collection and the clinical support of Dr. CK Payne

References

1. Abitbol, M.M.: Evolution of the ischial spine and of the pelvic floor in the Hominoidea. Am. J. Phys. Anthropol. **75**(1), 53–67 (1998)
2. Acton, P.D., Newberg, A.: Artificial neural network classifier for the diagnosis of Parkinson's disease using [(99m)Tc]TRODAT-1 and SPECT. Phys. Med. Biol. **51**(12), 3057–3066 (2006)
3. Artibani, W., Andersen, Ostergaard, D.R., Constantinou, C.E., Gajewski, J., Nitti, V., Klaskov, P., Tubaro, A.: Imaging and other investigations. In: Abrahms (ed.) Incontinence, pp. 401–445. WHO/UICC (1999)
4. Athanasiou, S., Khullar, V., et al.: Imaging the urethral sphincter with three-dimensional ultrasound. Obstet. Gynecol. **94**(2), 295–301 (1999)
5. Barbic, M., Kralj, B., et al.: Compliance of the bladder neck supporting structures: importance of activity pattern of levator ani muscle and content of elastic fibers of endopelvic fascia. Neurourol. Urodyn. **22**(4), 269–276 (2003)
6. Berghmans, L.C., Hendriks, H.J., et al.: Conservative treatment of stress urinary incontinence in women: a systematic review of randomized clinical trials. Br. J. Urol. **82**(2), 181–191 (1998)

7. Bhatikar, S.R., DeGroff, C., et al.: A classifier based on the artificial neural network approach for cardiologic auscultation in pediatrics. Artif. Intell. Med. **33**(3), 251–260 (2005)
8. Bo, K., Lilleas, F., et al.: Dynamic MRI of the pelvic floor muscles in an upright sitting position. Neurourol. Urodyn. **20**(2), 167–174 (2001)
9. Bo, K., Sherburn, M.: Evaluation of female pelvic-floor muscle function and strength. Phys. Ther. **85**(3), 269–282 (2005)
10. Buchsbaum, G.M., Duecy, E.E., et al.: Urinary incontinence in nulliparous women and their parous sisters. Obstet. Gynecol. **106**(6), 1253–1258 (2005)
11. Bump, R.C., Hurt, W.G., et al.: Assessment of Kegel pelvic muscle exercise performance after brief verbal instruction. Am. J. Obstet. Gynecol. **165**(2), 322–327 (1991), discussion 327–329
12. Christensen, L.L., Djurhuus, J.C., et al.: Imaging of pelvic floor contractions using MRI. Neurourol. Urodyn. 14(3): 209–216 (1995)
13. Comiter, C.V., Vasavada, S.P., et al.: Grading pelvic prolapse and pelvic floor relaxation using dynamic magnetic resonance imaging. Urology **54**(3), 454–457 (1999)
14. Constantinou, C.E.: Contribution of magnetic resonance imaging in the evaluation of pelvic floor function. In: Bourcier, McGuire (eds.) Pelvic Floor Disorders, pp. 176–182. Abrams Elsevier (2004)
15. Constantinou, C.E., Omata, S.: Direction sensitive sensor probe for the evaluation of voluntary and reflex pelvic floor contractions. Neurourol. Urodyn. **26**(3), 386–391 (2007)
16. Constantinou, C.E., Omata, S., Yoshimura, Y., Peng, Q.: Evaluation of the dynamic responses of female pelvic floor using a novel vaginal probe. Ann. NY. Acad. Sci. **1101**, 297–315 (2007)
17. Constantinou, C.E.: Dynamics of the Female Pelvic Floor. Int. J. Comput. Vision Biomech. (1), 69–81 (2007)
18. Constantinou, C.E., Govan, D.E.: Spatial distribution and timing of transmitted and reflexly generated urethral pressures in healthy women. J. Urol. **127**(5), 964–969 (1982)
19. Constantinou, C.E., Hvistendahl, G., et al.: Determining the displacement of the pelvic floor and pelvic organs during voluntary contractions using magnetic resonance imaging in younger and older women. BJU. Int. **90**(4), 408–414 (2002)
20. Constantinou, C.E., Omata, S.: Direction sensitive sensor probe for the evaluation of voluntary and reflex pelvic floor contractions. Neurourol. Urodyn. **26**(3), 386–391 (2007)
21. Constantinou, C.E.: Dynamics of female pelvic floor function using urodynamics, ultrasound and magnetic resonance imaging. Eur. J. Obstet. Gynecol. **144S**, 159–165 (2009)
22. Costantini, S., Esposito, F., et al.: Ultrasound imaging of the female perineum: the effect of vaginal delivery on pelvic floor dynamics. Ultrasound. Obstet. Gynecol. **27**(2), 183–187 (2006)
23. Deindl, F.M., Vodusek, D.B., et al.: Activity patterns of pubococcygeal muscles in nulliparous continent women. Br. J. Urol. **72**(1), 46–51 (1993)
24. Deindl, F.M., Vodusek, D.B., et al.: Pelvic floor activity patterns: comparison of nulliparous continent and parous urinary stress incontinent women. A kinesiological EMG study. Br. J. Urol. **73**(4), 413–417 (1994)
25. DeLancey, J.O.: The hidden epidemic of pelvic floor dysfunction: achievable goals for improved prevention and treatment. Am. J. Obstet. Gynecol. **192**(5), 1488–1495 (2005)
26. DeLancey, J.O., Strohbehn, K., et al.: Comparison of ureteral and cervical descents during vaginal hysterectomy for uterine prolapse. Am. J. Obstet. Gynecol. **179**(6 Pt 1), 1405–1408 (1998); discussion 1409–1410
27. Dietz, H.P.: Ultrasound imaging of the pelvic floor. Part II: three-dimensional or volume imaging. Ultrasound. Obstet. Gynecol. **23**(6), 615–625 (2004)
28. Dietz HP, Jarvis SK, et al. (2002). The assessment of levator muscle strength: a validation of three ultrasound techniques. Int Urogynecol J Pelvic Floor Dysfunct 13(3): 156–159; discussion 159
29. Dumoulin, C., Peng, Q., Stodkilde-Jorgensen, H., Shishido, K., Constantinou, C.E.: Changes in levator ani anatomical configuration following physiotherapy in women with stress urinary incontinence. J. Urol. **178**, 970–977 (2007)
30. Ferreira, P.H., Ferreira, M.L., et al.: Changes in recruitment of the abdominal muscles in people with low back pain: ultrasound measurement of muscle activity. Spine **29**(22), 2560–2566 (2004)

31. Fielding, J.R., Dumanli, H., et al.: MR-based three-dimensional modeling of the normal pelvic floor in women: quantification of muscle mass. AJR. Am. J. Roentgenol. **174**(3), 657–660 (2000)
32. Goh, V., Halligan, S., et al.: Dynamic MR imaging of the pelvic floor in asymptomatic subjects. AJR. Am. J. Roentgenol. **174**(3), 661–666 (2000)
33. Gousse, A.E., Barbaric, Z.L., et al.: Dynamic half Fourier acquisition, single shot turbo spin-echo magnetic resonance imaging for evaluating the female pelvis. J. Urol. **164**(5), 1606–1613 (2000)
34. Higuchi, K., Sato, K., et al.: Automated diagnosis of heart disease in patients with heart murmurs: application of a neural network technique. J. Med. Eng. Technol. **30**(2), 61–68 (2006)
35. Hodges, P.W., Richardson, C.A.: Altered trunk muscle recruitment in people with low back pain with upper limb movement at different speeds. Arch. Phys. Med. Rehabil. **80**(9), 1005–1012 (1999)
36. Howard, D., Miller, J.M., et al.: Differential effects of cough, valsalva, and continence status on vesical neck movement. Obstet. Gynecol. **95**(4), 535–540 (2000)
37. Jones, R.C., Peng, Q., et al.: Altered co-activation patterns of the pelvic floor muscles (PFM) during abdominal manoeuvres in stress urinary incontinent (SUI) women. 36th Annual Meeting of the International Continence Society (ICS) (2006)
38. Kara, S., Guven, A., et al.: Utilization of artificial neural networks in the diagnosis of optic nerve diseases. Comput. Biol. Med. **36**(4), 428–437 (2006)
39. Kessler, R., Constantinou, C.E.: Internal urethrotomy in girls and its impact on the urethral intrinsic and extrinsic continence mechanisms. J. Urol. **136**(6), 1248–1253 (1986)
40. Klutke, C., Golomb, J., et al.: The anatomy of stress incontinence: magnetic resonance imaging of the female bladder neck and urethra. J. Urol. **143**(3), 563–566 (1990)
41. Laycock, J., Brown, J., et al.: Pelvic floor reeducation for stress incontinence: comparing three methods. Br. J. Community. Nurs. **6**(5), 230–237 (2001)
42. Miller, J.M., Ashton-Miller, J.A., et al.: A pelvic muscle precontraction can reduce cough-related urine loss in selected women with mild SUI. J. Am. Geriatr. Soc. **46**(7), 870–874 (1998)
43. Miller, J.M., Perucchini, D., et al.: Pelvic floor muscle contraction during a cough and decreased vesical neck mobility. Obstet. Gynecol. **97**(2), 255–260 (2001)
44. Morin, M., Bourbonnais, D., et al.: Pelvic floor muscle function in continent and stress urinary incontinent women using dynamometric measurements. Neurourol. Urodyn. **23**(7), 668–674 (2004)
45. Neumann, P., Gill, V.: Pelvic floor and abdominal muscle interaction: EMG activity and intra-abdominal pressure. Int. Urogynecol. J. Pelvic. Floor. Dysfunct. **13**(2), 125–132 (2002)
46. Norton, C., Chelvanayagam, S., et al.: Randomized controlled trial of biofeedback for fecal incontinence. Gastroenterology **125**(5), 1320–1329 (2003)
47. Nygaard, I.: Physiologic outcome measures for urinary incontinence. Gastroenterology **126**(1 Suppl 1), S99–105 (2004)
48. Peng, Q., Jones, R.C., et al.: Characterization of the mechanical parameters associated with pelvic floor muscles contractions. 36th Annual Meeting of the International Continence Society (ICS) (2006)
49. Peng, Q., Jones, R.C., et al.: 2D Ultrasound image processing in identifying responses of urogenital structures to pelvic floor muscle activity. Ann. Biomed. Eng. **34**(3), 477–493 (2006)
50. Peng, Q., Jones, R.C., Shishido, K., Constantinou, C.E.: Ultrasound evaluation of dynamic responses of female pelvic floor muscles Ultrasound. Med. Biol. **33**(3), 342–352 (2007)
51. Peng, Q., Jones, R.C., Omata, S., Constantinou, C.E.: Spatial distribution of vaginal closure pressures of continent and stress urinary incontinent women. Physiologic. Measure. **28**(11), 1429–1450 (2007)
52. Pregazzi, R., Sartore, A., et al.: Perineal ultrasound evaluation of urethral angle and bladder neck mobility in women with stress urinary incontinence. Bjog **109**(7), 821–827 (2002)
53. Rahmanian, S., Jones, R., Peng, Q., Constantinou, C.E.: Visualization of biomechanical properties of female pelvic floor function using video motion tracking of ultrasound imaging. Technol. Informat. **132**, 390–395 (2008)

54. Reddy, A.P., DeLancey, J.O., et al.: On-screen vector-based ultrasound assessment of vesical neck movement. Am. J. Obstet. Gynecol. **185**(1), 65–70 (2001)
55. Sapsford, R.R., Hodges, P.W., et al.: Co-activation of the abdominal and pelvic floor muscles during voluntary exercises. Neurourol. Urodyn. **20**(1), 31–42 (2001)
56. Schaer, G.N., Perucchini, D., et al.: Sonographic evaluation of the bladder neck in continent and stress-incontinent women. Obstet. Gynecol. **93**(3), 412–426 (1999)
57. Shishido, K., Peng, Q., Jones, R., Omata, S., Constantinou, C.E.: Influence of pelvic floor muscle contraction on the profile of vaginal closure pressures of continent and stress urinary incontinent women. J. Urol. **179**(5), 1917–1922 (2008)
58. Smith, M.D., Russell, A., et al.: Disorders of breathing and continence have a stronger association with back pain than obesity and physical activity. Aust. J. Physiother. **52**(1), 11–16 (2006)
59. Stoker, J., Halligan, S., et al.: Pelvic floor imaging. Radiology **218**(3), 621–641 (2001)
60. Theofrastous, J.P., Wyman, J.F., et al.: Effects of pelvic floor muscle training on strength and predictors of response in the treatment of urinary incontinence. Neurourol. Urodyn. **21**(5), 486–490 (2002)
61. Yang, A., Mostwin, J.L.: Pelvic floor descent in women: dynamic evaluation with fast MR imaging and cinematic display. Radiology **179**(1), 25–33 (1991)

Population Exposure and Impact Assessment: Benefits of Modeling Urban Land Use in Very High Spatial and Thematic Detail

Christoph Aubrecht, Mario Köstl, and Klaus Steinnocher

Abstract This paper highlights the benefits that high-level geospatial modeling of urban patterns can provide for real-world applications in the field of population exposure and impact assessment. A set of techniques is described leading to identification of functional and socioeconomic relationships in a suburban environment. Diverse high resolution remote sensing data are classified using Object-Based Image Analysis in order to derive structural land cover information. Georeferenced address data then serve as essential link between this geometric framework and ancillary space-related information such as company and census data. The final very high resolution functional population model (i.e. broken down to address-based building part objects) is consulted for exposure and impact assessments exemplarily shown in two different fictitious scenarios: (1) earthquake hazard and (2) traffic noise propagation. High-detail spatial data sets including functional and socioeconomic information as derived in this study can be of great value in disaster risk management and simulation, but also in regional and environmental planning as well as geomarketing analyses.

Keywords Population disaggregation · Functional land use · Exposure · Earthquake hazard · Noise propagation

1 Introduction

In the context of disaster risk management and particularly for exposure and impact assessments the quality of available input data both in terms of spatial and thematic accuracy is one of the most important factors. Information on functional relationships in urban and suburban environments as well as high-level population distribution information is often not quickly available in case of emergency. Rapid mapping concepts mostly rely on Earth Observation data from different sensors as

C. Aubrecht (✉), M. Köstl, and K. Steinnocher
AIT Austrian Institute of Technology GmbH, Vienna, Austria
e-mail: christoph.aubrecht@ait.ac.at

J.M.R.S. Tavares and R.M.N. Jorge (eds.), *Computational Vision and Medical Image Processing: Recent Trends*, Computational Methods in Applied Sciences 19,
DOI 10.1007/978-94-007-0011-6_4,

e.g. provided by the International Charter of Space and Major Disasters.[1] Being independent of weather conditions Radar data are often considered as first-hand resource in order to delineate affected areas. Herrera-Cruz and Koudogbo [14] presented a rapid mapping workflow for flood events based on high-resolution TerraSAR-X data. Another study by Buehler et al. [7] showed that Radarsat-1 could however not provide a sufficient level of spatial detail for flood mapping, which was why eventually optical data (SPOT-5) was consulted. Following up with optical imagery applications Elvidge et al. [11] presented a study where DMSP nighttime lights data were used for near-real-time power outage detection and corresponding delineation of areas affected by natural phenomena such as earthquakes and hurricanes. Improving the usability of satellite derived products and improving the benefits of satellite data for disaster management support in general is still subject to ongoing research [8].

For building comprehensive urban data management systems and mapping the complex urban environment at a high level of detail diverse input data is required, with functional information such as socioeconomic and explicit demographic data on the one hand and 'real world' physical properties as derived from remote sensing on the other hand [19]. Earth Observation data classification is limited to physical characteristics of the analyzed objects but does not include process related information. With respect to manmade features this means that buildings can be detected as such, while building use and related socioeconomic activities cannot be derived that way.

Urban system modeling based on remote sensing and geoinformation technology often does not go beyond a certain spatial and thematic scale regarding the corresponding reference objects. Taking population and socioeconomic features into account and thus moving from land cover detection to land use assessment enables modeling of vulnerability and damage potential patterns. Integrative approaches considering remote sensing and ancillary information are therefore expected to further increase in importance in the future.

2 Data and Study Area

2.1 Study Area

The study area covering approx. 13 km^2 (3.7×3.5 km) is situated in the northern part of Linz (i.e. Linz-Urfahr), the state capital of Upper Austria with around 190,000 inhabitants (Fig. 1). In 2009 Linz was entitled 'European Capital of Culture' (www.linz09.at). This indicates the present designated focus of the city differing considerably from its former image of 'steel city', then primarily known for its industry leading steelworks company 'voestalpine'.

The suburban area in the north is widely dominated by fields and forest and agricultural use primarily including scattered detached houses whereas the beginning

[1] http://www.disastercharter.org (last accessed January 15, 2010)

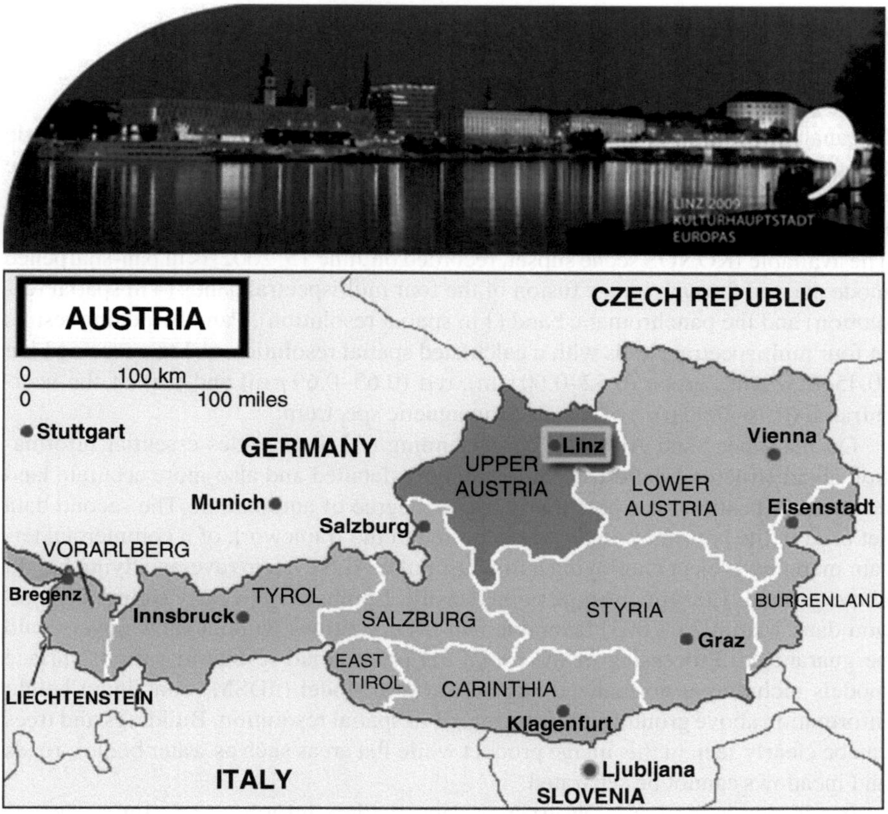

Fig. 1 Location of the study area in Upper Austria

urban area in the south is characterized by mixed residential and commercial use comprising large building blocks and semi-detached houses as well as shopping centers and recreational zones. An important identifying feature of Linz-Urfahr is the large educational complex including university and various other teaching institutions such as high schools and vocational schools.

In the south-east the landmark river Danube and the adjacent expressway A7 cross the study area. According to the 2008 traffic counts carried out by the Austrian Traffic Association (VCÖ Verkehrsclub Österreich) the part of the A7 in the urban area of Linz including the one crossing the test site is amongst the most frequented street sections in Austria, i.e. on working days featuring more than 100,000 cars per day. That is also why various plans exist on building an additional bypass expressway.

Featuring mixed land use with urban and rural characteristics the analyzed study area forms a heterogeneous suburban transition zone, thus being a perfect starting point for building a comprehensive knowledge base for further functional analyses.

2.2 *Remote Sensing Data and Ancillary Space-Related Information*

For analyzing land cover patterns in the study area and deriving sort of a geometric framework for further functional analyses two very high resolution (VHR) remote sensing data sets are used. On the one hand optical satellite imagery as provided by IKONOS-2 forms the basis for standard high resolution land cover classification. The available IKONOS scene subset, recorded on June 15, 2002, is in pan-sharpened mode derived through image fusion of the four multispectral bands (4 m spatial resolution) and the panchromatic band (1 m spatial resolution). Pan-sharpening results in four multispectral bands with a calculated spatial resolution of 1 m covering blue (0.45–0.52 μm), green (0.52–0.60 μm), red (0.63–0.69 μm) and part of the near-infrared (0.76–0.90 μm) of the electromagnetic spectrum.

On the other hand Airborne Laserscanning (ALS) provides essential information about structural patterns enabling a more detailed and also more accurate land cover classification on a potentially higher degree of automation. The second data set used in the presented study was acquired in the framework of a commercial terrain mapping project employing a first/last pulse ALS system (average flying height above ground: 1,000 m; average point density: 1 point/m^2). In early spring (acquisition date: March 24, 2003) favorable leaf-off conditions without snow cover could be guaranteed. Processing of the initial 3D point cloud results in various surface models including a normalized Digital Surface Model (nDSM) containing height information above ground and featuring a 1 m spatial resolution. Buildings and trees can be clearly seen in this image product while flat areas such as water bodies, roads and meadows cannot be separated.

In addition to the Earth Observation data ancillary information featuring diverse spatial and thematic characteristics are used in order to progress from land cover analysis to land use classification and specifically functional urban system analysis. These additional data sets include address point features, i.e. postal delivery addresses linked with precise geo-coordinates, as collected by the Austrian mail service Post AG. Distributed under the name Data.Geo[2] this data set is updated twice a year and comprises more than two million addresses in Austria using a standardized naming convention. About 3,700 discrete points are used in the presented study. Address data acts as the essential link between geometric framework and thematic information [3], i.e. enabling the integration of all kinds of address-related data such as company data (yellow pages) and census data (Austrian Census 2001).

3 Multi-Source Modeling of Functional Urban Patterns

The following paragraphs will give an overview of a set of various techniques finally resulting in a functional 3D building model, thus providing socioeconomic

[2] http://www.datageo.at (last accessed January 15, 2010)

information in addition to physical attributes. A more detailed description of this functional object grouping procedure including schematic model and ESRI ArcGIS implementation description can be found in Aubrecht et al. [2].

3.1 Object Based Image Analysis and Integrated Land Cover Classification

The availability of both optical satellite imagery and ALS data offers great potential for identifying urban land cover patterns. Due to the complexity of the heterogeneous urban transition zone analyzed in the presented study feature classification is a challenging task. VHR optical satellite imagery allows immediate visual discrimination of diverse spatial structures characterizing different urban and suburban zones. The implementation of LiDAR (Light Detection & Ranging) data significantly improves the land cover classification both in terms of accuracy and automation.

Object based image analysis (OBIA) as implemented in the software package Definiens Professional was considered to be the most promising technique (compared to standard pixel based classification algorithms) for handling the high spatial resolution and complexity as well as differing properties of the two available data sets [5, 16]. Just considering single pixels without accounting for the spatial context often leads to an unwanted 'salt-and-pepper effect' [23] which would not be suitable for the desired object identification (i.e. creation of a building layer).

The analysis can be divided into two processing steps: (1) segmentation of the data into homogeneous objects and (2) assignment of the segments to discrete classes. These steps can also be applied alternately, i.e. classification results of one processing step can serve as input for subsequent segmentation. Basic land cover classes such as vegetation, water and sealed surface can be distinguished just using the multispectral IKONOS image. Based on the additional height information provided by the ALS data, both sealed areas and vegetated areas can be further differentiated, which e.g. enables the exact separation of buildings and streets, which would not be possible by merely considering optical parameters [16]. Six land cover types are finally classified (buildings, streets, flat sealed area, trees, shrubs, water), while one additional class each is used for shadow and undefined areas (Fig. 2). With regard to the further steps of the urban system modeling procedure special attention is turned to the delineation of building objects later serving as the geometric basis for socioeconomic data integration.

3.2 Progressing from Land Cover to Land Use Assessment by Adding Ancillary Space-Related Information

The increasing availability of spatial and space related data enables integrative urban system modeling based on joint analysis of remote sensing data and ancillary

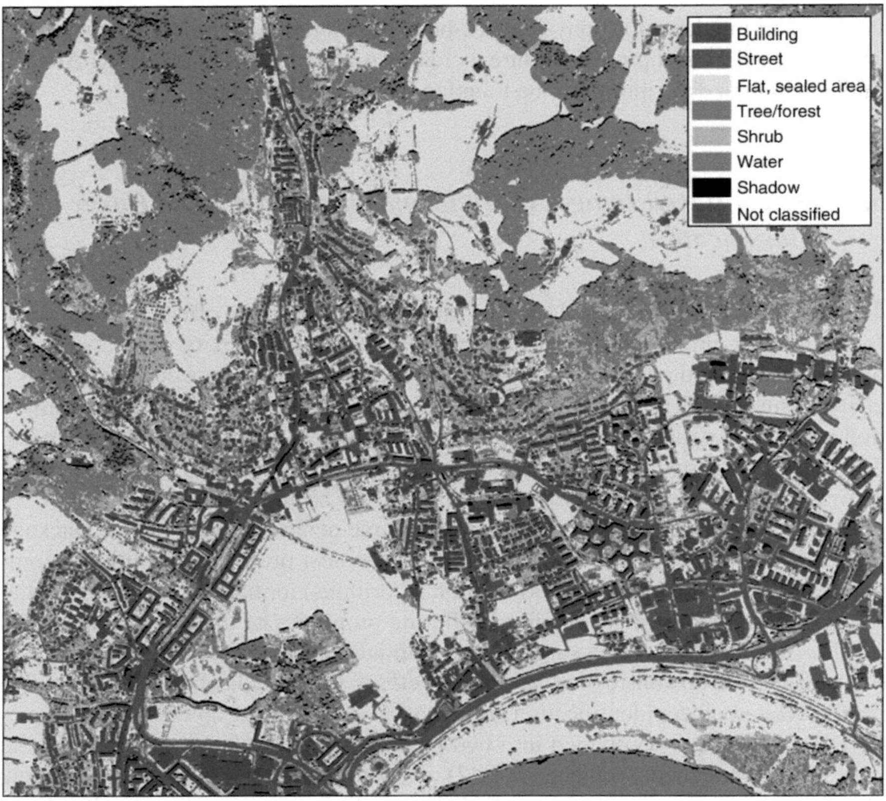

Fig. 2 Urban land cover classification

information [17]. Remote sensing approaches produce good results on physical properties of urban structures, while however functional information can hardly be identified that way.

In the presented study the available georeferenced address data (i.e. 'Data.Geo' postal address delivery points) is spatially linked to the building layer previously derived from remote sensing information (i.e. satellite imagery and Laserscanning data). Each address point is clearly related to one building. One building might however contain more than one postal address, e.g. apartment buildings and town houses, thus more than one point might be related to single buildings. A continuously unambiguous one-to-one relationship between address points and building objects is achieved through generation of Thiessen polygons being subsequently intersected with the building layer.

Attaching company information to the resulting sub-building model via their joint address attribute allows precisely locating those building parts in which economic activities take place and identifying those parts being in residential use only. The integration of company data serves not only for the detection of buildings hosting economic activities but also provides information about the type of activity. Based on the yellow pages inherent HIC (Herold Industrial Code) which groups branches of business to more general types functional object grouping can be carried out. This results in a building model providing feature information such as 'residential use', 'public use', 'commercial', 'agriculture', and others.

Being able to delineate functional patterns in an urban system and to identify concrete actual building use can be of utmost interest on various occasions. In case of emergency, e.g. due to a natural disaster, it is essential to quickly locate critical infrastructure as well as being able to perform first-pass damage potential assessments. Information on functional characteristics rather than mere physical information and consequently also information on population distribution is often indispensable in that context in order to effectively implement spatial disaster risk management concepts.

4 Spatial Analysis of Population Distribution Patterns

The final step in the urban system modeling process is therefore the integration of population data into the functional sub-building model. The backward projection of the available spatially aggregated census data is conducted by a method called spatial disaggregation of population [9] which is based on the previously derived actual building use and the resultant assessed potential residential capacity. For the presented project population data from the Austrian Census 2001 is available in raster format having a $125 \times 125\,\text{m}$ cell size.

In order to disaggregate population from the raster to sub-buildings, the latter have to be reduced to single points for being clearly linked to distinct census grid cells. As the specific address point data set serving as basis for the census raster creation is available in this study (i.e. population counts per address were summed up to get one value for each grid cell), it is possible to inversely re-trace the aggregation process. As in previous steps buildings were split into sub-buildings based on postal address information those objects can now easily be linked to the census address points. Aubrecht and Steinnocher [1] provide more detailed information on this procedure.

The availability of height information (from the Laserscanning data) and hence the possible use of building volume instead of area for the assessment of residential capacities significantly enhance the accuracy of the population distribution model. As just those buildings in residential use should be included in the disaggregation process an empirical weighting factor is introduced for the different building types in order to calculate the potential residential ratio of each sub building. Fully residential buildings are thus assigned a weighting factor of 1, i.e. 100% of the building volume is considered for the calculation, while non-residential buildings get a factor of 0. Calculating the mean volume density of each grid cell (i.e. population of one grid cell referred to the summed up relevant residential volume of all buildings

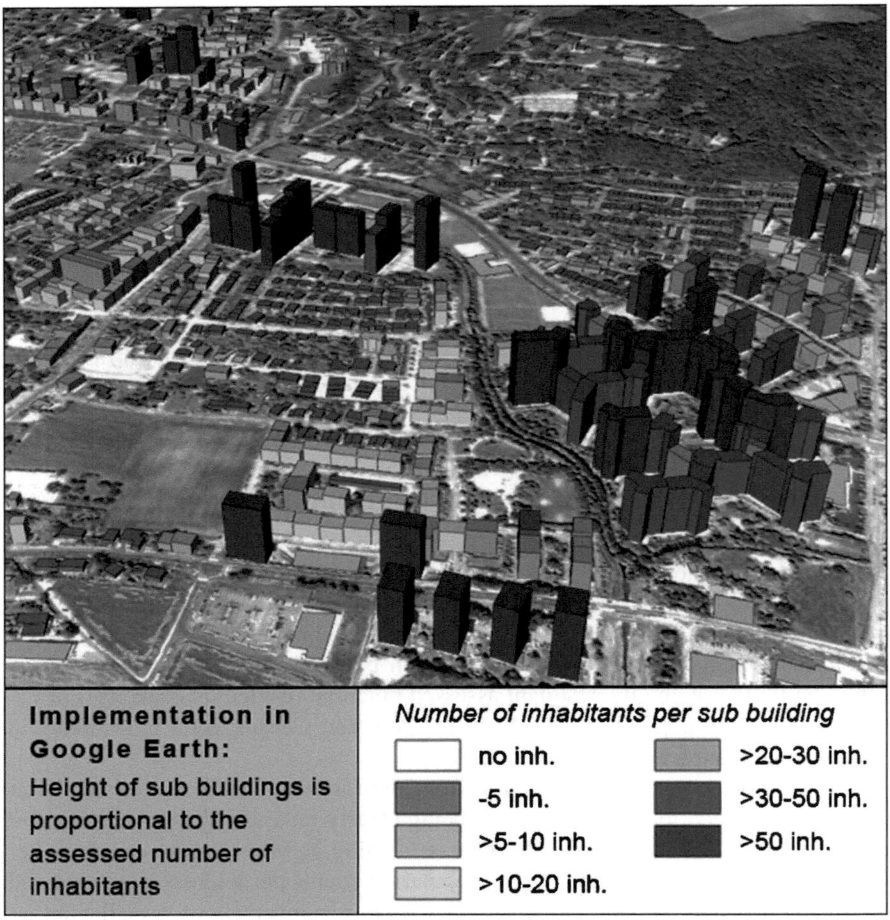

Fig. 3 3D visualization of population distribution patterns on sub-building level

in the same cell) results in sort of a '3D population density' (i.e. inhabitants/m^3). This value is then multiplied with the object's relevant volume finally resulting in an assessment of the number of inhabitants per sub-building (Fig. 3).

5 Exposure and Impact Assessment

In the following section of this paper two different scenarios are presented highlighting potential application areas of functional urban system models as described above. First is a fictitious earthquake (EQ) scenario, having the epicenter right in the center of the study area with the level of intensity decreasing towards the test site boundaries. Affected population as well as affected infrastructure can be reported with the possibility of specifically allocating emergency relevant objects such as nursing homes and playschools.

The second scenario shows two different levels of potential noise propagation surrounding the A7 expressway in the south of the study area. Assessed affected population numbers are given, whereas the essential improvement of the disaggregated population product in comparison to the initially available census raster is highlighted.

The list of potential application fields can be extended arbitrarily. Not only disaster risk management and spatial planning concepts can benefit from the availability of such high-level functional data sets. It is of high interest also for regional and local development strategies.

5.1 *Population Exposure to Earthquake Hazard*

Figure 4 shows a fictitious EQ scenario with the study area being categorized in five zones indicating varying levels of intensity around the theoretical epicenter (red and orange: high, yellow: medium, light and dark green: low). In real event analyses such intensity zones are often delineated using the Modified Mercalli Intensity (MMI) Scale [20], which is a subjective measure describing how strong a shock is

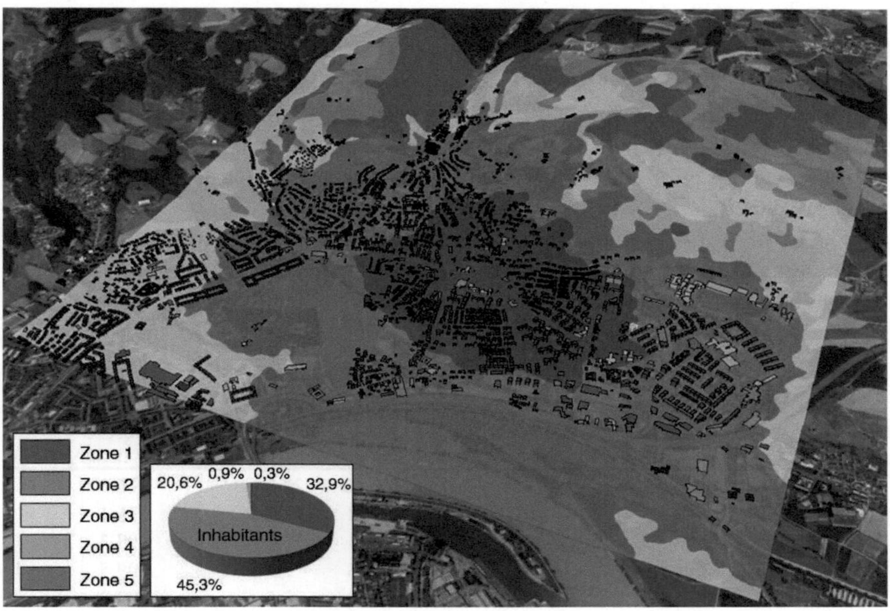

Fig. 4 Earthquake hazard zones and functional building model

felt at a particular location on a scale of I–XII. Buildings are visualized classified according to their land use, i.e. red indicating residential buildings, blue standing for commercial use and yellow for public use. Large parts of the residential area are located in the inner circle, i.e. the red zone of highest intensity, and only few built-up areas (mostly in the western part of the test site) are featuring medium to low intensities.

Having a closer look at the available modeled population numbers it becomes apparent that nearly half of the people living in the study area are related to buildings in Zone 2 (45.3%, cp. chart in Fig. 4). Table 1 also provides information on aggregated percentages, e.g. more than three quarters of the population (78.2%) is living in one of the two zones of highest intensity. Building ratio is slightly higher in Zone 2 than inhabitant ratio while in Zone 1 the contrary is observed. With Zone 1 being located somehow in the center of the study area the numbers confirm that this part is also featuring a higher population density (on average more inhabitants per building: 8.4) than the surrounding Zone 2 (inhabitants/building: 6.9). This fact also increases the overall vulnerability of that specific area. Regarding potential high financial damage we get the information that e.g. all car dealing companies are located in Zone 2 (selected blue buildings in the southeast of the study area). Also the biggest nursing home falls into the orange zone while the two major student homes are a bit farther away from the theoretical epicenter, thus being assigned to the yellow zone of medium intensity.

Given information on structural quality of buildings would additionally enhance risk assessment as e.g. standard EQ indices such as peak ground velocity (PGV, highest ground shaking velocity reached during an earthquake) and peak ground acceleration (PGA, largest recorded acceleration) can give an indication of potential building damage. PGA is measured in units of %g where g is the gravity-enforced acceleration. A PGA of 10 (0.1 g) may be enough to damage older buildings, while buildings constructed in line with EQ standards can even resist severe shaking up to 0.6 g without significant structural damage. The relationship between quantitative measures such as PGV and PGA with qualitative measures such as MMI is described e.g. by Wald et al. [21] and Wu et al. [24].

The fictitious EQ scenario showed how available functional information including building use and population distribution can help in getting an impression of risk exposure and damage potentials. It is also possible to identify certain hot spots (e.g.

Table 1 People/buildings located in the fictitious EQ zones

Zone	Inhabitants	Percentage (%)	Aggregated percentage (%)	Buildings	Percentage (%)	Aggregated percentage (%)
1	8,653	32.9	32.9	1,034	28.6	28.6
2	11,905	45.3	78.2	1,718	47.5	76.1
3	5,413	20.6	98.8	804	22.2	98.3
4	243	0.9	99.7	45	1.2	99.5
5	67	0.3	100.0	18	0.5	100.0
Σ	26,281	–	–	3,619	–	–

very high density, or specific critical building use) for search and rescue measures in case of emergency. Regarding real-time disaster management operations however, information on daytime versus nighttime population distribution as e.g. modeled by Freire [12] would be favored. Freire and Aubrecht [13] use exactly that kind of information for mapping spatio-temporal human exposure to earthquake hazard in Lisbon. Such efforts correlate with recent recommendations for improving vulnerability analyses [4, 6, 10, 18].

5.2 *Street Noise Propagation and Affected Population*

The second and for the analyzed study area more realistic scenario considers a simple linear street noise propagation model and integrates that information with the above described population distribution model in order to derive an assessment of the number of potentially affected persons. The model features two distance buffers around the expressway A7 which crosses the study area in the very south (Fig. 5).

As already mentioned this part of the A7 in the urban area of Linz is amongst the most frequented street sections in Austria featuring more than 100,000 cars per day on working days. Two potential noise propagation zones are simulated based on available Tele Atlas street network data (1) considering a 200 m neighborhood and (2) considering a 500 m neighborhood. Assessment of potentially affected

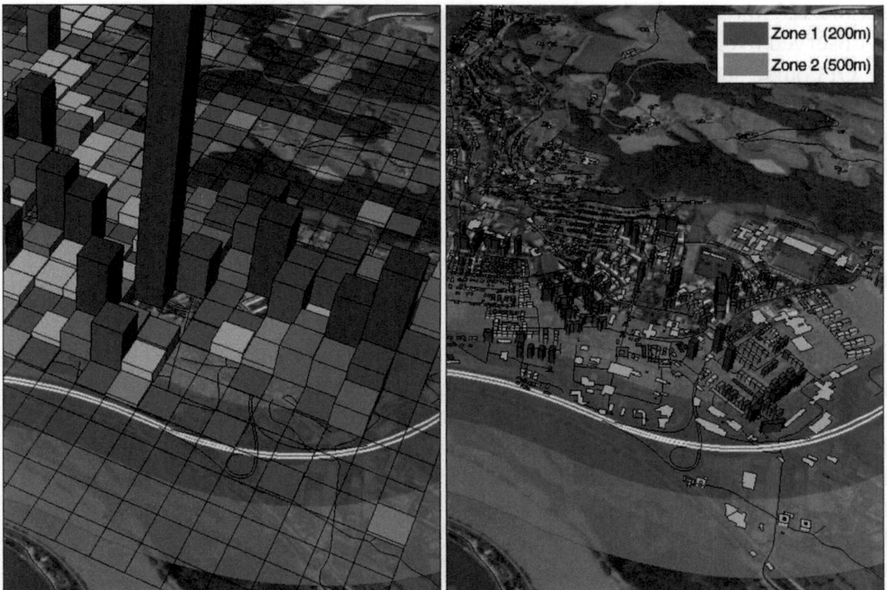

Fig. 5 Highway noise propagation and population model

Table 2 Differences in population number assessments based on different spatial reference

	Affected population		
Zone	250 m raster	125 m raster	Sub-buildings
1[a]	3,522 inh.	1,894 inh.	1,598 inh.
2[b]	8,489 inh.	7,414 inh.	6,199 inh.

[a]200 m buffer
[b]500 m buffer

population is indispensable for sustainable planning of noise control and protection measures. While modeling of real-world noise propagation involves more sophisticated parameters such as atmospheric and topographic characteristics [15] the present study shows how the integrated use of functional information increases population assessment accuracy in terms of general exposure analysis.

Comparison of the modeled population distribution on sub-building level with the initial census raster shows considerable differences in terms of resulting affected population numbers. Table 2 shows the results taking a 250 m census raster, a 125 m raster, and finally the sub-building population model as input. It is obvious that for such high-resolution analyses 250 m raster are just too coarse leading to an immense overestimation. In the inner zone the 250 m raster shows more than 3,500 people being affected. Taking the sub-building model estimate as reference (1,598 people), this is an overestimation of 120%. The 125 m raster already yields much better results with an overestimation of approximately 19%. Zone 2 shows a similar picture for the 125 m raster (20%), while a big improvement with regard to the 250 m raster is observed (37%).

Of course such estimates depend to a large extent on real-world population distribution patterns. Anyhow, the proposed results show the important role functional sub-building models can play in case high-resolution population data is needed as input or reference for high-level analyses.

6 Conclusion and Outlook

In this paper a model of a selected study area in Upper Austria (Linz-Urfahr) was presented with the objective of identifying functional and socioeconomic relationships in a suburban environment. Very high resolution satellite imagery and airborne Laserscanning data were considered in a joint classification using Object-Based Image Analysis which resulted in derivation of detailed structural land cover information. Georeferenced postal address data then enabled linking this geometric base data framework with ancillary spatial and space-related information such as yellow pages company data and population data from the census.

Integrating all available data sets resulted in a 3D population model on sub-building level which was finally consulted for exposure and impact assessments.

Two fictitious scenarios (earthquake, noise propagation) were discussed, whereas the high value and the gain in accuracy using such high-level spatial data sets including functional and socioeconomic information as compared to basic low-level data were highlighted.

As already mentioned the focus of this paper was on highlighting the asset functional urban system models can offer in terms of population related geospatial modeling. In real-world sophisticated impact analysis applications it is of course not sufficient to just have this part of the input available in very high detail. In terms of natural disasters this means that hazard zones need to be constantly improved and updated referring to the best available information (e.g. fault zones and general geological conditions for earthquake hazard modeling; slope stability and surface roughness for landslides and avalanches, etc.). When dealing with distribution models such as noise propagation and pollutant dispersal a lot of input factors need to be considered such as atmospheric conditions, wind fields and topographic features as well as shadowing effects. Figure 6 shows an exemplary traffic noise propagation

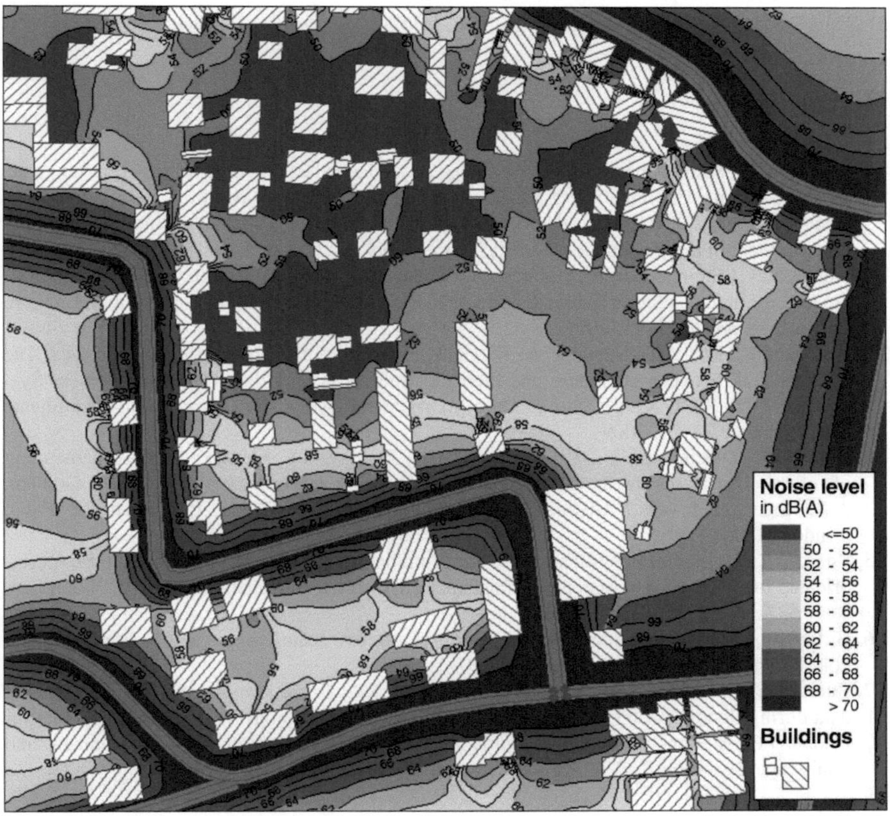

Fig. 6 Modeled traffic noise propagation including building object barrier considerations

model as derived in the software package SoundPLAN,[3] which is widely used in road and traffic management. Tools and strengths of this software are described by Wasserthal [22] when presenting a state-wide ambient noise mapping project for Germany. Besides other input factors also building barrier effects are considered for the analysis. It is obvious that noise levels behind large building objects are much reduced which plays an important role in planning considerations of noise control measurements. Of course also for population related exposure assessments such realistic models result in significant quality improvement and refinement of derived numbers of affected persons.

Results as presented in this study can be of utmost interest in disaster risk management and simulation, but also in regional and environmental planning as well as local development concepts.

Acknowledgment The presented work was funded by the Austrian Research Promotion Agency (FFG) in the frame of the Austrian Space Applications Programme (ASAP). The ALS data was provided by the Department of Geoinformation und Real Estate of the Federal State Government of Upper Austria. The georeferenced address data was provided by Tele Atlas Austria and the demographic data was provided by Statistik Austria.

References

1. Aubrecht, C., Steinnocher, K.: Der Übergang von Bodenbedeckung über urbane Struktur zu urbaner Funktion – Ein integrativer Ansatz von Fernerkundung und GIS. In: Schrenk, Popovich, Benedikt (eds) CORP2007: 12th International Conference on Urban Planning and Regional Development in the Information Society. Proceedings, pp. 667–675 (2007)
2. Aubrecht, C., Steinnocher, K., Hollaus, M., Wagner, W.: Integrating earth observation and GIScience for high resolution spatial and functional modeling of urban landuse. Comput. Environ. Urban Syst. **33**(1), 15–25 (2009)
3. Aubrecht, C., Köstl, M., Steinnocher, K., Hackner-Jaklin, N.: Georeferenced address data: The essential link between geometric and thematic features in an Urban Data Management System. In: UDMS'09: XXVII. Urban Data Management Symposium. Proceedings. Ljubljana, Slovenia, June 24–26, 2009
4. Balk, D.L., Deichmann, U., Yetman, G., Pozzi, F., Hay, S.I., Nelson, A.: Global mapping of infectious diseases: methods, examples and emerging applications. In: Hay, S.I., Graham, A.J., Rogers, D.J. (eds.) Advances in Parasitology, vol. 62, pp. 119–156. Academic Press, London (2006)
5. Benz, U.C., Hofmann, P., Willhauck, G., Lingenfelder, I., Heynen, M.: Multiresolution, object-oriented fuzzy analysis of remote sensing data for GIS-ready information. ISPRS J. Photogram. Remote Sens. **58**, 239–258 (2004)
6. Birkmann, J.: Risk and vulnerability indicators at different scales: Applicability, usefulness and policy implications. Environ. Hazards **7**, 20–31 (2007)
7. Buehler, Y.A., Kellenberger, T.W., Small, D., Itten, K.I.: Rapid mapping with remote sensing data during flooding 2005 in Switzerland by object-based methods: A case study. In: Martin-Duque, J.F., Brebbia, C.A., Emmanouloudis, D.E., Mander, U. (eds.) Geo-Environment and Landscape Evolution II. WIT Press, Southampton, UK (2006)

[3] http://www.soundplan.eu (last accessed January 15, 2010)

8. Buehler, Y. A., Kellenberger, T. W.: Development of processing chains for rapid mapping with satellite data. In: Li, J., Zlatanova, S., Fabbri, A. (eds.) Geomatics Solutions for Disaster Management. Lecture Notes in Geoinformation and Cartography, pp. 49–60. Springer, Berlin, Heidelberg (2007)
9. Chen, K.: An approach to linking remotely sensed data and areal census data. Int. J. Remote Sens. **23**(1), 37–48 (2002)
10. Cutter, S.: GI science, disasters, and emergency management. Trans. GIS **7**(4), 439–445 (2003)
11. Elvidge, C., Aubrecht, C., Baugh, K., Tuttle, B., Howard, A.T.: Satellite detection of power outages following earthquakes and other events. In: Third International Geohazards Workshop. Group of Earth Observations (GEO) & Integrated Global Observing Strategy (IGOS) Geohazards. Proceedings. ESA/ESRIN, Frascati (Rome), Italy, 6–9 November 2007
12. Freire, S.: Modeling of spatio-temporal distribution of urban population at high-resolution – Value for risk assessment and emergency management. In: Konecny, M., Zlatanova, S., Bandrova, T., Friedmannova, L. (eds.) Cartography and Geoinformatics for Early Warning and Emergency Management: Towards Better Solutions. Proceedings, pp. 42–50. Springer, Heidelberg (2009)
13. Freire, S., Aubrecht, C.: Towards improved risk assessment – Mapping spatio-temporal distribution of human exposure to earthquake hazard in Lisbon. In: Boccardo, P., et al. (eds.) Gi4DM 2010, Geomatics for Crisis Management. Proceedings, CD-Rom. Torino, Italy, 2–4 February 2010
14. Herrera-Cruz, V., Koudogbo, F.: TerraSAR-X rapid mapping for flood events. In: ISPRS Hannover Workshop 2009: High-Resolution Earth Imaging for Geospatial Information. Hannover, Germany, 2–5 June 2009
15. Hritonenko, N., Yatsenko, Y.: Modelling of Traffic Noise Propagation. Chapter 4.2 in Applied mathematical modelling of engineering problems, pp. 125–129. Springer, Netherlands (2003) (see http://books.google.at/books?id=3FUf81s7oSwC&printsec=frontcover)
16. Kressler, F., Steinnocher, K.: Object-oriented analysis of image and LiDAR data and its potential for a dasymetric mapping application. In: Blaschke, T., Lang, S., Hay, G.J. (eds.) Object-based image analysis. Spatial concepts for knowledge-driven remote sensing applications. Lecture Notes in Geoinformation and Cartography, XVIII, pp. 611–624. Springer, Heidelberg (2008)
17. Mesev, V.: Identification and characterization of urban building patterns using IKONOS imagery and point-based postal data. Comput. Environ. Urban Syst. **29**, 541–557 (2005)
18. NRC (National Research Council): Tools and Methods for Estimating Populations at Risk from Natural Disasters and Complex Humanitarian Crises. Report by the National Academy of Sciences, 264 pp. National Academy Press, Washington, DC (2007)
19. Steinnocher, K., Köstl, M.: Mapping urban functions by integrating socioeconomic information, address data, and remote sensing. In: 2007 Urban Remote Sensing Joint Event, Paris, France, 11–13 April 2007
20. USGS United States Geological Survey: The severity of an earthquake. USGS General Interest Publication. http://pubs.usgs.gov/gip/earthq4/severitygip.html, last modified 04/29/2009 (2009)
21. Wald, D.J., Quitoriano, V., Heaton, T.H., Kanamori, H.: Relationships between peak ground acceleration, peak ground velocity, and modified Mercalli intensity in California. Earthquake Spectra **15**(3), 557–564 (1999)
22. Wasserthal, I.: Bundesweite Umgebungslärmkartierung. 4th GeoForum MV 2008. Rostock-Warnemünde, Germany, 28–29 April 2008
23. Willhauck, G.: Comparison of object oriented classification technique and standard image analysis for the use of change detection between SPOT multispectral satellite images and aerial photos. Int. Arch. Photogram. Remote Sens.**XXXIII**(Suppl B3), 35–42 (2000)
24. Wu, Y.-M., Teng, T.-L., Shin, T.-C., Hsiao, N.-C.: Relationship between peak ground acceleration, peak ground velocity, and intensity in Taiwan. Bull. Seismol. Soc. Am. **93**(1), 386–396 (2003)

Dynamic Radiography Imaging as a Tool in the Design and Validation of a Novel Intelligent Amputee Socket

George Papaioannou, Dimitris Tsiokos, Goeran Fiedler, Christos Mitrogiannis, Ilya Avdeev, Jake Wood, and Ray McKinney

Abstract It is apparent that socket fit is the most common source of dissatisfaction in amputees and part of a growing medical and socioeconomic problem. Even the most up to date trans-tibial socket designs are not capable of coping with the issue of continuous stump volume change that is apparent within a day, week, month or season of socket use. Intelligent sockets integrating variable volume (VVSS) with elevated vacuum (EV) systems hold that promise but have yet to reach completion in feasibility studies. This is mainly due to delays in the relevant technological maturity, cost and poor assessment methodologies. These challenges can be overcome by current advantages in dynamic radiography imaging. These advantages are presented with an example of a novel socket design as: a) solutions to problems of direct socket-stump motion measurement, and b) as tools for calibrating socket control hardware and computer aided socket design. Imaging can therefore be integrated as part of an expert clinical system for imaging-driven computer-aided socket design and evaluation (cost-labor effective).

Keywords Intelligent transtibial socket · Elevated vacuum · Variable volume · Dynamic radiography · CAD-CAE

1 The Need for Novel Socket Designs in a Constantly Increasing Amputee Population

Limb loss is obviously a severe medical condition that has potentially life changing consequences. Prevalence of amputation has been addressed by analyzing a large number of US hospital discharge records (20% of total in US) issued between 1988

G. Papaioannou (✉), D. Tsiokos, G. Fiedler, C. Mitrogiannis, I. Avdeev, J. Wood, and R. McKinney
Wisconsin Institute for Biomedical Health Technology, Director of "MOVE Center", Department of Civil Engineering and Mechanics, College of Engineering and Applied Science and Department of Occupational Therapy, College of Health Sciences, University of Wisconsin, Milwaukee, P.O. Box 784, Milwaukee, WI 53201-0784 414 326 0665

J.M.R.S. Tavares and R.M.N. Jorge (eds.), *Computational Vision and Medical Image Processing: Recent Trends*, Computational Methods in Applied Sciences 19,
DOI 10.1007/978-94-007-0011-6_5,

and 1996 [18]. The average annual number of limb-loss-related hospital discharges is 133,325 nationwide (~3% increase per year). Vascular conditions were by far the most common cause with 82% overall (46.19 per 100,000 persons in 1996). Corrected for population effects, the total number of amputations increased by 27% over the period of the study. Incidence rates for lower limb amputations vary between 0.1 and 1.9/10,000 for most western countries [19]. Amputation rates are by trend increasing around the world. In the US this rate increased from 63 per 10,000 diabetics in 1980 to 81 per 10,000 diabetics in 1987. *An estimated 1.6 million Americans were living with limb loss in 2005, (estimated to become 3.6 million by the year 2050)* (total cost of Amputee healthcare exceeds 4.5 Billion annually in US [20, 75]. Continuous research was also conducted to establish how well prostheses are perceived by their respective users [45]. Of the participants (1538 persons: 18–84 years old) 94.5% had prosthesis and used it extensively. However, only 75.7% were overall satisfied with their prosthesis, *where the socket fit was least acceptable (75.5%)* behind appearance (80.4%) and weight (77.1%). *It is apparent that socket fit is a major challenge in Prosthetics and Orthotics (P&O), the most common source of dissatisfaction in amputees and part of a growing medical and socioeconomic problem.*

2 Current State-of-the-Art Socket Evaluation Methodologies Are Inefficient in Assessing Trans-Tibial (TT) Socket Problems

Trans-tibial amputations have a clear advantage over higher-level leg amputations since the knee joint remains functional and less mass is substituted by the artificial leg. Nonetheless, the bony structure and the low soft tissue coverage make it susceptible to pressure and friction related injuries. Long established and still commonly used designs are the *Patellar Tendon Bearing Socket (PTB) and the "Kondylen Bettung Muenster" (KBM)* socket. However, a well working PTB or KBM socket will inevitably spark a deflection related patellar reflex every time the user steps on the prosthesis with an ever so slightly flexed knee disrupting the natural walking pattern and inducing a range of undesired consequences, such as exaggerated metabolism. Alternative socket concepts can be summarized under the category *Total Surface Bearing sockets* (TSB). The intention is essentially that weight transfer, controllability, and suspension are realized by improved evenly distributed contact pressure with the aid of silicon liners and locking mechanisms to provide full skin-material contact and design flexibility [69]. Comparative studies [32, 69] confirmed that "a more physiological walking pattern with the TSB socket is apparent, and is therefore recommended as to "be used effectively in the rehabilitation of trans-tibial amputees"." *However these studies suggest that the TSB socket is not capable of coping with the issue of continuous stump volume change that is apparent within a day, week, month or season of socket use. Many amputees end up having several socket rectification sessions every year.*

Most patients experience stump volume changes within a single day or over the course of seasons and in response to temperature, activity, nutrition and pressure.

Most promising, and best established approaches to address that problem today are *elevated vacuum (EV) suspension sockets.* The principle of elevated vacuum is to achieve a better pressure distribution either mechanically (e.g. Otto Bock Harmony trans-tibial [68] or by means of an electric pump). Negative pressure is deployed, to *"expand the soft tissue and bring it closer to the socket wall"*, avoiding soft tissue compression. All *vacuum assisted socket systems (VASS)* work with a silicon or gel liner with or without a pin lock, and a pump mechanism that provides the desired negative pressure over ideally the entire stump surface (Fig. 1q). The first comparison studies with the Harmony system [7] found that the stump volume decreases by 6.5% on average in a custom made TSB socket after 30 min of walking,

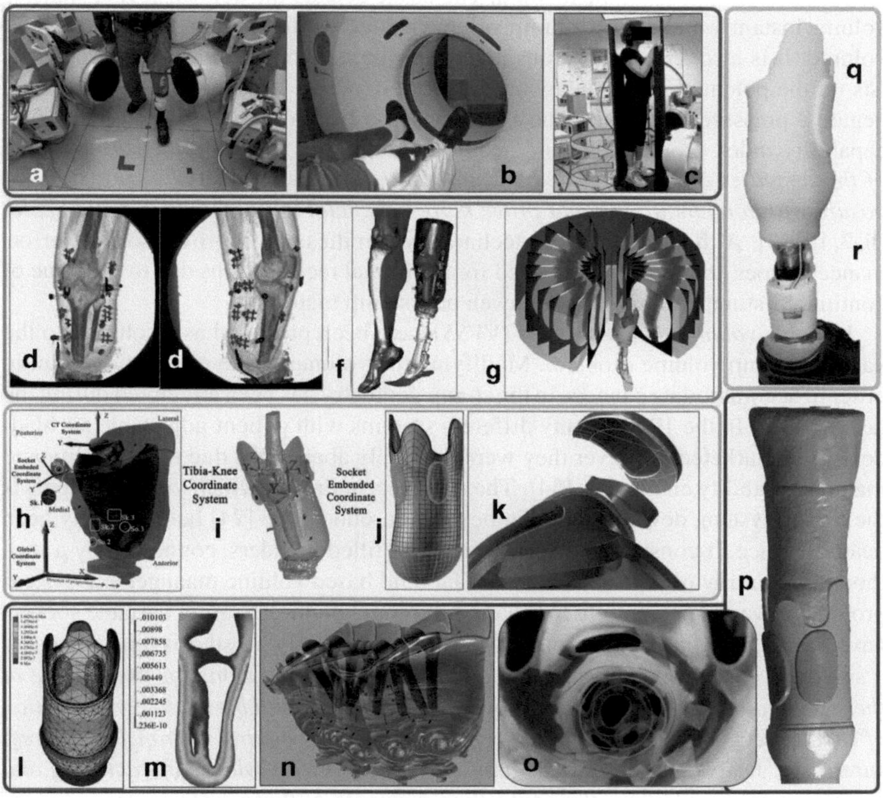

Fig. 1 The role of imaging in SMARTsocket's overall reverse engineering approach to socket design and evaluation is critical. The procedural steps to any socket rectification protocol are presented in Fig. 5. Imaging modalities for amputee screening include (**a**) DRSA, (**b**) CT, (**c**) turn table dynamic radiography. Samples of images obtained of the three modalities are shown is (**d–g**) respectively. Note the abundance of skin-socket markers and that a careful data fusion protocol is used to co-register 2D and 3D information from all scans in (**h, i**). Finally the socket rectification protocol (**j–k**) with CAD-CAE tools precedes the virtual fitting in (**p**) while an iterative computational modeling evaluation process is under way in (**l–n**). Rapid prototyping of the final virtual prototype is warranted in (**o, q, r**) to establish the SMARTsocket integration with the prosthetic parts

whereas it was maintained and even increased by 3.7% when elevated vacuum was used. The tibia displacement was also clearly less with the vacuum pump and a more tight suspension of the prosthesis was achieved as the participants confirmed. A follow-up study [23] concluded that *a socket that is 4–6% undersized with no deep voids is recommended for the fitting of trans-tibial amputees*. It has been also reported that the measurable reduction in positive pressure aids the level of compliance of TT sockets [5]. The study also reported that changes in contact pressure over the step cycle were of different range for different subjects – something that could not be explained in the article, but might hint at the necessity to vary the socket volume anyway for optimized fit. The aforementioned studies used casting and water displacement procedure to assess stump-volume which poses questions on the clinical validity of the method. The tissue outside the donned socket changes volume instantly and donned stump volume is much different than undonned stump volume. It is also a very laborious and messy procedure. Another controversy exists on the potential disadvantageous effect of exposure of tissue to just prolonged negative pressure. In a later study [10], the use of VASS sockets and locomotor capability index promoted wound healing in amputees with skin ulceration. *In all of these studies it was suggested that alternate positive and negative pressure exposure within boundaries could prove more beneficial to tissue healing and health* [5, 7, 10, 23]. Although EV-VASS technology significantly improves socket performance, it does not eliminate the need for additional rectifications due to the issue of continuous stump volume change (even past stump maturity).

Variable volume socket systems (VVSS) have been proposed as a solution to the variable stump volume problem. Modifying the volume of the prosthetic socket in order to accommodate changes in the stump geometry has been attempted during the last decades. In the 1990s, many different systems with patient-adjustable air bladders were marketed, however they were gradually abandoned due to feasibility and manufacturability challenges [54]. The most recent project which yielded patents is the SVGS system, developed by Simbex LLC around 2003 [24] but has rarely been heard of since. It consists of a variety of water filled bladders, connected by a well thought-out array of pipes and valves. The fluid based volume management system provides a way of accounting for changing stump volumes. Similar variable sockets have been used in the field of interim-fittings, where early prosthesis must allow for a swift and uncomplicated adaptation [27]. *Most likely reasons for the decline of these technologies (VVSS) are lack of feasibility due to bulkiness, no consideration of shear effects, lack of accurate and precise real-time control of transferred pressure/shear, weight, leakage, wear and tear and problems with manufacturing and maintenance. In addition, the controlling elements of these systems are yet to be fully calibrated with real life input from strenuous activities. This would require a sophisticated in-vivo unobtrusive indirect stump-socket measurement method, which could be used to calibrate a real-time continuous feedback mechanism (sensor-to-actuator) that returns information of the socket-stump interface (pressure and shear magnitude and direction) to the VVS system.*

This accurate calibration leads to successful socket fit involving pressure, shear, deformation and slippage measurement and monitoring between the subject's skin, the residual limb tissues and the socket. These measurements have been conducted for about 50 years involving fluid-filled sensors, pneumatic sensors, diaphragm deflection strain gauge [67], cantilever/beam strain gauge [55] and printed circuit sheet sensors [14,29,67,74]. *In-vivo* socket-pressure measurements are also possible with commercial capacitive, piezoelectric, ink-film based products [11,14,46]. *However, these sensors possess many disadvantages such as accuracy, hysteresis, signal drift, response to curvature, spatial resolution, temperature sensitivity, installation instability* [3] *and unknown shear coupling effects* [11,16,44,46,49]. An ideal system should be able to monitor real interfacial stresses continuously, both the normal (pressure) and shear component (dynamic slippage). The challenge of measuring slippage within the socket is yet to be efficiently tackled by the prosthetist in and outside the laboratory.

In this direction, research in Computed tomography (CT) allowed the incorporation of patient-specific stump-socket geometry into a CAD/CAM system, performing modifications, and milling a plaster positive likeness. Despite being static analyses, these studies offered high image quality and the benefit of seeing below the skin. However, significant CT disadvantages from movement artifacts were reported. A number of spiral X-ray computed tomography (SXCT) studies [13,25,61,62,64,65] demonstrated that the SXCT scanner is sufficiently precise and accurate for distance and static volumetric quantitative socket-fitting studies. Simpler methods involving ordinary radiographs analyzed different static 2D positions between bone and socket during different parts of a gait cycle. The next level of static, yet 3D analysis, is the use of Roentgen Stereogrammetric Analysis (RSA) to completely characterize socket and stump interactions in all six degrees of freedom with a biplane (stereo) imaging three dimensional (3D) configuration [8,30]. RSA socket-stump motion studies have reported variation of 10–30mm in the vertical motion and 0–15 mm in the AP motion [63]. Ultrasound techniques were also used to assess femur movements within trans-femoral sockets [15]. Similarly, conventional gait analysis cannot "see" below the skin or past the socket and its accuracy cannot effectively address dynamic movement [37,39]. *Currently there is no way of accurately addressing the rate of slippage, shear and stump pistoning and their direction during the performance of dynamic tasks by amputees.* There is, therefore, a need to identify new methods for quantification of the dynamic interaction between the residual limb and the prosthetic socket with visualization paradigms that the clinician is trained to interpret.

3 Integrating Dynamic Radiographic Imaging with Computer-Aided Design and Computational Modeling in Socket Evaluation

In recent years these state-of-the-art-and-Science perspectives of technology integration are starting to be employed in the P&O arena to increase yield and reduce labour and cost. According to a National survey [50] of US Prosthetists and

Orthotists, the development of "smart" prosthetics will require development of basic knowledge and understanding of the mechanics of socket fitting as well as technological advancements in soft tissue characterization. As such, *dynamic imaging-driven, template-based computer aided design (CAD-CAE) tools employing fast-track learning offer great promise in the process of socket rectification at the virtual environment with the associated reductions in cost and labour*. As of recently, Dynamic Roentgen Stereogrammetric Analysis (DRSA) has been introduced as an accurate tool for dynamic in-vivo measurement of stump/socket kinematics [37, 38, 41, 42]. The method allows direct observation of tissue deformations during activities of daily life, such as walking or stepping down stairs, and during more strenuous higher-speed activities such as jumping or running. The DRSA method (Fig. 1a) is one order of magnitude more accurate that current conventional *in-vivo* motion analysis techniques (socket-stump and residual bone pistoning motion can be assessed with as much as 0.03mm translational and 1.3° rotational accuracy [37–39]). Shear forces, and the so called stump pistoning information can be derived from the dynamic slippage between the residual bone, skin and socket wall using the 3D displacement history of tantalum markers tracked from the DRSA data. Absolute and relative displacements between residual bone, skin and socket wall have been reported in several studies for several below knee amputees using DRSA [37–39].

This patient specific accurate kinematics information can also improve the efficiency of computational modeling. Computational modeling can in turn reduce the iterative cycles between experimental testing and socket fabrication-prototyping. Finite element methods (FEM) are becoming more common ground in socket engineering for two major methodological reasons: (1) FEM models produce full field information on the stress, strain, and motion anywhere within the modeled objects and (2) Parametric analysis for an optimal design is possible. To date, prescribing the displacement boundary conditions at the nodes on the outer surface of the socket or liner is the protocol used for most socket rectification simulations [9, 52, 59, 72, 73]. Similar studies suggest that only qualitative identification of the tolerant and sensitive areas is possible with current methods. Dynamic imaging could also address this issue in addition to calibrating the patient specific FE models with respect to material properties [6, 43, 71]. *A fully scalable patient specific FE model driven by high accuracy in-vivo internal residual bone-stump-socket DRSA kinematics would be the ideal engineering analysis method for this problem.*

From a biomechanics perspective these analyses could help resolve some current state of the art contradictions of fairly common beliefs and everyday practices, suggesting that some stump areas are designated for higher load bearing purposes than others. They suggest that these areas are patient specific so customization of socket is necessary. Apart from that, these studies do not conclusively answer how to translate the result into practical applications. In addition, there are remaining questions regarding the practicability of the necessary technical effort, and the consideration of shear forces, which are believed to contribute significantly to most socket comfort problems. *Dynamic imaging, offers, due to its accurate, indirect non-invasive and unobtrusive characteristics a solution to these problems of direct measurement (relying on kinematics assessment of the outside of socket only) and computational modeling. It can therefore be integrated as part of an expert clinical system for imaging-driven computer-aided socket design and manufacturing (cost effective electronic as opposed to actual prototype based socket rectification).*

4 SMARTsocket: An Example of Integration of Dynamic Imaging, CAD-CAE and FE Methods in Socket Evaluation

An example of performance validation with the synergy of the three methodologies is presented for an intelligent socket system that combines variable volume socket system (VVSS) technology with an elevated vacuum system. Although the EV socket component is in the process of undergoing full feasibility study and has been fitted to hundreds of amputees by our prosthetists, the integration of the two systems is yet to see the fruits of a complete feasibility study. The novel system proposed here (acronym: SMARTsocket) intends to complete the advanced performance of EV sockets *by dealing with the variable stump volume problem* that occurs during prolonged use of the socket or at very strenuous activities such as athletic endeavors or heavy-duty work. The new socket and the new methodologies for each efficient validation intend to give amputees an advanced level of autonomy in terms of enabling them in conditions of demanding strenuous mobility [28, 34, 35, 66].

SMARTsocket combines two technologies (EV+VVSS) thus offering for the first time *real-time* controllability of socket elevated vacuum and overall socket volume by incorporating counter-shear actuators for readjusting the pressure/shear distribution across the stump-socket interface. All parts are fabricated by Lincolnshire Manufacturers SA and assembled by our prosthetists. The feasibility study includes sensitivity, operability, safety, durability and efficiency (structural, functional) testing. Functional tests in clinical trials are currently under way for the validation of the new system. We use reverse engineering methodologies in our approach to tackle this complex problem (Fig. 1). A summary of the main tested hypotheses justifying the rationale behind the integration of the elevated vacuum socket and the adaptable volume socket being tested is presented next:

1) *Hypothesis 1: Vacuum equalizes stump pressures*. It is known that a vacuum system equalizes pressures, stabilizes fluid levels and helps vaporize perspiration [1,4,5,21,22,26]. Carl Caspers, a prosthetist in St. Cloud, Minnesota along with Dr. Glenn Street at St. Cloud State University [7, 12, 17] are the inventors of one of the first mechanical vacuum pumps. The major limitation of the conventional prosthesis, referred to as a PTB type socket is that it employs varying pressurized areas within the sockets. Upon stump volume reduction the prosthetist advises the patient to add socks or pads to tighten the socket. However, by applying more pressure to the limb, more volume changes occur (fluid compression) and the cycle will repeat itself. Stump volume reduction is a result of the properties of the soft tissue (the interstitial fluid is very pressure sensitive). It is common ground that basic fitting of a PTB socket requires some compression [4, 5]. The reasons

those sockets are made somewhat snug are to prevent rotation of the prosthesis, to keep it from falling off, and to support body weight, among other functions. It has been reported [14] that it takes approximately 10.544 gr of positive pressure per square mm to perform these functions. The mere act of an amputee applying the prosthesis to the remaining limb places approximately *6.803 gr of positive pressure* that one would otherwise not be subjected to. The interstitial fluids are very pressure sensitive. This complex non-linear and viscous phase of deformation will depend mainly upon the rate of loading (anisotropy and non-homogeneity are also very difficult to control when planning for the cast). The body reacts by "releasing" some of the fluid. This is somewhat like letting a little air of a balloon. When enough fluid is released, the internal pressure drops down to its normal settings. The body "wins this battle" every time.

We hypothesize that it is initial application of positive pressure that creates the change in the volume of the interstitial fluid with an escapade of undesired events after that. It has been shown that with the conventional socket, the average below-the-knee amputee can shrink 6–7% of their limb volume a day and 12–13% on an above-the-knee amputee [7, 56]. Of course, this varies with the size and makeup of the patient's limb. However, in a properly fit vacuum system, the change is typically <1%. Our previous work suggests that patients do not experience significant problems in a fitting until they reach a 3–4% level of change but quantification of this change is yet to be effectively addressed with conventional methods. Typically, our prosthetists take the casting under 558.8 mm of vacuum (Fig. 1). The plaster is not molded or shaped, as is done with the conventional PTB. Patients have their own unique shape and this method is not trying to change that. As a matter of fact, wherever a modification is applied with bare hands, a pressure gradient is created and that will be the likely area where patients might expect strange interactions. After a cast has been taken with the 558.8 mm of mercury in vacuum, it is simply removed and then a global reduction of 4% around the entire cast [7, 12, 17] is sculpted. In other words, it is not any tighter or looser in anyone spot over another.

2) *Hypothesis 2: Choosing an appropriate liner is necessary for socket performance*. The next item that is crucial to our method of fitting is the use of the *urethane liner* (Fig. 2). The liner can change shape slightly become thicker or thinner, become quite firm or very soft. For a below-the-knee amputee, if we simply roll on the modified urethane liner and allow them to step into the socket, it will be fairly tight. It is the exact shape of the patient's limb, but with the thickness of the liner, it is then compressed 4%. As the patient puts the limb into the socket, the material will move towards the path of least resistance. This means that since it is a new socket and there are not any loose areas or voids at the socket, the liner will move up and out of the socket. Typically on a below-the-knee patient it will move about 5/8″ and closer to 1″ on an above-the-knee patient. *Again this value is empirically estimated and not possible to quantify with conventional measurement technologies*. This is expected since this donning process is patient specific. This value also differs even between donning sessions for the same patient. When the patient stands in that socket, as their

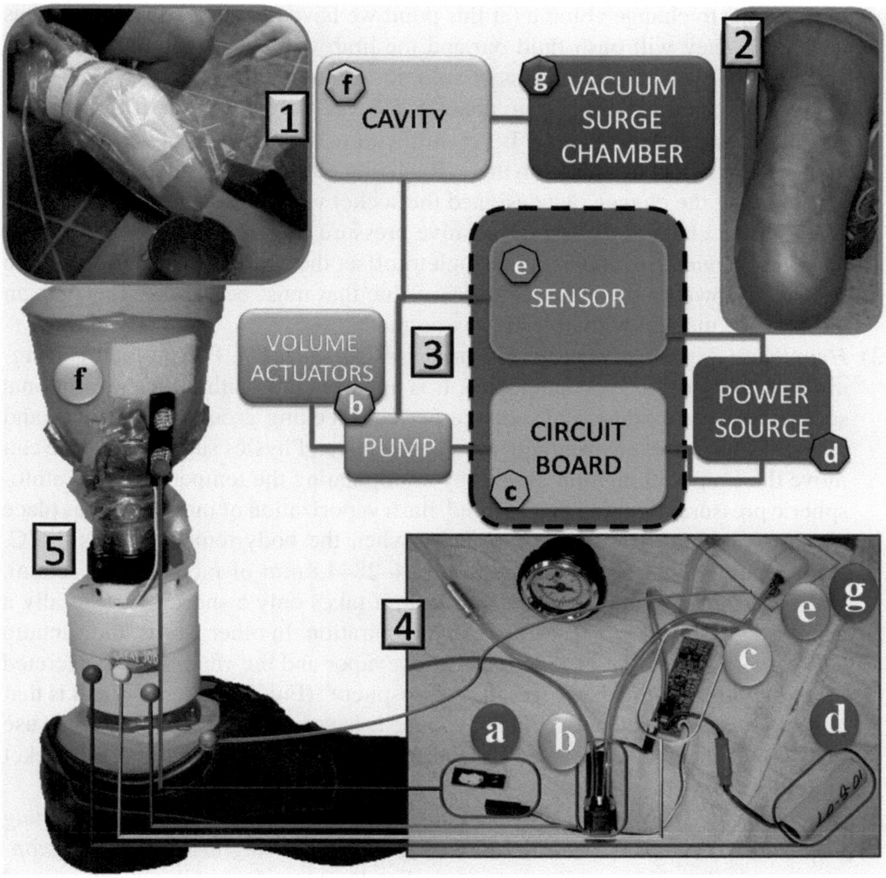

Fig. 2 (1) The SMARTsocket casting method uses the principle of vacuum and minimal sculpting by the prosthetist. The cast assumes the contour of the stump with negative pressure applied equally everywhere in the segment; (2) The Urethane liner that forms the negative cavity with the socket; (3) Flowchart of the operational components of the SMARTsocket system. SMARTsocket comprises of an elevated vacuum system for maintaining a negative pressure in a cavity between a socket of a prosthetic device and a positive pressure system of actuators that can change the overall socket volume if necessary. (4) The system (parts are fabricated by Lincolnshire Manufacturers SA and assembled by our prosthetists) comprises of a concealable vacuum surge chamber: 20.41 g (**g**), a vacuum and inflating reversible pump: 24.66 g (**b**), a variable positive pressure actuator (**b**), a power source: 21.97 g, (**d**) and microcontroller: 5.67 g (**c**), USB switch: 1.70 g (**a**), housing tubing, tubing connectors: 45.54 gr, and means for sensing pressure (**b**) and actuating (**g**) the system. The sensor triggers an actuation event when the negative pressure decays to a predetermined differential from atmospheric pressure. This actuates the vacuum pump to increase the negative pressure in the cavity and the opposite actuation event when the negative pressure reaches a predetermined threshold (de-activation of the vacuum pump). Similarly the positive pressure pump inflates the air-bladders to increase the stiffness of the socket locally or change the socket volume (increase or decrease it)

limb begins to change volume (at this point we have not added vacuum) and as they walk, they will push fluid out and the limb will shrink. The urethane absorbs partially the change in loss of volume. Although this is very dynamic, the adjustment can only come up to about 4–5%, i.e. only a portion of the average shrinkage. Again this estimate is very difficult to quantify objectively. The vacuum system will take over from there. Realizing that it was positive pressure that was creating the change, we designed the socket with enough negative pressure to offset the changes caused by positive pressure. A minimum of *457.2 mm of mercury vacuum (or higher)* is enough to offset the negative effects of positive pressure. However this is an empirical value that must be validated against an unobtrusive method with objective assessments.

3) *Hypothesis 3: The vacuum system vaporizes perspiration*. Perspiration is a significant problem for most amputees. It is apparent that within the conventional socket, it is warm, dark and moist, a perfect breeding ground for bacteria and the undesired onset environment for a blister-ulcer. Physics suggests that we can move the evaporation point around by manipulating the temperature and atmospheric pressure. Keeping that in mind, flash vaporization of moisture takes place at approximately 711.2 mm of mercury when the body temperature is 37 °C. With a pump that can deliver up to 660.4–2844.8 mm of mercury of vacuum, while it is not instantaneous and not flash, it takes only a short time (literally a small fraction of a second) to vaporize perspiration. In other words, the vacuum socket can convert that excess liquid into a vapor and the vapor can be excreted through ports of pump back into the "atmosphere" (Fig. 2). The end result is that the patient's limb is kept dry. This hypothesis is very easy to test; prolonged use of EV sockets can be assessed by simply undonning them and test for socket humidity with a humidity tester.
4) *Hypothesis 4: The vacuum system cannot solve the volumetric changes resulting from very strenuous activities (running, jumping, bearing heavy weights, stopping suddenly)*. The current system applies to every day walking and normal ambulation. We have shown that when patients are involved in heavy labor and athletic endeavors, they will be subjected to higher rates of loading that challenge the vacuum system technology. To this end we integrated the variable volume socket (VVS) to the EV principle. At the proof-of-concept stage of the prototype the system is static (no real time operation). The user inflates or deflates the actuator based bladders in the socket before performing a strenuous task (running) that requires higher socket suspension and stiffness. This system is not yet capable of responding to real-time changes in volume but it can still allow us to change the positive pressure and the overall socket volume if necessary before the EV functionality kicks in.

A miniaturized electronic pump (Fig. 2) (about the size of a pen 4 cm long, 15–20 gr), can be fitted inside the shin tubs or inside feet-shoe. Figure 2 presents the full technical characteristics of the system. This pump can be hidden for cosmetic reasons but its size helps eliminate the weight and increase the application of volume to these patients. The advantage of the electronic system, besides the cosmesis and weight is the fact that it does not require, as the mechanical ones (Harmony), to be walked on and compress a piston to draw up the vacuum. The patient can actually be sitting all day and the circuit board and the motor will make sure the patient stays within a very therapeutic range. The socket's pressure boundaries have been set at 190.5–546.1 mm of mercury. We know that we need to have vacuum of at least 381 mm (or higher) in order to control some of the shrinkage of the limb and vaporize the moisture. This is one of the highest values of vacuum to be obtained to our knowledge. For this function most of the systems require between 200 and 300 mA and several volts per day and the unit has to be charged every night. Our system is a very low voltage system requiring only 15 μV for daily operation. That means that the power that is used to operate one of these other systems in a day will power our system for the better part of several months.

The major challenges in tackling hypotheses 1, 4 are related to (a) accurate 3D volumetric imaging of the socket stump interface and (b) accurate 4D imaging of stump-skin slippage and pistoning. Stump-skin slippage and pistoning within the socket can cause discomfort, internal limb pain and eventually skin ulcers as a result of the excessive pressure and shear within the socket. Classical 3D CT methodologies present *three challenges*: (1) the image matrix must be higher than the commonly used clinical 512 × 512 resolution matrix which produces poor socket-stump geometry information particularly when defending hypotheses 1, 2, 4; (2) the issue of patient irradiation. The expected equivalent dose for the CT scan of the full socket-stump for above knee amputees is 2 mSv [57] with about two-thirds of this corresponding to the below knee scan; and (3) the CT can only convey static information on stump-socket geometry and cannot assess its dynamics behavior.

To overcome challenges one and two our group has been using a turntable technology that is introducing a low irradiation method for volumetric imaging. It combines the method of Biplane Dynamic Roentgen Stereogrammetric Analysis (DRSA) instrumentation with a turntable configuration that allows 3D scanning of extremities during load bearing at a fraction of the irradiation [37, 39] (Bioimerosin Laboratories SA, WI, USA) (Figs. 1c and 3). The system functions as a fluoroscopic or digital radiography device with the exception that the patient is rotated (180–360°) while standing on a supportive turntable. Although normal fluoroscopy or digital radiography is limited in high-speed acquisition, DRSA due to its high end camera and lens systems is capable of acquiring images at a high resolution matrix (1150 × 1150) and high data acquisition rate (up to 1000 Frames/s). This capability offers sampling of sequences of high resolution of images of the amputee extremity in less than 3 s (360° rotation). This axisymmetric cone-beam stack of image sequences (Fig. 3b) (the high sampling rate offers a very small sampling interval solving the issue of blurring due to motion artifacts and resulting in very high out of plane resolution) can be reconstructed during post-processing using COBRA software (Exxim Computing Corporation, CA, USA). Both one plane and biplane DRSA (which requires half the rotation period) configurations can be used. The software offers efficient ways to register the DRSA X-ray system in 3D, using the projection data [31, 39]. This is essential for Cone Beam Tomography with C-Arms or unconstrained biplane radiography. The most important aspect of this technology is that during a single DRSA turntable scan an exposure of 110 mR is estimated

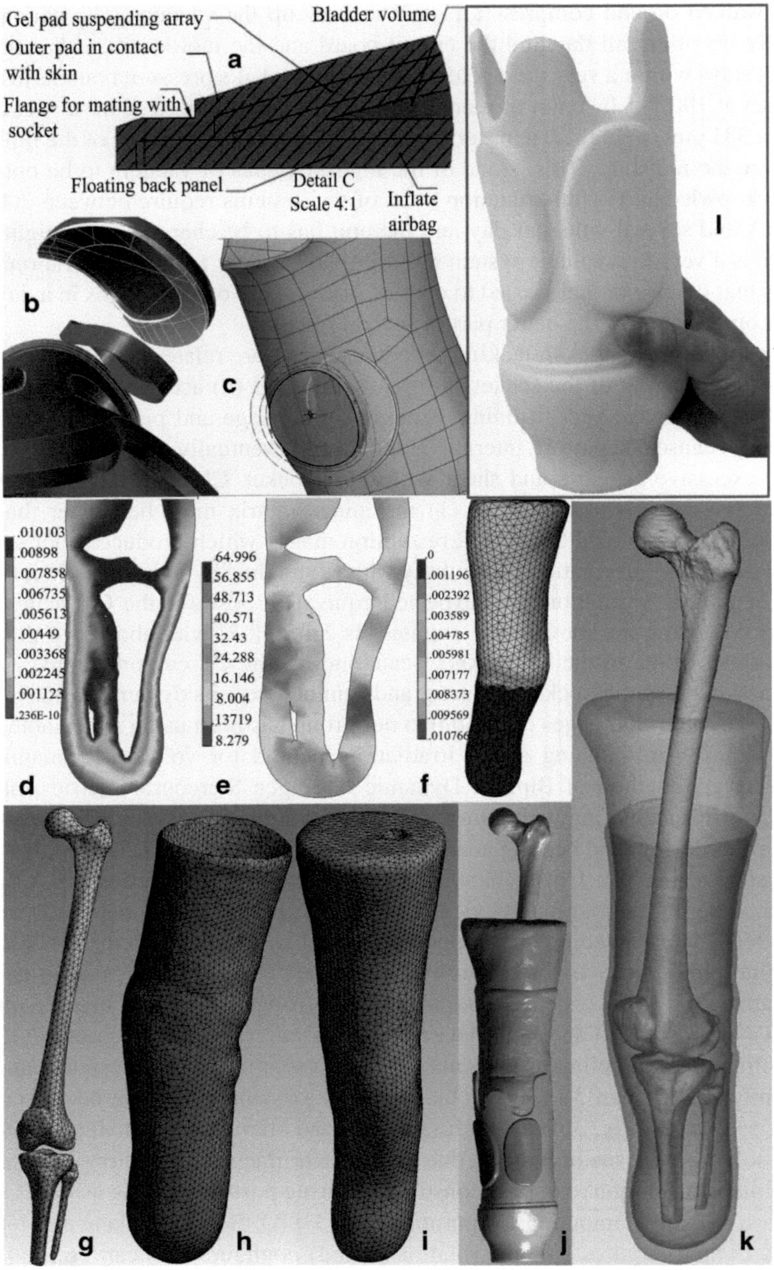
Gel pad suspending array
Outer pad in contact
with skin
Flange for mating with
socket
Bladder volume
a
Floating back panel
Detail C
Scale 4:1
Inflate
airbag
b
c
l
.010103
.00898
.007858
.006735
.005613
.00449
.003368
.002245
.001123
.236E-10
64.996
56.855
48.713
40.571
32.43
24.288
16.146
8.004
13719
8.279
0
.001196
.002392
.003589
.004785
.005981
.007177
.008373
.009569
.010766
d
e
f
g
h
i
j
k

[70] which translates into an equivalent dose of approximately 0.2–0.3 mSv. The expected equivalent dose for the CT scan of the pelvis is 2 mSv [57].

The third challenge is overcome with our new in-vivo method of assessment of three-dimensional (3D) direct, unobtrusive socket-stump kinematics/slippage of strenuous activities (high speed of motion) using Biplane DRSA instrumentation [37–41]. During these studies our group screened 50 patients (20 EV, ten TSB and ten SMARTsocket trans-tibial socket wearers). Results from the ten amputees with SMARTsocket sockets enrolled in the study approved by the University of Wisconsin Milwaukee IRB committee (see papers [37–41] for detailed methods and protocols) are presented here. The subjects were asked to perform several strenuous activities (fast walking, fast stop, running, jumping, ascending/descending stairs, pivoting) while their socket-stump kinematics was assessed with DRSA. The DRSA method is one order of magnitude more accurate that current conventional *in-vivo* motion analysis techniques (socket-stump and residual bone pistoning motion was assessed with as much as 0.03mm translational and 1.3° rotational accuracy [37–39]. The method is capable of assessing skin strain and engineering shear (between clusters of tantalum paint skin markers and socket markers) with the same accuracy. A model-based (markerless) method (MBT) for tracking of the residual limb was also demonstrated. Quantitative measurement bias between DRSA (marker based) and the MBT method ranged from −0.012 to −0.11 mm (depending on coordinate axis) for the residual bone and from 0.004 to 0.048 mm for the socket [38]. The above studies produced mixed results that stress the patient specificity in socket fitting. The methods offer a more holistic representation of the downward slippage trend of proximal side of stump with respect to the socket and an even more characteristic and of higher magnitude downward – and anterioposterior – slippage at the distal side.

Maximum slippage at strenuous tasks reached values of *151 mm for fast-stop tasks and 19 mm for the step-down task* (all patients) in the distal stump side after the impact phase of these strenuous activities. Displacement between skin-to-skin marker pairs reached maximum values of approximately 10 mm for the step-down

Fig. 3 Taking a 3D, high-resolution scan by a laser digitizer (Minolta 910) and fusing it with CT and the DRSA turntable volumetric data allows manipulation of the socket geometry using computer-aided design tools. (**a–c**) Steps of the CAD method using templates that significantly reduces the time needed to add bladders (**a**) shows a sagittal cut in the bladder pad of the SMART-socket; Note the different bladder virtual components in (**b**) and (**l**). A virtual socket fitting process follows in (**g–k**): The surface data is improved first and molding of the patient-specific socket data onto a "solid" socket template with the bladders, circuitry and conduits follows. After creating a solid model of mesh data, a (drug and drop) pad data (airbag) can be inserted and a modifiable model, based on existing template-based airbag/pad database, (**b–c**) is obtained. A 3D FEA is then generated; (**d–f**) show the residual limb deformation under the vertical displacement imposed on the truncated bones. The soft muscle tissues are modeled as a Neo-Hookean hyperelastic material. (**d**) Total displacement (Vertical deformation field) of the residual limb soft tissue inside the socket (centimeter). Graph (**f**) shows the 3-D structural mesh (24,895 tetrahedral elements) and (**e**) the Vertical normal stress distribution (kPa); photo (**l**) shows the final rapid prototyping of the computationally validated socket trials and up to 24 mm for the fast stop trials. Maximum skin strain was dependent on the position of the skin markers. Distally positioned skin marker-pairs demonstrated mainly anterioposterior displacement between each other (maximum relative strain: 13–14%). Maximum relative strain for the proximal side was 8–10%. In the worst case relative engineering shear (γ) between selected skin marker clusters that form orthonormal meshes ranged between 81.5° and 129° for the sudden stop trial. Figure 4 shows a visualization paradigm of stump-socket-residual limb kinematics of the ten BK amputees wearing the SMARTsocket. Switching the vacuum pump off had a detrimental effect is socket suspension and slippage leading to excess pistoning effect (approx. 20–30% increase). It is obvious though that even with the vacuum on the system cannot handle the accelerations due to the loading rates of the strenuous activities. Our work in-progress is looking into the crucial question of: “what would be the effect of repeating these tasks with the actuator bladders on,

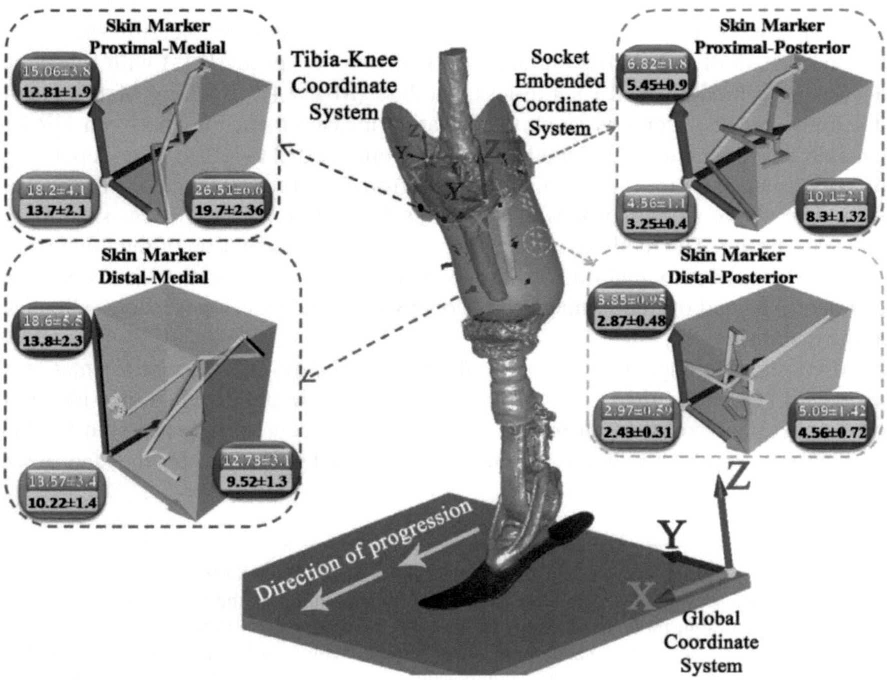

Fig. 4 Fusion of DRSA, CT and turntable radiography data produces these 3D slippage maps (distances in millimeter) between stump-skin markers and socket during a step-down trial for ten patients. Switching the vacuum pump off (*gray line*) had a detrimental effect in socket suspension and slippage leading to excess pistoning effect as compared to vacuum pump on (*black line*). It is obvious that even with the vacuum-on the system strangles with the accelerations due to the loading rates of this strenuous activity. Note also that the maximum values of the X, Y, Z axes are given for the no-vacuum (*top*) and vacuum-on (*bottom*) trials (six trials for all ten patients ±SD). The magnitude of skin perturbations in selected areas of the stump was clearly larger (20–30%) when the vacuum was switched off

i.e. having the internal socket volume reduced and then reapply the vacuum effect?" *In brief, this highly-accurate, in- vivo, patient-specific, unobtrusive dynamic information, presented using 3D visualization tools that were up to now unavailable to the clinician-prosthetist, is part of our novel core reverse engineering approach is expected to impact the iterative cycle of socket fitting and evaluation.*

The protocol for DRSA assessment includes two to four visits in total to the imaging laboratory which means minimum four to maximum ten DRSA turntable/dynamic radiography trials. The total amount of radiation exposure that the patient will receive over the two years of the study is about 1.4–1.8 mSv or 1400–1800 mrem focused on knee-shank area. This dose is approximately equivalent to the exposure that one is expected to receive from normal daily living activities over 4.6 years. This level of radiation has not been shown to cause harmful effects in adults. The expected equivalent dose for an ordinary clinical CT scan of the pelvis is 2 mSv [57]. With an overall number of six DRSA tests (=three with each socket) which is on average the amount of visits, exposure will sum up to an equivalent dose of 2.0 mSv. This amount is in the range of a one fourth of the exposure of a clinical CT scan of the trunk [57], with 20 mSv being the TLV (threshold limit value) for annual average dose for radiation workers, averaged over five years (ACGIH – American Conference of Governmental Industrial Hygienists).

A static and dynamic 3D imaging based performance index (virtual socket fitting and strain-deformation maps for all types of strenuous activities) using this 3D visualization tools is constructed for each patient. This index is crucial in our effort to optimize socket performance and reduces the overall socket rectification labor and cost (almost 50% less visits to the prosthetist).

The detailed socket rectification protocol is shown in Fig. 5 (also Fig. 1). After the first DRSA patient screening (with original socket) and after taking the patient new (or first ever interim) cast a virtual process of socket rectification takes place. Taking a 3D high-resolution scan by a 3D laser digitizer (Minolta 910) and fusing it with CT or the DRSA turntable volumetric data allows us to manipulate the socket

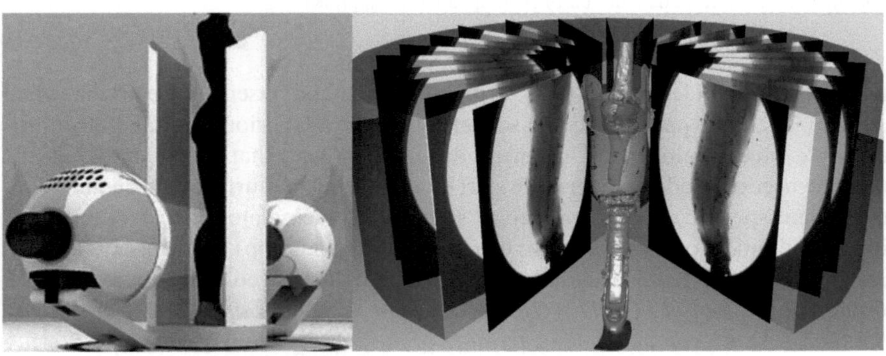

Fig. 5 (**a**) (*Left*) The DRSA turntable digital radiography scanner (see also Fig. 1 in use) and (**b**) (*right*) the axisymmetric cone-beam stack of image sequences that can be reconstructed during post-processing by registering the DRSA X-ray system in 3D, using the projection data [31, 39]

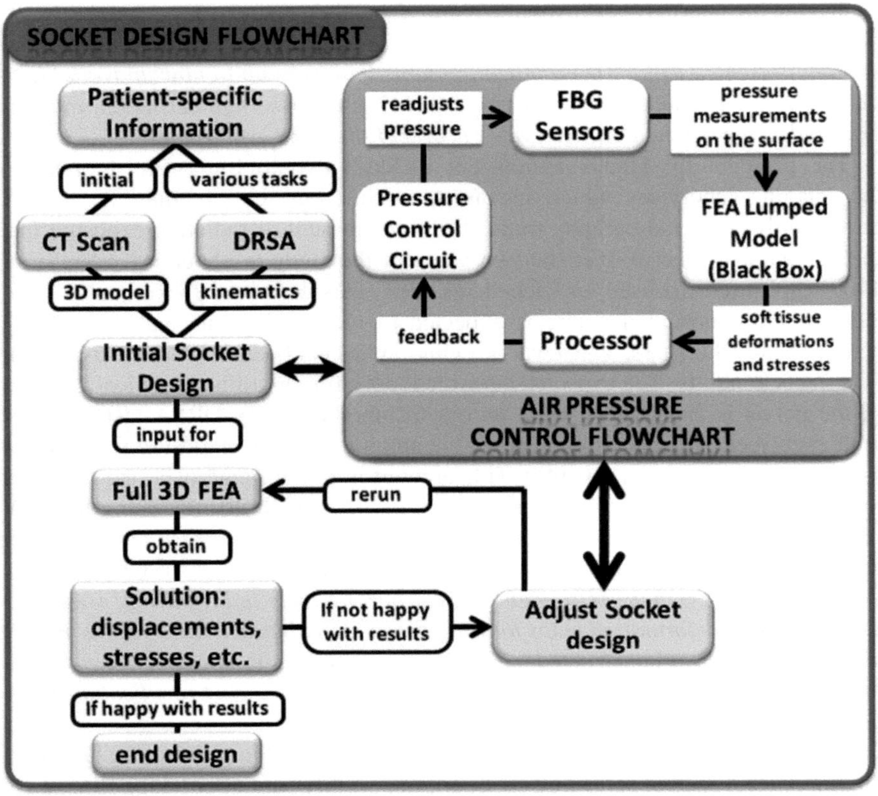

Fig. 6 Socket design and rectification flowchart showing the initial scanning of the amputee with all imaging modalities followed by the first socket design (with virtual and actual prototyping and fitting) and the iterative computational fitting process. The intermediate flowchart (*in green*) contains the tuning of the air-pressure hardware protocol based on the dynamic measurements obtained using a DRSA data driven FEA lumped model approach

using computer-aided design tools. Without this method, inserting the urethane and air bladders in the patient-specific sockets would be a laborious trial-and-error process. We have developed a CAD method using templates that significantly reduces the time needed to add bladders. We start by improving the surface data and molding the patient-specific socket data onto a "solid" socket template (Fig. 6). After creating a solid model of mesh data, we can insert (drug and drop) pad data (airbag) and create a modifiable model based on existing template-based airbag/pad database. *Using the flex tool of SOLID WORKS (Dassault Systèmes SolidWorks Corp. Santa Monica, CA), we can match the curvature of the socket to that of the pad, allowing for a perfect fit between socket and pad, thereby laying the foundation for geometry creation to remove indent in socket for pad insertion*. Once the SMARTsocket virtual prototype (mesh) is finished, the finite element model preparation begins.

The models are currently used to study the structural integrity of the socket (Fig. 6) using parameterization for the choice of material properties and boundary conditions from the high–accuracy, in-vivo kinematics acquired by the DRSA patient trials. Accurate socket models and fully validated patient-specific finite element (FE) models of the lower extremity are being developed for all patients [36, 43]. The current computational efforts focus on accurate characterization of strains and stresses in both the soft tissues of the residual limb and at the limb/socket interface. Early parametric finite element analysis (FEA) studies were used to qualitatively describe the behavioral trends rather than specific stress values (see review in [60]). Simplified, axisymmetric 2-D representations of the residual limb were proposed in the early 1990s to examine the effects of socket rectification, friction between the residual limb and prosthetic socket, and socket material properties on the interface pressures [51, 52]. Later, more complex, but geometrically generic 3-D models were proposed to investigate the influence of prosthetic design parameters and limb geometry on the interface stress distribution [58]. The models treated the socket and the bones as rigid, non-deformable bodies. The soft residual limb tissues were assumed to behave like linear elastic isotropic homogeneous materials. Recently, the simplified 2-D FEA models showed to be useful for developing real-time FEA modeling tools, which could be used in the clinical environment [47]. The simplified models also showed importance of such factors as (a) patient-specific geometry of the limb/socket, (b) non-linear material properties of soft tissues and liners, and (c) accurate kinematic tracking of limb/socket relative motion. Patient-specific FE modeling allows us to obtain qualitative and quantitative results, such as limb/socket interface stresses [48], temperatures, soft tissue strains and stresses [48], and mechanical response of the socket. Greater understanding of muscle tissue non-linear material behavior led to the development of 3-D, patient-specific, non-linear FEA models for computing internal stresses and strains in the muscle flap of residual limbs [48]. An MRI analysis of a patient used in the study determined the patient had a relatively thin muscle flap layer and almost no fat tissue [48]. The patient-specific stress state depends on the stump geometry (both soft and hard tissues), mechanical loading (patient's weight and type of physical activity), and the socket response (geometry, deformation, and pressure feedback in elevated vacuum (EV) sockets). In addition, many amputees wear silicone inserts to improve the fit, which adds an extra design parameter. *The goal of this part of the socket evaluation work is to supplement and significantly enhance the physical socket fitting with virtual fitting*. We present here also an exempt of a methodology of using 3D static and dynamic imaging data to perform 3-D, non-linear finite element analysis (FEA) for fitting TTA sockets, which is driven by high-accuracy dynamic radiography. The preliminary FE models include the socket, the silicone liner, and the residual stump (soft tissues, fibula, and tibia bones). The socket is assumed to be made of homogeneous isotropic linear elastic material (Modulus of Elasticity of 1.1 GPa and Poisson's ratio of 0.38). Both bones are considered to be rigid. The soft tissues are assumed to be homogeneous isotropic and compressible. We are comparing various material models of the soft tissues: linear elastic, hyperelastic [2] and viscoelastic [33, 48]. The urethane liner is represented by a linear elastic material model (Modulus of Elasticity of 0.004 GPa). We also assume that there is no slip between bones and soft tissues, while the coefficient of friction between the liner and the socket is set to 0.7 [53]. Time-transient kinematic boundary conditions are applied to the rigid bone surfaces using data obtained from the high-accuracy dynamic radiography (DRSA) (Fig. 5). The socket is kinematically constrained at the bottom. A series of quasi-static, non-linear numerical experiments is conducted by varying bone displacements from the unloaded limb stage to the full weight (the most compressed) stage. The analysis gives us: (1) surface stress distributions (both pressure and shear) (Fig. 5), (2) soft tissue internal strains and stresses, (3) boundary slip conditions, and (4) internal socket stresses for various loading scenarios. The fully transient analysis, which accounts for impact and other inertial effects, is considered next. As a rule if the parameterization and modeling is successful, a rapid prototyping procedure begins for the socket (Fig. 5). *This analysis offers for the first time a full patient-specific analysis of stresses and deformations towards an optimum virtual socket that can be prototyped faster with less expense and less labor*. We then incorporate the results of the patient-specific FE analysis into the design of the vacuum control system. The dynamics of the limb/socket system is very complex, but we are in the process of constructing a reduced-order dynamic model from a series of 3-D analyses. We are currently developing a methodology to automatically generate a transfer function between external loads (applied displacements and external pressures) and system response (e.g., point deformations, maximum stresses) using polynomial functions.

5 Conclusion

Delays in technological maturity, cost and poor assessment methodologies in novel socket designs prevent their adoption in the clinic. Current advantages in dynamic radiography (DR) imaging were used here to remedy the problems of direct socket-stump motion measurement, and socket calibration for a new socket design. The results showed that the socket with elevated vacuum functionality always outperforms competition when assessed with high accuracy imaging information. *This overall reverse engineering approach is expected to impact the iterative cycle of socket fitting and evaluation*.

Acknowledgements *U.S. ARMY MEDICAL RESEARCH & MATERIEL COMMAND, "MOVE" CENTER Award: # 07-2-01; European Commission EC FP7: IASiS, contract #: 232479*; and SMARTsocket: FP7-PEOPLE- 2009-IAPP.

References

1. Arndt, B.: Case study: use of a partial foot prosthesis under elevated vacuum. The American Academy of Orthotists and Prosthetists. 36th Annual Meeting and Scientific Symposium Chicago, IL, USA, 24–27 Feb 2010

2. Avril, S., Bouten, L., Dubuis, L., et al.: Mixed experimental and numerical approach for characterizing the biomechanical response of the human leg under elastic compression. J. Biomech. Eng. (2010). doi:132/031006-1
3. Bansal, C., Scott, R., Stewart, D., et al.: Decubitus ulcers: a review of the literature. Int. J. Dermatol. **44**, 805–801 (2005)
4. Beil, T.L., Street, G.M.: Comparison of interface pressures with pin and suction suspension systems. J. Rehabilit. Res. Develop. **41**, 821–828 (2004)
5. Beil, T.L., Street, G.M., Covey, S.J.: Interface pressures during ambulation using suction and vacuum-assisted prosthetic sockets. J. Rehabilit. Res. Develop. **39**, 693–700 (2002)
6. Beillas, P., Papaioannou, G., Yang, K.H., et al.: A new method to investigate in-vivo knee behavior using a finite element model of the lower limb. J. Biomech. **37**, 1019–1030 (2004)
7. Board, W.J., Street, G.M., Caspers, C.: A comparison of trans-tibial amputee suction and vacuum socket conditions. Prosthet. Orthot. Int. **25**, 202–209 (2001)
8. Bocobo, C.R., Castellote, J.M., MacKinnon, D., et al.: Videofluoroscopic evaluation of prosthetic fit and residual limbs following transtibial amputation. J. Rehabil. Res. Dev. **35**, 6–13 (1998)
9. Brennan, J.M., Childress, D.S. Finite element and experimental investigation of above-knee amputee limb/prosthesis systems: a comparative study. ASME Adv. Bioengi. **20**, 547–550 (1991)
10. Brunelli, S., Averna, T., Delusso, S., et al.: Vacuum assisted socket system in trans-tibial amputees: clinical report. Orthopädie-Technik Quart. (English edn) **2**, 2–8 (2009)
11. Buis, A.W., Covery, P.: (1997) Calibration problems encountered while monitoring stump/socket interface pressures with force sensing resistors: techniques adopted to minimise inaccuracies. Prosthet. Orthot. Int. **21**, 179–182 (2009)
12. Caspers, C.A.: Vacuum apparatus and method for managing residual limb volume in an artificial limb (2004). Patent No:US 2004/0181290 Al
13. Commean, P.K., Smith, K.E., Cheverud, J.M., et al.: Precision of surface measurements for below-knee residua. Arch. Phys. Med. Rehabil. **77**, 477–486 (1996)
14. Convery, P., Buis, A.W.: Socket/stump interface dynamic pressure distribution recorded during the prosthetic stance phase of gait of a trans-tibial amputee wearing a hydrocast socket. Prosthet. Orthot. Int. **23**, 107–112 (1999)
15. Convery, P., Murray, K.D.: Ultrasound study of the motion of the residual femur within a transfemoral socket during gait. Prosthet. Orthot. Int. **24**, 226–232 (2000)
16. Cork, R.: XSENSOR technology: a pressure imaging overview. Sens. Rev. **27**, 24–28 (2007)
17. Danzig, M., Bush, H., McKinney, R.: A prosthetic vacuum system (2009). Patent No:US 2008/0147202 A1
18. Dillingham, T.R., Pezzin, L.E., MacKenzie, E.J.: Limb amputation and limb deficiency: epidemiology and recent trends in the United States. South. Med. J. **95**, 875–883 (2002)
19. Ephraim, P., Dillingham, T., Sector, M., et al.: Epidemiology of limb loss and congenital limb deficiency: a review of the literature. Arch. Phys. Med. Rehabil. **84**, 747–761 (2003)
20. Frost, Sullivan: U.S. lower extremity prosthetics markets (2007)
21. Gerschutz, M.J.: Elevated vacuum suspension: outcome measures evaluating patient preferences and vacuum pressure & evaluation of residual limb movement in a prosthetic socket. Am. Acad. Orthot. Prosthet. 36th Annual Meeting and Scientific Symposium Chicago, IL, USA, 24–27 Feb 2010
22. Gerschutz, M.J.: Elevated vacuum suspension: the effects on an amputees residual limb volume. Am. Acad. Orthot. Prosthet. 36th Annual Meeting and Scientific Symposium Chicago, IL, USA, 24–27 Feb 2010
23. Goswami, J., Lynn, R., Street, G., et al.: Walking in a vacuum-assisted socket shifts the stump fluid balance. Prosthet. Orthot. Int. **27**, 107–113 (2003)
24. Greenwald, R.M.: Volume management: smart variable geometry socket (SVGS) technology for lower-limb prostheses. J. Prosthet. Orthort. **15**, 107–112 (2003)
25. Kalender, W.A., Seissler, W., Klotz, E., et al.: Spiral volumetric CT with single-breath-hold technique, continuous transport, and continuous scanner rotation. Radiology **176**, 181–183 (1990)

26. Klute, G.K.: Vacuum suspension: fit and function. Am. Acad. Orthot. Prosthet. 36th Annual Meeting and Scientific Symposium Chicago, IL, USA, 24–27 Feb 2010
27. Kokegei, D.: Survey of possible socket designs for old age amputated persons. Orthopädie-Technik **9**, 625–633 (2001)
28. Krohg, N.O.: Apparatus and methods for surface contour measurements (2009). Patent No:6, 270 and 7,242,484
29. Lee, V.S.P., Solomonidis, S.E., Spence, W.D.: Stump–socket interface pressure as an aid to socket design in prostheses for trans-femoral amputees – a preliminary study. Proceedings of the Institution of Mechanical Engineers. Part H. J. Engi. Med. **211**, 167–180 (1997)
30. Lilja, M., Johansson, T., Oberg, T.: Movement of the tibial end in a PTB prosthesis socket: a sagittal X-ray study of the PTB prosthesis. Prosthet. Orthot. Int. **17**, 21–26 (1993)
31. Mitrogiannis, C., Fiedler, G., Papadopoulos, C., et al.: Validation of 3D fluoroscopy image distortion correction and calibration algorithms. 9th International Conference on Information Technology and Applications in Biomedicine Larnaca. Cyprus. Nov. **5–7** (2009)
32. Narita, H., Yokogushi, K., Ship, S., et al.: Suspension effect and dynamic evaluation of the total surface bearing (TSB) trans-tibial prosthesis: a comparison with the patellar tendon bearing (PTB) trans-tibial prosthesis. Prosthet. Orthot. Int. **21**, 175–178 (1997)
33. Palevski, A., Glaich, I., Portnoy, S., et al.: Stress relaxation of porcine gluteus muscle subjected to sudden transverse deformation as related to pressure sore modeling. J. Biomech. Eng. **128**, 782–787 (2006)
34. Papaioannou, G.: Non-invasive wound prevention, detection and analysis (2008). Patent No:025369–9002
35. Papaioannou, G.: Adaptable surface with variable pneumatic pressure control (2009). Patent No:025369-9004-00
36. Papaioannou, G., Demetropoulos, K.C., King, H.Y.: Predicting the effects of knee focal articular surface injury with a patient-specific finite element model. The Knee **17**, 61–68 (2009)
37. Papaioannou, G., Mitrogiannis, C., Nianios, G., et al.: Assessment of amputee socket-stump-residual bone kinematics during strenuous activities using Dynamic Roentgen Stereogrammetric Analysis. J. Biomech. **43**, 871–878 (2010)
38. Papaioannou, G., Mitrogiannis, C., Nianios, G., et al.: Assessment of internal and external prosthesis kinematics during strenuous activities using Dynamic Roentgen Stereogrammetric Analysis. J. Prosthet. Orthot. **22**, 1–15 (2009)
39. Papaioannou, G., Mitrogiannis, C., Nianios, G., et al.: Tracking high speed arthrokinematics using a new and high resolution Biplane Dynamic Roentgen Stereogrammetric method. Int. J. Imag. **2**, 66–85 (2009)
40. Papaioannou, G., Mitrogiannis, C., Nianios, G., et al.: Assessment of internal and external prosthesis kinematics during strenuous activities using Dynamic Roentgen Stereogrammetric Analysis (DRSA). 36th Academy Annual Meeting and Scientific Symposium, American Academy of Orthotics and Prosthetics Chicago, IL, USA, 24–27 Feb 2010
41. Papaioannou, G., Mitrogiannis, C., Nianios, G., et al.: (2010) Bilateral below knee amputee socket-stump kinematics using Biplane Dynamic Roentgen Stereogrammetric Analysis 56th Annual Meeting Orthopaedic Research Society New Orleans, Louisiana, 6–9 March 2010
42. Papaioannou, G., Mitrogiannis, C., Nianios, G., et al.: Dynamic Roentgen-Stereogrammetric Analysis (DRSA) of Socket-Tissue Kinematics during high impact activities in trans-femoral amputees. 36th Anuual meeting of the American Avademy of Orthotists and Prosthetists Chicago, IL, USA, 24–27 Feb 2010
43. Papaioannou, G., Nianios, G., Mitrogiannis, C., et al.: Patient-specific knee joint finite element model validation with high-accuracy kinematics from biplane Dynamic Roentgen Stereogrammetric Analysis. J. Biomech. **41**, 2633–2638 (2008)
44. Papaioannou, G., Protopappas, C.V., Tsopelas, P., et al.: A new Method for pressure sensor Equilibration and conditioning. Brazil. J. Biomotric. **2**, 176–195 (2008)
45. Pezzin, L.E., Dillingham, T.R., MacKenzie, E.J., et al.: (2004) Use and satisfaction with prosthetic limb devices and related services. Archiv. Phys. Med. Rehabilit. **85**, 723–729 (2008)
46. Polliack, A.A., Sieh, R.C., Craig, D.D., et al.: Scientific validation of two commercial pressure sensor systems for prosthetic socket fit. Prosthet. Orthot. Int. **24**, 63–73 (2000)

47. Portnoy, S., Yarnitzky, G., Yizhar, Z., et al.: Real-time patient-specific finite element analysis of residual limb stresses in transtibial amputees during treadmill walking. J. Biomech. **39**, S539 (2007)
48. Portnoy, S., Yizhar, Z., Shabshin, N., et al.: Internal mechanical conditions in the soft tissues of a residual limb of a trans-tibial amputee. J. Biomech. **41**, 1897–1909 (2008)
49. Pramanik, C., Saha, H., Gangopadhyay, U.: Design optimization of a high performance silicon MEMS piezoresistive pressure sensor for biomedical applications. J. Micromech. Microeng. **16**, 2060–2066 (2006)
50. Report on the State-of-The-Science meeting in prosthetics and orthotics. Research in P&O: Are We Addressing Clinically-Relevant Problems. Northwestern University Feinberg School of Medicine Chicago, USA (2006)
51. Reynolds, D.: Shape design and interface load analysis for below-knee prosthetic sockets. Ph.D dissertation, University of California, Berkeley, USA (1988)
52. Reynolds, D.P., Lord, M.: Interface load analysis for computer-aided design of below-knee prosthetic sockets. Med. Biol. Eng. Comput. **30**, 419–426 (1992)
53. Sanders, J.E., Bell, D.M., Okumura, R.M., et al.: Effects of alignment changes on stance phase pressures and shear stresses on transtibial amputees: measurements from 13 transducer sites. IEEE Trans. Rehabil. Eng. **6**, 21–31 (1998)
54. Sanders, J.E., Cassisi, D.V.: Mechanical performance of inflatable inserts used in limb prosthetics. J. Rehabil. Res. Dev. **38**, 365–374 (2001)
55. Sanders, J.E., Daly, C.H.: Measurement of stresses in the three orthogonal directions at the residual limb-prosthetic socket interface. IEEE Trans. Rehabil. Eng. **1**, 79–85 (1993)
56. Sanders, J.E., Greve, J.M., Clinton, C., et al.: Clinical study: Changes in interface pressure and stump shape over time: Preliminary results from a trans-tibial amputee subject. Prosthet. Orthot. Int. **24**, 163–168 (2000)
57. Shrimpton, P.C., Hillier, M.C., Lewis, M.A., et al.: National survey of doses from CT in the UK: 2003. Br. J. Radiol. **79**, 968–980 (2006)
58. Silver-Thorn, M.B.: Generic, geometric finite element analysis of the transtibial residual limb and prosthetic socket. J. Rehabil. Res. Dev. **34**, 171–186 (1997)
59. Silver-Thorn, M.B., Childress, D.C.: Parametric analysis using the finite element method to investigate prosthetic interface stresses for persons with trans-tibial amputation. J. Rehabil. Res. Dev. **33**, 227–238 (1996)
60. Silver-Thorn, M.B., Steege, J.W., Childress, D.S.: A review of prosthetic interface stress investigations. J. Rehabil. Res. Dev. **33**, 253–266 (1996)
61. Smith, K.E., Commean, P.K., Vannier, M.W.: In vivo 3D measurement of soft tissue change due to lower limb prostheses using spiral computed tomography. Radiology **200**, 843–850 (1996)
62. Smith, K.E., Vannier, M.W., Commean, P.K.: Spiral CT volumetry of below knee residua. IEEE Trans. Rehabil. Eng. **3**, 235–241 (1995)
63. Soderberg, B., Ryd, L., Person, B.M.: Roentgen stereogrametric analysis of motion between the bone and the socket in the transtibial amputation prosthesis: a case study. J. Prosthet. Orthot. **15**, 95–99 (2003)
64. Vannier, M.W., Commean, P.K., Brunsden, B.S., et al.: Visualization of prosthesis fit in lower-limb amputees. IEEE Comput. Graph. Appl. **17**, 16–29 (1997)
65. Vannier, M.W., Commean, P.K., Smith, K.E.: 3D Lower- extremity residua measurement systems error analysis. J. Prosthet. Orthot. **9**, 67–76 (1997)
66. Verni, J.: ComScan 3D scanning semispherical work envelope. Application No # 11/438, 181. filed: 05/22/2006 (2006)
67. Williams, R.B., Porter, D., Roberts, V.C.: Triaxial force transducer for investigating stresses at the stump/socket interface. Med. Biol. Eng. Comput. **1**, 89–96 (1992)
68. Otto Bock: www.ottobock.com (2010). Accessed 15 Jan 2010
69. Yiğiter, K., Sener, G., Bayar, K.: Comparison of the effects of patellar tendon bearing and total surface bearing sockets on prosthetic fitting and rehabilitation. Prosthet. Orthot. Int. **26**, 206–212 (2002)

70. You, B.-M., Siy, P., Anderst, W., et al.: In-vivo measurement of 3D skeletal kinematics from sequences of biplane radiographs: application to knee kinematics. IEEE Trans. Med. Imaging **20**, 514–525 (2001)
71. Zhang, M., Lee, W.: Quantifying the regional load bearing ability of trans-tibial residual limbs. Prosthet. Orthot. Int. **30**, 25–34 (2006)
72. Zhang, M., Lord, M., Turner-Smith, A.R., et al.: Development of a nonlinear finite element modeling of the below-knee prosthetic socket interface. Med. Eng. Phys. **17**, 559–566 (1995)
73. Zhang, M., Mak, A.F.: A finite element analysis of the load transfer between an above-knee residual limb and its prosthetic socket – roles of interfacial friction and distal-end boundary conditions. IEEE Trans. Rehabil. Eng. **4**, 337–346 (1996)
74. Zhang, M., Turner-Smith, A.R., Tanner, A., et al.: Clinical investigation of the pressure and shear stress on the trans-tibial stump with a prosthesis. Med. Eng. Phys. **20**, 188–198 (1998)
75. Ziegler-Graham, K., MacKenzie, E., Ephraim, P., et al.: Estimating the prevalence of limb loss in the United States: 2005 to 2050. Arch. Phys. Med. Rehabil. **89**, 422–429 (2008)

A Discrete Level Set Approach for Texture Analysis of Microscopic Liver Images

Daniela Iacoviello

Abstract In this paper the analysis of microscopic liver tissue images is addressed to identify abnormal zones due to the presence of tissue with necrosis, or to malignant lymphoma; the study is performed by texture analysis. A discrete level set approach is considered, applying the well know segmentation algorithm to a new data constituted by a linear combination of the matrices of Uniformity, Contrast and Entropy. The proposed method makes use of the classification capability of the discrete level set analysis applied to a suitable transformation of the original data. The algorithm is applied to a significant set of liver tissue, showing encouraging results.

Keywords Texture analysis · Level set · Microscopic liver images

1 Introduction

Image analysis of liver is particularly difficult because of the physical characteristics of the organ; there are several adjacent organs, such as the pancreas and the stomach, that have signal levels similar to the liver. A solution may be the use of contrast agent to obtain contrast enhancements; also in this case image analysis may be difficult: the main problem is related to the features of the liver consisting of soft tissue. The major modalities commonly used for hepatic diagnosis are X-ray computed tomography (CT), the ultrasound (US) images, the magnetic resonance (MR) images and the positron emission tomography (PET). In particular, the US images, though have limitation in imaging range and quality, enjoy the advantage in real time imaging; the dynamic CT has short acquisition time, wide imaging range and high spatial resolution. In multi-phase CT images the time lag between one phase and the other allow the deformation of the liver, due, for example, to the respiratory movement

D. Iacoviello (✉)
Department of Computer and System Sciences, Sapienza University of Rome,
Via Ariosto 25, 00185 Rome, Italy
e-mail: iacoviel@dis.uniroma1.it

J.M.R.S. Tavares and R.M.N. Jorge (eds.), *Computational Vision and Medical Image Processing: Recent Trends*, Computational Methods in Applied Sciences 19,
DOI 10.1007/978-94-007-0011-6_6, © Springer Science+Business Media B.V. 2011

of the patient [11]. Microscopic images of liver tissue are useful to recognize, for example, metastatic carcinoma, or lesion, or micronodular cirrhosis.

Liver diseases may be roughly divided into two categories, focal diseases, where the abnormality is concentrated in small area of liver tissue, and diffused diseases, where the abnormality is distributed all over the liver volume [8]. The focal lesions may be differentiated by the echo texture patterns; hence texture analysis is efficient to avoid biopsy test and to obtain an early non invasive identification method of different focal lesions types. To identify liver fibrosis 2D wavelet transform appears to be useful. The wavelet transform possesses the property of multiresolution and in [10] a multiresolution technique for color medical image representation for liver fibrosis identification is proposed. In [1] diffused liver diseases are detected using Gabor wavelets; the aim was to classify ultrasonic liver images into three classes of liver diseases, normal, hepatitis and liver cirrhosis. In [2] focal lesions in ultrasound liver are automatically classified using principal component analysis and neural network; four classes (normal, cyst, benign and malignant masses) are considered and the texture features considered are extracted by spectral and statistical methods. The problem of classification of cirrhotic liver is faced in [13] using shape and texture analysis; the degree of cirrhosis was obtained as the output of an artificial neural network. In [12] segmentation results from three different texture extraction methods, co-occurrence matrices, Gabor filters and Markov Random Fields, are compared for CT liver images.

Texture analysis is an important topic in image processing; it is considered in many application and, of course, in medical image analysis. There isn't a unique method that suits for any kind of medical images, since the possible textures of interest may be very different. Basically we may distinguish between statistical, spectral and structural analysis of texture. As noted in [1], in texture analysis one of the most difficult aspect is to define a set of feature that adequately describes the characteristics of the texture.

In this paper microscopic images of liver tissue are considered; in these images irregular regions corresponding to metastatic infiltrations, or to granuloma, or to lymphoma may be present; what really distinguishes these different regions is their texture. The problem of identifying different texture is faced in this paper applying the discrete level set theory [4] to a suitable transformation of the data. In the level set formulation for image segmentation the basic idea is to find a function that, with its evolution, allows the optimal partition of the image into regions homogeneous with respect to some properties, for example the gray level. The optimality is related to the minimization of a suitable cost index that usually takes into account the fit error and the regularity of the segmented regions' boundary. The method proposed in this paper makes use of the classification capability of the discrete level set analysis applied to a transformation of the original data. It is important to choose the transformation that better describes the texture characteristics of the considered images. The method proposed in this paper may be considered in the framework of the papers [3] and [9]; the differences rely mainly in the choice of the cost index. In particular, in [9] a region based segmentation of textured sonar images within a level set approach is presented. Texture-based and angle-dependent similarity measure are defined and sonar images are segmented into homogeneous textural regions.

The paper is organized as follows. In Sect. 2 the mathematical formulation of the proposed method is presented; in particular three subsections are present: the outline of the discrete level set theory, the texture analysis and the proposed algorithm. In Sect. 3 the texture parameters along with the morphological ones are analyzed. In Sect. 4 numerical results are presented and conclusions with further developments are discussed in Sect. 5.

2 Mathematical Formulation

In this section the discrete level set theory developed in [4] is briefly recalled, subsection 2.1. The texture analysis is presented with reference to liver tissue in subsection 2.2 whereas in the subsection 2.3 the discrete level set theory is applied to a function that suitable describes the texture content of the data.

2.1 Discrete Level Set Theory

In the discrete level set theory the image $f \longrightarrow [0, 1]$ is defined on a grid of points

$$D = \{(i, j),\ i = 1, \ldots, \bar{N}\ ;\ j = 1, \ldots, \bar{M}\}$$

For simplicity, let assume that in the image domain D the two regions D_1 and D_2 constitute a partition into regions homogeneous with respect to some properties, for example the gray level. A piece wise constant segmentation I_S of the considered image is defined as follows:

$$I_S = c_1 \aleph_{D_1} + c_2 \aleph_{D_2} \tag{1}$$

where

$$\aleph_{D_k} = \begin{cases} 1 & for\ (i, j) \in D_k \\ 0 & otherwise \end{cases}, \quad k = 1, 2$$

The sub domains D_1 and D_2 may be defined through the level sets of a function $\phi = \{\phi_{i,j}\} : D \rightarrow R$:

$$D_1 = \{(i, j) : \phi_{i,j} \geq 0\} \quad D_2 = \{(i, j) : \phi_{i,j} < 0\}$$

The segmentation with respect to the chosen homogeneity property is provided by the minimization of the following cost index:

$$E(c_1, c_2, \phi) = \lambda \sum_{i,j} H(\phi_{i,j})(f_{i,j} - c_1)^2 + \lambda \sum_{i,j} \left(1 - H(\phi_{i,j})\right) \left(f_{i,j} - c_2\right)^2 + \frac{1}{2} \sum_{i,j} \phi_{i,j}^2 \tag{2}$$

where $\lambda > 0$ and H is the Heaviside function

$$H(z) = \begin{cases} 1 & z \geq 0 \\ 0 & z < 0 \end{cases}$$

In the cost index (2) the first two terms are the fit errors, whereas the third term has not a physical meaning but is important for the existence of the solution. In the level set theory in the cost index other two terms are usually present: one is related with the regularity of the contours and the second with the area of the sub domains. Is has been shown in [5] that the influence of these two terms is not as high as the fit errors' ones; for this reason in the cost index (2) these two terms are not considered.

To avoid complex analysis a smooth version of cost index (2) is obtained considering the Heaviside function H as the weak limit of a sequence of integrable functions

$$H_\varepsilon(z) = \frac{1}{2}\left(1 + \frac{2}{\pi} \tan^{-1}\left(\frac{z}{\varepsilon}\right)\right).$$

As shown in [5], the optimal solution of the minimization problem (2) is obtained solving the Euler-Lagrange equation and is given by:

$$c_1 = \frac{\sum_{i,j} H_\varepsilon(\phi_{i,j}) f_{i,j}}{\sum_{i,j} H_\varepsilon(\phi_{i,j})} \tag{3}$$

$$c_2 = \frac{\sum_{i,j} \left(1 - H_\varepsilon(\phi_{i,j})\right) f_{i,j}}{\sum_{i,j} \left(1 - H_\varepsilon(\phi_{i,j})\right)} \tag{4}$$

$$\alpha\phi_{i,j} + \lambda\left[\left(f_{i,j} - c_1\right)^2 - \left(f_{i,j} - c_2\right)^2\right]\delta_\varepsilon\left(\phi_{i,j}\right) = 0 \tag{5}$$

where the limit $\varepsilon \to 0$ of the function $\delta_\varepsilon(z) = \frac{1}{\pi}\frac{\varepsilon}{\varepsilon^2+z^2}$ is the Dirac function. The obtained values c_i represent the mean values of the function f in the sub domain D_i. Equation (5) is solved introducing a fictitious time variable; it has been shown that it has a unique bounded solution [5].

The described level set procedure may be applied hierarchically to obtain a 2n-th levels segmentation. In [4] the discrete level set theory has been successfully applied to segment images with respect to gray levels.

2.2 Texture Analysis of Liver Tissue

For the liver images that are considered in this paper what really distinguish a damaged region from the normal ones is not in general the gray level but its texture. For example, in Fig. 1a an image with typical granuloma with necrosis is shown; it is important to automatically identify the presence of the granuloma and its characteristics. In the considered images the main texture properties that distinguish normal tissue from suspect one are the Entropy, the Uniformity and the Contrast.

Let z denotes the gray level, L the number of distinct gray levels and $p(z_i),\ i = 0, 1, 2, \ldots, L-1$ the corresponding histogram; we now recall the definitions of Entropy, Uniformity and Contrast in a chosen sub domain, for example a square of size q [6]. The average entropy measure is defined as follows:

$$\bar{E} = -\sum_{i=0}^{L-1} p(z_i) \log_2 p(z_i) \tag{6}$$

For constant images the value of Entropy is equal to zero; it is a measure of variability of the gray level. The Uniformity is given by:

$$\bar{U} = \sum_{i=0}^{L-1} p^2(z_i) \tag{7}$$

It is maximum in the regions in which all gray levels are equal. The Contrast is given by the standard deviation of the pixels intensity:

$$\bar{C} = \sqrt{\frac{(I - I_m)^2}{q^2 - 1}} \tag{8}$$

where I_m is the mean value of the image I in the considered sub domain. Therefore, where the images are constant the entropy is equal to zero, the uniformity assumes its maximum value and the contrast is minimum.

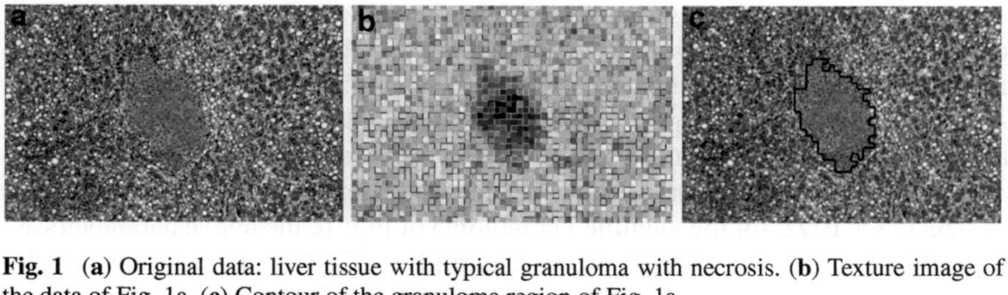

Fig. 1 (**a**) Original data: liver tissue with typical granuloma with necrosis. (**b**) Texture image of the data of Fig. 1a. (**c**) Contour of the granuloma region of Fig. 1a

2.3 The Proposed Algorithm

The image is divided into non overlapping squares with side of length q. In each of these sub domains the above quantities Entropy, Uniformity and Contrast are evaluated. The obtained constant values $\bar{E}$, $\bar{U}$ and $\bar{C}$ are assigned to each pixel constituting the considered $q \times q$ square and are computed for each square in which the image is divided. Therefore we obtain three new matrices, the matrices of Energy, of Uniformity and of Contrast that we denote by E, U and C, respectively. We then apply the discrete level set approach described in the previous subsection 2.1, not to the original image, but to the weighted sum of the Uniformity matrix, the Entropy matrix and the Contrast matrix:

$$f = \alpha_1 (1 - U) + \alpha_2 E + \alpha_3 C, \quad \alpha_1, \alpha_2, \alpha_3 \in R \tag{9}$$

This texture function will assume its maximum value where the gray level of the image varies more than in other regions; in Fig. 1b the texture image of the data of Fig. 1a is shown. On the function f the cost index (2) is applied and the solution (3)–(5) is obtained. The values c_i represent the mean values of the texture function f in the sub domains $D_i, i = 1, 2$, that constitute a partition of the image into domain homogeneous with respect to the tissue texture properties that it has been decided to consider. Therefore, the procedure allows to distinguish zones with different texture properties.

3 Morphological and Texture Parameters Identification

With the procedure developed in Sect. 2 any image may be partitioned into n regions that show different textures. Therefore there will be n distinct values c_i describing the mean values of the texture function f in each of the n identified regions.

In the liver tissue images considered a two levels segmentation is sufficient to identify the irregular regions corresponding, for example, to metastatic infiltrations, or to granuloma, or to lymphoma.

In Fig. 1c the contour of the granuloma present in Fig. 1a is shown. It has been determined applying the described procedure; the numerical details with the choice of the parameters will be discussed in the next section. In this section some morphological and texture parameters evaluated on the identified regions will be analysed. Among the morphological parameters it may be useful to characterize the irregular region by its extension (i.e. the number of pixels), its shape (i.e. eccentricity, solidity, and orientation), its position by the centroid. For example, in the image of Fig. 1a of size 728×1092, for the identified granuloma of Fig. 1c the above parameters assume the values: Area = 66,103 pixels, Centroid = (521 369), Eccentricity = 0.75, Solidity (that is the ratio Area/Convex_Area) = 0.85, Orientation = −65. These properties may help in a more precise classification of the regions identified by the proposed discrete level set procedure applied to the texture function.

Table 1 Comparison between entropy, uniformity and contrast values evaluated inside and out side the irregular region of image of Fig. 1c

	Granuloma region	Background	E_{irr}	E_{reg}
Entropy	0.30	0.82	0.62	0.04
Uniformity	0.83	0.44	0.74	0.03
Contrast	0.03	0.04	0.42	0.10

Table 2 Haralick properties evaluated inside and outside the granuloma region of image of Fig. 1c

	Granuloma region	Background	E^H_{irr}	E^H_{reg}
Contrast	0.30	0.45	0.21	0.16
Correlation	0.71	0.88	0.19	0.002
Energy	0.24	0.09	1.18	0.18
Homogeneity	0.86	0.81	0.03	0.01

For a comparison of the considered properties (Entropy, Uniformity and Contrast) inside and outside the irregular region see Table 1. In the last two columns the normalized errors between these values inside and outside the irregular regions with respect to a reference zone in the background (i.e. outside the irregular region) are shown and are indicated with E_{irr} and E_{reg} respectively.

Moreover also texture properties such as those related to the co-occurrence matrix may be evaluated for the two identified regions, [7]. The co occurrence matrix calculates how often a pixel with gray level value i occurs in the neighbour (for example adjacent horizontally) of a pixel with gray level value j; the contrast, the correlation, the energy and the homogeneity may be evaluated on the co-occurrence matrix (these properties are commonly referred to as Haralick properties). The identification of these properties may be useful to further classify the different tissues that are present in the image, especially if more than two regions D_1 and D_2 with different texture are present and have been identified with the application of the proposed algorithm with an n-th level texture-based segmentation. In Table 2 an example of the chosen Haralick properties evaluated inside and outside the irregular region are shown along with the absolute values of errors between these values inside $\left(E^H_{irr}\right)$ and outside $\left(E^H_{reg}\right)$ the irregular regions, with respect to the reference zone in the background.

From the previous analysis performed on different liver tissues the main difference between the irregular tissue and the background is related with the Energy. In the next section the results reported in Tables 1 and 2 will be analyzed.

4 Numerical Results

In this Section the proposed algorithm for texture identification is applied to test images from Brodatz database and to liver tissue images with different pathologies.

The algorithm (3)–(5) depends on the choice of the parameter λ in the cost function (2). In [5] it has been shown that the choice of λ mainly depends on the image contrast; values ranging from 10^2 to 10^5 have proven to give satisfactory results in general applications. We assumed $\lambda = 10^4$ for all the images.

The proposed algorithm depends also on the values of the weights α_i, $i = 1, 2, 3$ in the texture function f in (9), on the size q of the squares in which the image is partitioned to evaluate the matrices of Entropy, Uniformity and Contrast and on the value L representing the number of distinct gray level to be considered for the calculus of the histogram. The idea of considering Uniformity, Entropy and Contrast to build the new image f given by the (9) is based on a preliminary analysis performed on some liver tissue images used to calibrate the algorithm and therefore to set a range in which it would be advisable to choose the above parameters α_i, $i = 1, 2, 3$, q and L. For example, let us consider the image of Fig. 1a in which a malignant lymphoma is present; it is evident the presence of two regions with different texture. The values of the considered texture properties (the Entropy, the Uniformity and the Contrast) are shown in Table 1; the absolute values of the errors with respect to a reference zone show significant difference inside the granuloma region and outside. The same test has been performed on a significant set of microscopic liver images. Generally, the Uniformity and the Entropy are particularly robust and discriminating; this is the reason for which in the weighted function f the following values were chosen: $\alpha_1 = 0.5$, $\alpha_2 = 0.4$, $\alpha_3 = 0.1$, for all the real images considered.

The choices of q and L influence the matrices E, U and C and, therefore, the texture function f. The more suitable value of q is related to the extension of the zones with different texture; roughly speaking, a small value of q (2, 3 pixels) would not highlight the texture's characteristics of the square sub domains, whereas a larger value (30, 40 pixels) should mix them excessively.

The choice of the value of L is mainly related with the number of gray levels more frequent in the image; a large value of L (more than ten) generally introduces in the segmentation process false detections (i.e. new regions with different texture).

In real images with domains with similar texture properties a filter on detected small regions is advisable; therefore we introduced a filter on regions with area less than 3% than the total image extension.

Preliminarily the proposed algorithm has been tested on images from Brodatz database. For example let us consider the image of Fig. 2a; it is constituted by two test images with different texture. The algorithm has been applied with the following choices for the parameters: $L = 6$, $q = 10$; in this case, since we had no reason to weight more one texture matrix over the others, in the texture function f the weights α_i, $i = 1, 2, 3$ have been chosen equal. In Fig. 2b the contour of the identified smaller region is superimposed to the original image; the error in the separation of the two domains is less than 5% evaluated on the area of the identified regions. The result is quite satisfactory.

Now we discuss the application of the algorithm on liver tissue data. For the image of Fig. 1a the following values have been assumed: $q = 20$ and $L = 4$. The

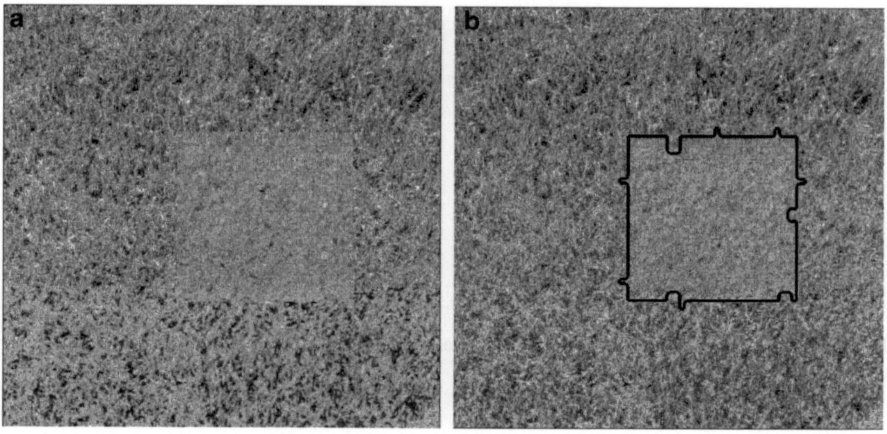

Fig. 2 (**a**) Brodatz image composed of two regions with different texture properties. (**b**) Contour of the inner region of Fig. 2a

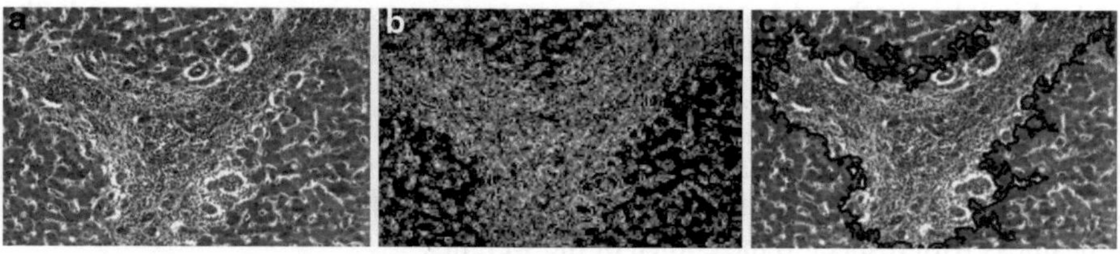

Fig. 3 (**a**) Original data: liver tissue with malignant lymphoma. (**b**) Texture image of the data of Fig. 3a. (**c**) Contour of the granuloma region of Fig. 3a. Some of its morphological properties are: the area equal to 380,347 pixels, its eccentricity equal to 0.69, its solidity equal to 0.63

result of Fig. 1c is obtained: the contour of the granuloma is well identified and, as already discussed in the previous section, morphological properties of this region may be found.

We then applied the described algorithm to images not considered in the calibration process. In Fig. 3a an image of liver tissue is shown. A malignant lymphoma is present; typical portal area infiltration appears as small cell lesion. The aim is to automatically identify the malignant lymphoma along with its morphological properties. A γ-correction preprocessing with $\gamma = 2$ is advisable. On the corrected image the level set algorithm is applied: the image is divided into non overlapping squares with side of length $q = 6$. For each of the obtained square the Energy, the Uniformity and the Contrast are evaluated and then the new data f is built (Fig. 3b). On this data the level set segmentation algorithm (3)–(5) is applied and the irregular region constituting the malignant lymphoma is identified (see Fig. 3c). In the caption of Fig. 3c some useful morphological properties of the lymphoma are shown; in this case it is useful to notice the solidity value that is equal to 0.635, whereas in the previous example was about 0.85. This parameter well describes the irregularity of the contour of the identified region in this second

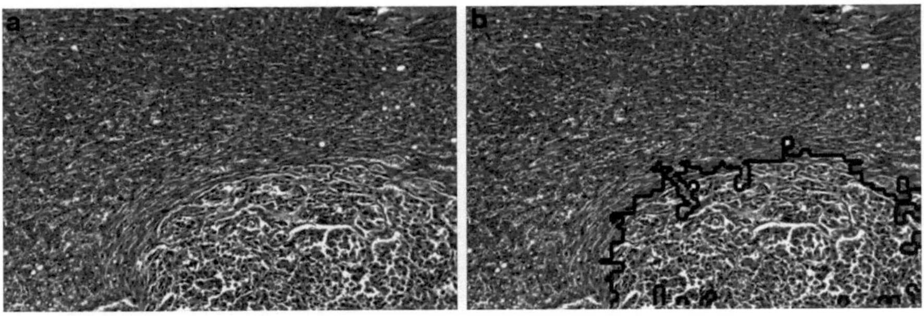

Fig. 4 (**a**) Original data: liver tissue with metastatic carciroma. (**b**) Contour of the carcinoma of Fig. 4a

example. Also for this image the texture properties from the co-occurrence matrix may be evaluated; in particular the Energy, that is equal to one for constant image, is almost double in the background with respect to the value in the irregular region.

In Fig. 4a another liver tissue with metastatic carcinoma is presented; the algorithm has been applied with the same choice of weights α_i, $i = 1, 2, 3$ of the previous example and $q = 10$ and $L = 4$. The result is shown in Fig. 4b. An a-posteriori analysis on the texture properties of the two regions in the image showed that in this particular example the most discriminating properties was the contrast. Nevertheless the obtained result is quite satisfactory as well, showing its robustness with respect to the choice of the weights.

The proposed texture segmentation algorithm has been applied to a significant set of liver tissue images, showing the power of its classification capability also in situation in which the analysis based only on the co-occurrence matrix would have not yield a univocal conclusion.

5 Conclusions

In this paper the problem of liver tissue image analysis is addresses. In liver tissue, the presence of metastatic carciroma, granuloma with necrosis, lymphoma, and fibrosis in micronodular cirrhosis may be identified by a level set segmentation applied to a suitable transformation of the original data. The adopted transformation is a linear combination of three matrices, the Entropy, the Uniformity and the Contrast. In particular a two-levels segmentation is considered; therefore the original data is partitioned according to the different texture content. The algorithm is tested showing good classification capability in distinguishing zones with different texture content. Future development will be the analysis of different texture properties to be included in the texture function. Moreover the extension to other kind of medical images is an on-going study.

References

1. Ahmadian, A., Mostafa, A., Abolhassani, M.D., Salimpou, Y.: A texture classification method for diffused liver diseases using Gabor wavelets. In: Proceedings of the IEEE Engineering in Medicine and Biology 27th Annual Conference, pp. 1567–1570, Shanghai, China (2005)
2. Balasubramanian, D., Srinivasan, P., Gurrupatham, R.: Automatic classification of focal lesions in ultrasound liver images using principal component analysis and neural networks. In: Proceedings of the 29th Annual International Conference of the IEEE EMBS, pp. 2134–2137, Lyon (2007)
3. Besson, S.J., Barlaud, M., Aubert, G.: Image segmentation using active contours: calculus of variations for shape gradients? SIAM J. Appl. Math. **63**, 2128–2154 (2003)
4. De Santis, A., Iacoviello, D.: A discrete level set approach for image segmentation. Signal Image Video Process. **1**, 303–320 (2007)
5. De Santis, A., Iacoviello, D.: Robust real time eye tracking for computer interface for disabled people. Comput. Methods Programs Biomed. **96**, 1–11 (2009)
6. Gonzales, R.C., Woods, R.E.: Digital Image Processing. Prentice hall Inc, NJ. SMC-3 **6**, 610–621 (2002)
7. Haralick, R.M., Shanmugam, K., Dinstein, I.: Textural features for image classification. IEEE Trans. Syst. Man Cybern. SMC-3 **6**, 610–621 (1973)
8. Horng, M.H.: An ultrasonic image evaluation system for assessing the severity of chronic liver disease. Comput. Med. Imag. Graph. **31**, 485–491 (2007)
9. Imen, K., Fablet, R., Boucher, J.M., Augustin, J.M.: Region- based and incidence angle dependent segmentation of seabed sonar images using a level set approach combined to local texture statistics. Asia Pacific Oceans **2006**, 1–7 (2007)
10. Lu, Z., Song, E., Wang, Q., Wang, X.: The liver fibrosis identification based on color 2D wavelet transform for the medical image. In: Proceedings of the International Conference on Wavelet Analysis and Pattern Recognition, pp. 205–208, Hong Kong (2008)
11. Masutani, Y., Uozumi, K., Akahane, M., Ohtomo, K.: Liver CT image processing: a short introduction of the technical elements. Eur. J. Tadiol. **58**, 246–251 (2006)
12. Pham, M., Susomboon, R., Disney, T., Raicu, D., Furst, J.: A comparison of texture models for automatic liver segmentation. In: Proceedings of SPIE Medical Imaging (2007)
13. Zhang, X., Fujita, H., Kanematsu, M., Zhou, X., Hara, T., Kato, H., Yokoyama, R., Hoshi, H.: Improving the classification of cirrhotic liver by using texture features. In: Proceedings of the 2005 IEEE Engineering in Medicine and Biology 27th Annual Conference, pp. 867–870, Shanghai, China (2005)

Deformable and Functional Models

Demetri Terzopoulos

Abstract This article summarizes most of the material on deformable and functional models that the author covered in an invited plenary lecture presented at the 2009 VIPIMAGE Conference. Following the organization of the presentation, the first part of the article reviews deformable models, particularly, active contours and surfaces, topologically-adaptive active contours and surfaces, and deformable organisms, focusing on their applications in medical image analysis, while the second part of the article reviews functional models, particularly realistic biomechanical models of the human face and body.

Keywords Deformable models · Active contours (snakes) · Active surfaces · Deformable organisms · Medical image analysis · Biomechanical modeling and simulation · Human face modeling · Human body modeling

1 Introduction

The modeling of biological structures and the model-based interpretation of medical images present many challenging problems. This article summarizes most of the material comprising my invited plenary lecture at the VIPIMAGE 2009 Conference, in which I discussed and demonstrated how one can tackle such problems through physics-based and biomechanical modeling.

In the first part of the article, Sect. 2, I review our work on a powerful paradigm that combines geometry, physics, and estimation theory, known as *deformable models*. Mathematically formulated in terms of variational principles and partial differential equations governed by the continuum mechanical principles of flexible materials, deformable models evolve in response to simulated forces that, for the purposes of image analysis, are derived from images. The presentation focuses on

---

D. Terzopoulos
University of California, Los Angeles
e-mail: dt@cs.ucla.edu; see www.cs.ucla.edu/~dt

J.M.R.S. Tavares and R.M.N. Jorge (eds.), *Computational Vision and Medical Image Processing: Recent Trends*, Computational Methods in Applied Sciences 19,
DOI 10.1007/978-94-007-0011-6_7,

several biomedical image analysis applications, including image segmentation using dynamic, finite element and topologically-adaptive deformable models, as well as recent work on "deformable organisms" which aims to automate the segmentation process by augmenting deformable models with behavioral and cognitive control mechanisms.

In the second part of the article, Sect. 3, I briefly review the recent focus of our research on *functional models*, which emulate physics (and oftentimes biology) with enough accuracy that they may be used in visually realistic simulations. I specifically present our work on functional models aimed at the realistic biomechanical simulation of the human body, particularly facial modeling, modeling and controlling the neck-head-face complex, and confronting the challenge of modeling and controlling more or less all of the relevant articular bones and skeletal muscles in the body, as well as simulating the physics-based deformations of its soft tissues.

2 Deformable Models

This section reviews deformable models. First, I will summarize the mathematics of planar *active contour models*, also known as "snakes", including energy-minimizing snakes and dynamic snakes. I will discuss the discretization and numerical simulation of snakes, as well as their probabilistic interpretation. I will then review higher-dimensional generalizations of snakes, in particular, *deformable surfaces*. Next, I will review *topology-adaptive deformable models*, which provide the topological flexibility of level set methods[1] without sacrificing the explicit geometric substrate upon which the classic deformable model formulations are based. Finally, I will review *deformable organisms* and their application to fully-automated medical image segmentation. Much of the material in this section has also appeared in [18].

2.1 Energy-Minimizing Snakes

Snakes are planar deformable contours that are useful in a variety of image analysis tasks [5]. They are often used to approximate the locations and shapes of object boundaries in images, based on the assumption that boundaries are piecewise continuous or smooth (Fig. 1a). In its basic form, the mathematical formulation of snakes draws from the theory of optimal approximation involving functionals.

Geometrically, a snake is an explicit, parametric contour embedded in the image plane $(x, y) \in \Re^2$. The contour is represented as $\mathbf{v}(s) = (x(s), y(s))^\top$, where x and

[1] In image analysis, the introduction of level set methods (refer, e.g., to the volume in which reference [18] appears) was motivated by the success of (Lagrangian) deformable models and the need for a related (Eulerian) technique that makes no prior assumption about the topology of the underlying structure of interest.

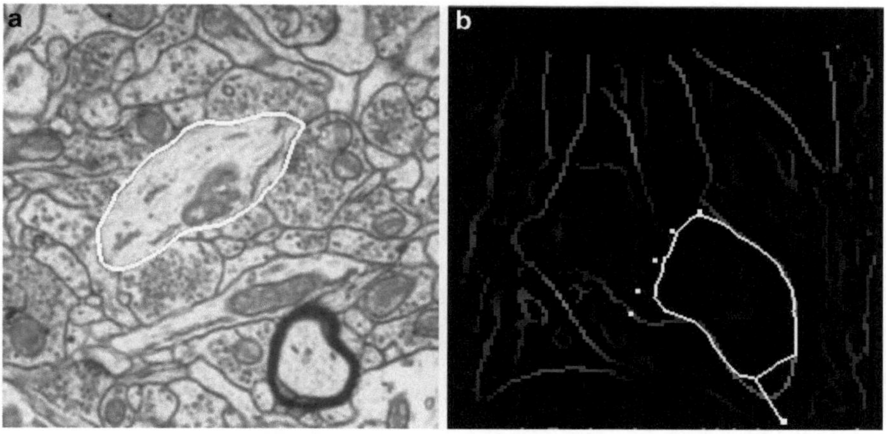

Fig. 1 Medical image analysis with snakes. (**a**) Snake (*white*) segmenting a cell in an EM photomicrograph [1]. The snake is attracted to the dark cell membrane. (**b**) Snake deforming towards high gradients in a processed cardiac image, influenced by "pin" constraints and an interactive "spring" with which the user pulls the contour towards an edge [10]

y are the coordinate functions and $s \in [0, 1]$ is the parametric domain (the symbol $^\top$ denotes transposition). The shape of the contour subject to an image $I(x, y)$ is dictated by the functional

$$\mathscr{E}(\mathbf{v}) = \mathscr{S}(\mathbf{v}) + \mathscr{P}(\mathbf{v}), \tag{1}$$

which represents the energy of the contour. The final shape of the contour corresponds to the minimum of this energy.

The first term in (1),

$$\mathscr{S}(\mathbf{v}) = \frac{1}{2}\int_0^1 w_1(s)\left|\frac{\partial \mathbf{v}}{\partial s}\right|^2 + w_2(s)\left|\frac{\partial^2 \mathbf{v}}{\partial s^2}\right|^2 ds, \tag{2}$$

is the internal deformation energy. It characterizes the deformation of a stretchy, flexible contour. Two physical parameter functions, the non-negative functions $w_1(s)$ and $w_2(s)$, dictate the simulated physical characteristics of the contour at any point s on the snake: $w_1(s)$ controls the "tension" of the contour while $w_2(s)$ controls its "rigidity". For example, increasing the magnitude of $w_1(s)$ tends to eliminate extraneous loops and ripples by reducing the length of the snake. Increasing $w_2(s)$ makes the snake smoother and less flexible. Setting the value of one or both of these functions to zero at a point s permits discontinuities in the contour at s.

The second term in (1) couples the snake to the image. Traditionally,

$$\mathscr{P}(\mathbf{v}) = \int_0^1 P(\mathbf{v}(s))ds, \tag{3}$$

where $P(x, y)$ denotes a scalar potential function defined on the image plane. To apply snakes to images, external potentials are designed whose local minima coincide with intensity extrema, edges, and other image features of interest. For example, the contour will be attracted to intensity edges in an image $I(x, y)$ by choosing a potential $P(x, y) = -c|\nabla[G_\sigma * I(x, y)]|$, where c controls the magnitude of the potential, ∇ is the gradient operator, and $G_\sigma * I$ denotes the image convolved with a (Gaussian) smoothing filter whose characteristic width σ controls the spatial extent of the local minima of P.

In accordance with the calculus of variations, the contour $\mathbf{v}(s)$ which minimizes the energy $\mathcal{E}(\mathbf{v})$ must satisfy the Euler–Lagrange equation

$$-\frac{\partial}{\partial s}\left(w_1 \frac{\partial \mathbf{v}}{\partial s}\right) + \frac{\partial^2}{\partial s^2}\left(w_2 \frac{\partial^2 \mathbf{v}}{\partial s^2}\right) + \nabla P(\mathbf{v}(s,t)) = \mathbf{0}. \tag{4}$$

This vector-valued partial differential equation (PDE) expresses the balance of internal and external forces when the contour rests at equilibrium. The first two terms represent the internal stretching and bending forces, respectively, while the third term represents the external forces that couple the snake to the image data. The usual approach to solving (4) is through the application of numerical algorithms (see Sect. 2.3).

2.2 *Dynamic Snakes*

While it is natural to view energy minimization as a static problem, a potent approach to computing the local minima of a functional such as (1) is to construct a dynamical system that is governed by the functional and allow the system to evolve to equilibrium. The system may be constructed by applying the principles of Lagrangian mechanics. This leads to dynamic deformable models that unify the description of shape and motion, making it possible to quantify not just static shape, but also shape evolution through time. Dynamic models are valuable for, e.g., time-varying medical image analysis, since most anatomical structures are deformable and continually undergo nonrigid motion *in vivo*. Moreover, dynamic models exhibit intuitively meaningful physical behaviors, making their evolution amenable to interactive guidance from a user (Fig. 1b).

A simple example is a dynamic snake which can be represented by introducing a time-varying contour $\mathbf{v}(s,t) = (x(s,t), y(s,t))^\top$ along with a mass density $\mu(s)$ and a damping density $\gamma(s)$. The Lagrange equations of motion for a snake with the internal energy given by (2) and external energy given by (3) is

$$\mu \frac{\partial^2 \mathbf{v}}{\partial t^2} + \gamma \frac{\partial \mathbf{v}}{\partial t} - \frac{\partial}{\partial s}\left(w_1 \frac{\partial \mathbf{v}}{\partial s}\right) + \frac{\partial^2}{\partial s^2}\left(w_2 \frac{\partial^2 \mathbf{v}}{\partial s^2}\right) = -\nabla P(\mathbf{v}(s,t)). \tag{5}$$

The first two terms on the left hand side of this partial differential equation represent inertial and damping forces. As in (4), the remaining terms represent the internal stretching and bending forces, while the right hand side represents the external forces. Equilibrium is achieved when the internal and external forces balance and the contour comes to rest (i.e., $\partial \mathbf{v}/\partial t = \partial^2 \mathbf{v}/\partial t^2 = 0$), which yields the equilibrium condition (4).

2.3 Discretization and Numerical Simulation

In order to compute numerically a minimum energy solution, it is necessary to discretize the energy $\mathscr{E}(\mathbf{v})$. The usual approach is to represent the continuous geometric model $\mathbf{v}$ in terms of linear combinations of local-support or global-support basis functions. Finite elements, finite differences, and geometric splines are local representation methods, whereas Fourier bases are global representation methods. The continuous model $\mathbf{v}(s)$ is represented in discrete form by a vector $\mathbf{u}$ of shape parameters associated with the basis functions. The discrete form of energies such as $\mathscr{E}(\mathbf{v})$ for the snake may be written as

$$E(\mathbf{u}) = \frac{1}{2}\mathbf{u}^\top \mathbf{K}\mathbf{u} + \mathrm{P}(\mathbf{u}), \tag{6}$$

where $\mathbf{K}$ is called the *stiffness matrix*, and $\mathrm{P}(\mathbf{u})$ is the discrete version of the external potential. The minimum energy solution results from setting the gradient of (6) to $\mathbf{0}$, which is equivalent to solving the set of algebraic equations

$$\mathbf{K}\mathbf{u} = -\nabla \mathrm{P} = \mathbf{f}, \tag{7}$$

where $\mathbf{f}$ is the generalized external force vector.

Finite elements and finite differences generate local discretizations of the continuous snake model, hence the stiffness matrix will have a sparse and banded structure. To illustrate the discretization process, suppose we apply the finite difference method to discretize the energy (2) on a set of nodes $\mathbf{u}_i = \mathbf{v}(ih)$ for $i = 0, \ldots, N-1$ where $h = 1/(N-1)$ and suppose we use the finite differences $\mathbf{v}_s \approx (\mathbf{u}_{i+1} - \mathbf{u}_i)/h$ and $\mathbf{v}_{ss} \approx (\mathbf{u}_{i+1} - 2\mathbf{u}_i + \mathbf{u}_{i-1})/h^2$. For cyclic boundary conditions (i.e., a closed contour), we obtain the following symmetric pentadiagonal matrix (unspecified entries are 0):

$$\mathbf{K} = \begin{bmatrix} a_0 & b_0 & c_0 & & & & c_{N-2} & b_{N-1} \\ b_0 & a_1 & b_1 & c_1 & & & & c_{N-1} \\ c_0 & b_1 & a_2 & b_2 & c_2 & & & \\ & c_1 & b_2 & a_3 & b_3 & c_3 & & \\ & & \ddots & \ddots & \ddots & \ddots & \ddots & \\ & & & c_{N-5} & b_{N-4} & a_{N-3} & b_{N-3} & c_{N-3} \\ c_{N-2} & & & & c_{N-4} & b_{N-3} & a_{N-2} & b_{N-2} \\ b_{N-1} & c_{N-1} & & & & c_{N-3} & b_{N-2} & a_{N-1} \end{bmatrix}, \tag{8}$$

where

$$a_i = (w_{1\,i-1} + w_{1\,i})/h^2 + (w_{2\,i-1} + 4w_{2\,i} + w_{2\,i+1})/h^4, \tag{9}$$

$$b_i = -w_{1\,i}/h^2 - 2(w_{2\,i} + w_{2\,i+1})/h^4, \tag{10}$$

$$c_i = w_{2\,i+1}/h^4, \tag{11}$$

assuming that $w_{1\,i} = w_1(ih)$ and $w_{2\,i} = w_2(ih)$ are sampled at the same nodes. All indices in these expressions are interpreted modulo N.

The discretized version of the Lagrangian dynamics equation (5) may be written as a set of second order ordinary differential equations (ODEs) for $\mathbf{u}(t)$:

$$\mathbf{M}\ddot{\mathbf{u}} + \mathbf{D}\dot{\mathbf{u}} + \mathbf{K}\mathbf{u} = \mathbf{f}, \tag{12}$$

where $\mathbf{M}$ is the mass matrix and $\mathbf{D}$ is a damping matrix. In a finite difference discretization, the mass and damping matrices are diagonal matrices.

To simulate the snake dynamics, the system of ordinary differential equations (12) in the shape parameters $\mathbf{u}$ must be integrated forward through time. The finite element literature offers several suitable explicit and implicit direct integration methods, including the central difference, Houbolt, Newmark, or Wilson methods. We can illustrate the basic idea with a semi-implicit Euler method that takes time steps Δt. We replace the time derivatives of $\mathbf{u}$ with the backward finite differences $\ddot{\mathbf{u}} \approx (\mathbf{u}^{(t+\Delta t)} - 2\mathbf{u}^{(t)} + \mathbf{u}^{(t-\Delta t)})/(\Delta t)^2$, and $\dot{\mathbf{u}} \approx (\mathbf{u}^{(t+\Delta t)} - \mathbf{u}^{(t-\Delta t)})/2\Delta t$, where the superscripts denote the quantity evaluated at the time given in parentheses. This yields the update formula

$$\mathbf{A}\mathbf{u}^{(t+\Delta t)} = \mathbf{b}^{(t)}, \tag{13}$$

where $\mathbf{A} = \mathbf{M}/(\Delta t)^2 + \mathbf{D}/2\Delta t + \mathbf{K}$ is a pentadiagonal matrix and the vector $\mathbf{b}^{(t)} = (2\mathbf{M}/(\Delta t)^2)\mathbf{u}^{(t)} - (\mathbf{M}/(\Delta t)^2 - \mathbf{D}/2\Delta t)\mathbf{u}^{(t-\Delta t)} + \mathbf{f}^{(t)}$. The pentadiagonal system can be solved efficiently ($O(N)$ complexity) by factorizing $\mathbf{A}$ into lower and upper triangular matrices, then solving the two resulting sparse triangular systems. We compute the unique normalized factorization $\mathbf{A} = \mathbf{LYU}$ where $\mathbf{L}$ is a lower triangular matrix, $\mathbf{Y}$ is a diagonal matrix, and $\mathbf{U} = \mathbf{L}^\top$ is an upper triangular matrix. The solution $\mathbf{u}^{(t+\Delta t)}$ to (13) is obtained by first solving $\mathbf{Ls} = \mathbf{b}^{(t)}$ by forward substitution, then $\mathbf{Uu} = \mathbf{Y}^{-1}\mathbf{s}$ by backward substitution. For the linear snakes described above, only a single factorization is necessary, since $\mathbf{A}$ is constant. Note that the factorization and forward/backward substitutions are inherently sequential, recursive operations.

Researchers have investigated alternative approaches to numerically simulating snake models, including dynamic programming and greedy algorithms (see [12] for a survey in the context of medical image analysis).

2.4 Probabilistic (Bayesian) Interpretation

An alternative view of deformable models emerges from casting the model fitting process in a probabilistic framework. This permits the incorporation of prior model and sensor model characteristics in terms of probability distributions. The probabilistic framework also provides a measure of the uncertainty of the estimated shape parameters after the model is fitted to the image data.

Let $\mathbf{u}$ represent the deformable model shape parameters with a prior probability $p(\mathbf{u})$ on the parameters. Let $p(I|\mathbf{u})$ be the imaging (sensor) model – the probability of producing an image I given a model $\mathbf{u}$. Bayes' theorem

$$p(\mathbf{u}|I) = \frac{p(I|\mathbf{u})p(\mathbf{u})}{p(I)} \tag{14}$$

expresses the posterior probability $p(\mathbf{u}|I)$ of a model given the image, in terms of the imaging model and the prior probabilities of model $p(\mathbf{u})$ and image $p(I)$.

It is easy to convert the internal energy measure (2) of the deformable model into a prior distribution over expected shapes, with lower energy shapes being the more likely. This is achieved using a Boltzmann (or Gibbs) distribution of the form

$$p(\mathbf{u}) = \frac{1}{Z_s} \exp(-S(\mathbf{u})), \tag{15}$$

where $S(\mathbf{u})$ is the discretized version of $\mathscr{S}(\mathbf{v})$ in (2) and Z_s is a normalizing constant (called the partition function). This prior model is then combined with a simple sensor model based on linear measurements with Gaussian noise

$$p(I|\mathbf{u}) = \frac{1}{Z_I} \exp(-\mathrm{P}(\mathbf{u})), \tag{16}$$

where $\mathrm{P}(\mathbf{u})$ is a discrete version of the potential $\mathscr{P}(\mathbf{v})$ in (3), which is a function of the image $I(x, y)$.

Models may be fitted by finding $\mathbf{u}$ which locally maximize $p(\mathbf{u}|I)$ in (14). This is known as the maximum a posteriori solution. With the above construction, it yields the same result as minimizing (1), the energy configuration of the deformable model given the image.

The probabilistic framework can be extended by assuming a time-varying prior model, or system model, in conjunction with the sensor model, resulting in a Kalman filter. The system model describes the expected evolution of the shape parameters $\mathbf{u}$ over time. If the equations of motion of the physical snakes model (12) are employed as the system model, the result is a sequential estimation algorithm known as "Kalman snakes" [22], which is useful for tracking objects in video.

2.5 Higher-Dimensional Generalizations

Snakes are a special case within the general framework of continuous (multidimensional) deformable models in a Lagrangian dynamics setting that is based on deformation energies in the form of (controlled-continuity) generalized splines [16].

In a p-dimensional domain $\mathbf{x} = (x_1, \ldots, x_p) \in \Re^p$, the natural generalization of the smoothness functional (2) defined on a q-dimensional vector of coordinate functions $\mathbf{v}(\mathbf{x}) = [v_1(\mathbf{x}), \ldots, v_q(\mathbf{x})]$ is

$$\mathcal{S}_n(\mathbf{v}) = \frac{1}{2} \int_{\Re^p} \sum_{m=1}^{n} \sum_{|j|=m} \frac{m!}{j_1! \ldots j_p!} w_j(\mathbf{x}) \left| \frac{\partial^m \mathbf{v}(\mathbf{x})}{\partial x_1^{j_1} \ldots \partial x_p^{j_p}} \right|^2 d\mathbf{x}. \quad (17)$$

Here, $j = (j_1, \ldots, j_p)$ is a multi-index with $|j| = j_1 + \ldots + j_p$. Note that this functional offers higher-order smoothness by generalizing (2) beyond second-order derivatives, to derivatives of order n. Analogous to equation (4), assuming that the control functions $\mathbf{w}(\mathbf{x})$ are differentiable to order p, the Euler–Lagrange equation is:

$$\sum_{m=1}^{n} (-1)^m \Delta_w^m \mathbf{v}(\mathbf{x}) + \nabla P(\mathbf{v}(\mathbf{x})) = \mathbf{0}, \quad (18)$$

where

$$\Delta_w^m = \sum_{|j|=m} \frac{m!}{j_1! \ldots j_p!} \frac{\partial^m}{\partial x_1^{j_1} \ldots \partial x_p^{j_p}} \left(w_j(\mathbf{x}) \frac{\partial^m}{\partial x_1^{j_1} \ldots \partial x_p^{j_p}} \right) \quad (19)$$

is a spatially weighted mth-order iterated Laplacian operator.

2.5.1 Deformable Surfaces

In the special case $n = 2$, $q = 3$, and $p = 2$, where we define $\mathbf{x} = (x_1, x_2) = (x, y)$ for notational convenience and restrict the two-dimensional domain to the unit square, (17) can be written as

$$\begin{aligned} \mathcal{S}(\mathbf{v}) = \frac{1}{2} \int_0^1 \int_0^1 & w_{10} \left| \frac{\partial \mathbf{v}}{\partial x} \right|^2 + w_{01} \left| \frac{\partial \mathbf{v}}{\partial y} \right|^2 \\ & + w_{20} \left| \frac{\partial^2 \mathbf{v}}{\partial x^2} \right|^2 + 2 w_{11} \left| \frac{\partial^2 \mathbf{v}}{\partial x \partial y} \right|^2 + w_{02} \left| \frac{\partial^2 \mathbf{v}}{\partial y^2} \right|^2 dx\, dy, \end{aligned} \quad (20)$$

where the subscripts on $\mathbf{v}$ denote its partial derivatives with respect to x and y. This functional, the natural, two-dimensional generalization of the snake energy (2), pertains to the problem of deformable surfaces. The physical parameter functions

$w_{10}(x, y)$ and $w_{01}(x, y)$ control the tension of the surface, while $w_{20}(x, y)$, $w_{11}(x, y)$, and $w_{02}(x, y)$ control its "rigidity".

This *thin plate under tension* functional has seen considerable application, notably to 2.5D (visible-surface) and three-dimensional surface reconstruction in computer vision [17, 24].

2.6 Topology-Adaptive Deformable Models

As physics-based models of nonrigid solids, deformable models have had an enormous impact in medical image analysis [12]. The complexity of human anatomy, comprising numerous nonrigid organs with intricate substructures at multiple scales of resolution, means that deformable models must generally be able to deal with non-simple and even non-constant topologies; for example, in serial reconstruction the topology of a segmented cross-section can vary dramatically as the image data are sliced in different ways. Unfortunately, without additional machinery, classic, Lagrangian deformable models cannot alter their prescribed topology.

Level set image segmentation methods (see footnote 1 on page 126) were motivated by the need for a related technique that makes no prior assumption about the topology of the underlying object of interest. To this end, level-set methods formulate boundary curve or surface estimation as an Eulerian problem defined over the entire image domain. The dimensionality of the Eulerian problem typically is one greater than the dimensionality of the associated Lagrangian problem for deformable models. The primary feature of this approach is that the higher-dimensional hypersurface remains a simple function, even as the level set changes topology (or ceases to be simply connected). Hence, topological changes are handled naturally.

Topology-adaptive deformable models are an alternative approach to non-fixed topology [13, 14]. They circumvent the increased dimensionality of the level set methods while retaining the strengths of standard parametric deformable models, including the explicit geometric representation, the natural user interaction mechanisms, and the constraint mechanisms implemented through energy or force functions. Topology-adaptive deformable models can segment and reconstruct some of the most complex biological structures from two-dimensional and three-dimensional images. In this section, I will first review *topology-adaptive snakes*, or T-snakes, followed by *topology-adaptive deformable surfaces*, or T-surfaces.

2.6.1 Topology-Adaptive Snakes

T-snakes are hybrid models that combine Lagrangian, parametric snakes with aspects of the Eulerian, level set approach. They employ an Affine Cell Image Decomposition (ACID) of the image domain. The ACID extends the abilities of

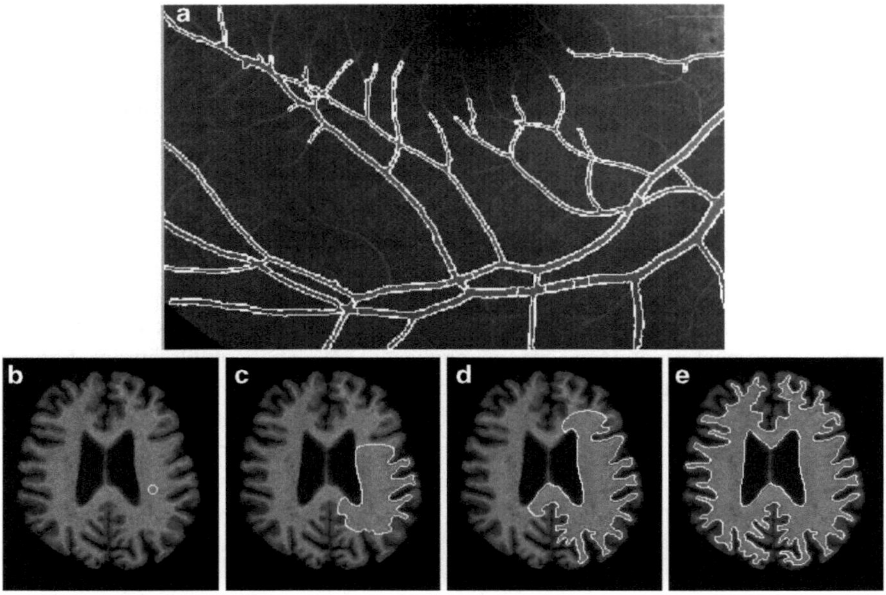

Fig. 2 Segmentation with T-snakes. (**a**) T-snakes segmenting blood vessels in a retinal angiogram. Geometric flexibility allows the T-snakes to grow into the complex vessel shapes. (**b–e**) T-snake segmenting gray-matter/white-matter interface and ventricles in an MR brain image slice. The initially circular T-snake (**b**) changes its topology to a highly deformed annular region (**e**)

conventional snakes, enabling topological flexibility, among other features [14]. In particular, the ACID framework enables a novel snake reparameterization mechanism, which enables snakes to "flow" into geometrically complex objects, conforming to the object boundaries (Fig. 2a). One or more T-snakes can be dynamically created or destroyed and can seamlessly split or merge as necessary in order to adapt to object topology (Fig. 2b–e). See reference [11] for numerous additional examples of T-snakes applied to images.

As a T-snake deforms under the influence of external and internal forces, it is systematically reparameterized with a new set of nodes and elements. This is done by efficiently computing the intersection points of the model with the superposed affine cell grid; for example, the Coxeter–Freudenthal decomposition (Fig. 3a). At the end of each deformation step, the nodes have moved relative to the grid cell edges (Fig. 3b–d). In Phase I of the reparameterization algorithm, the intersection points between the T-snake elements and the grid cell edges are computed. These intersection points will become the nodes of the new T-snake. In Phase II, grid cell vertices that have moved from the exterior to the interior of the T-snake are marked as "on"; in this manner, the interior of a T-snake is continuously tracked.

A closed T-snake defines a region. When a T-snake bounded region collides with itself or with another T-snake region, or splits into two or more subregions, (or

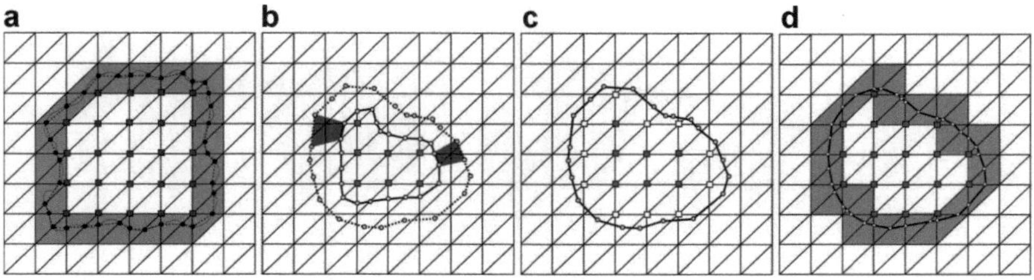

Fig. 3 (**a**) Simplicial approximation (*dashed-line*) of an object contour (*solid-line*) using a Freudenthal triangulation. The model nodes (intersection points) are marked and the boundary triangles are shaded. (**b–d**) Illustration of the T-snake reparameterization process. (**b**) Shaded regions show examples of grid vertices that are turned on by the expanding contour, (**c**) new inside grid vertices (*white*) added to current inside vertices (*dark*), (**d**) new contour after one deformation step showing new grid intersections, inside grid vertices, and boundary grid cells (*gray shaded*)

shrinks and disappears,) a topological transformation must take place. Topology changes are performed automatically via the ACID (Fig. 2b–e). The boundary can always be determined unambiguously by keeping track of the inside grid vertices (and hence the boundary grid cells) and re-establishing the correspondence of the T-snake boundary with the grid after every deformation step. New elements are constructed based on the "signs" (i.e., inside or outside) of the grid vertices in each boundary cell and from the intersection points computed in Phase I, such that the inside and outside grid vertices in these cells are separated by a single line.

Compared to conventional snakes, the T-snake is relatively insensitive to its initial placement within regions of interest in the image. It flows into complex shapes, modifying its topology as necessary in order to fit the relevant image data. The ACID provides a principled, computational geometry framework for topological transformations, but disabling the ACID reduces the T-snakes model to a conventional parametric snake model. Consequently, T-snakes also incorporate shape constraints in the form of energy functionals and applied forces. An important advantage of the latter is user control, which caters to medical image analysis, where it is often essential for an expert user to be able to control and refine the segmentation process in an interactive manner.

2.6.2 Topology-Adaptive Deformable Surfaces

The main components of the three-dimensional T-surfaces formulation (see [13] for the details) are analogous to those for the two-dimensional T-snakes. The first component is a discrete form of the conventional parametric deformable surfaces [10]. The second component is the extension of the ACID framework to three dimensions

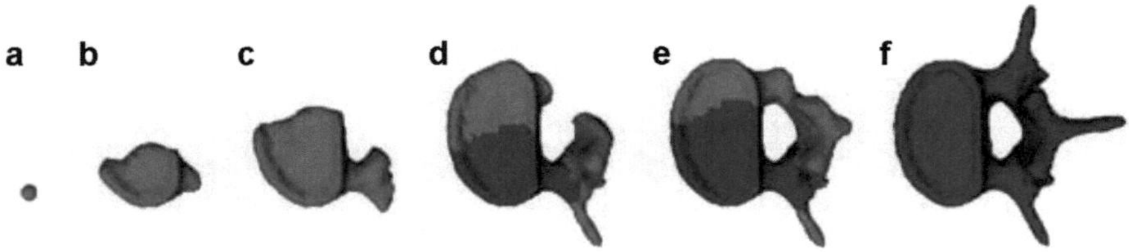

Fig. 4 T-surface segmenting vertebra phantom from CT volume image [13]. The images illustrate the temporal progression of the segmentation process from the initial spherical deformable model (**a**) to the final toroidal segmented surface (**f**)

using simplicial (tetrahedral) cells or nonsimplicial (e.g. hexahedral) cells.[2] The third component of T-surfaces is a reparameterization process analogous to the one for T-snakes. To determine if a T-surface triangular element intersects a grid cell edge, a standard ray-triangle intersection algorithm is used and local neighborhood searches are employed to speed up the process. The user can interact with a T-surface by applying three-dimensional interaction forces, by applying two-dimensional interaction forces to cross-sections of the surface that are overlaid on image slices thorough the three-dimensional dataset.

Figure 4 demonstrates the topological adaptability of a T-surface when applied to a $120 \times 128 \times 52$ CT volume image of a human vertebra phantom. This example uses a $32 \times 30 \times 13$ cell grid (where each cubical cell is divided into six tetrahedra).

2.7 Deformable Organisms

In medical images, the general shape, location and orientation of an anatomical structure is known and this knowledge may be incorporated into the deformable model in the form of initial conditions, data constraints, constraints on the model shape parameters, or into the model fitting procedure. The use of implicit or explicit anatomical knowledge to guide shape recovery is especially important for robust automatic interpretation of medical images. For automatic interpretation, it is essential to have a model that not only describes the size, shape, location and orientation of the target object but that also permits expected variations in these characteristics. Automatic interpretation of medical images can relieve clinicians from the labor intensive aspects of their work while increasing the accuracy, consistency, and reproducibility of the interpretations [12].

An extreme example of incorporating prior knowledge, aspiring toward fully automated medical image segmentation, is *deformable organisms* [3, 9]. This recent

[2] Most nonsimplicial methods employ a rectangular tessellation of space. The formulation of T-surfaces using a non-simplicial grid is essentially identical to its simplicial counterpart except for the addition of the disambiguation scheme.

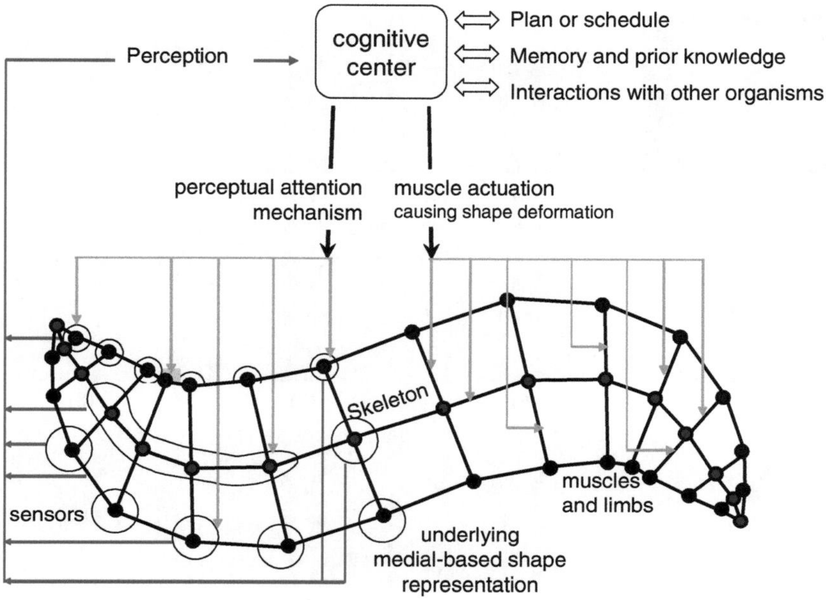

Fig. 5 A deformable organism. The organism's brain issues muscle actuation and perceptual attention commands. The organism's body deforms and senses image features, whose characteristics are conveyed to the brain. The brain makes decisions based on sensory input, information in memory and prior knowledge, and a pre-stored plan, which may involve interaction with other organisms

paradigm for automatic image analysis combines deformable models and concepts from artificial life modeling. The goal is to incorporate and exploit all the available prior knowledge and global contextual information in any specific medical image analysis task. Analogous to natural organisms capable of voluntary movement, deformable organisms possess deformable bodies with distributed sensors, as well as (rudimentary) brains with motor, perception, behavior, and cognition centers (Fig. 5). Deformable organisms are perceptually aware of the image analysis process. Their behaviors, which manifest themselves in voluntary movement and body shape alteration, are based upon sensed image features, stored structural knowledge, and a cognitive plan. The organism framework separates global top-down, model-fitting control functionality from the local, bottom-up, feature integration functionality. This separation enables the definition of model-fitting controllers or 'brains' in terms of the high-level structural features of objects of interest, rather than the low-level image features. The result is an 'intelligent agent' that is continuously 'aware' of the progress of the segmentation process, allowing it to apply prior knowledge about target objects in a deliberative manner (Fig. 6). Three-dimensional physics-based deformable organisms have recently been developed and software is available [4].

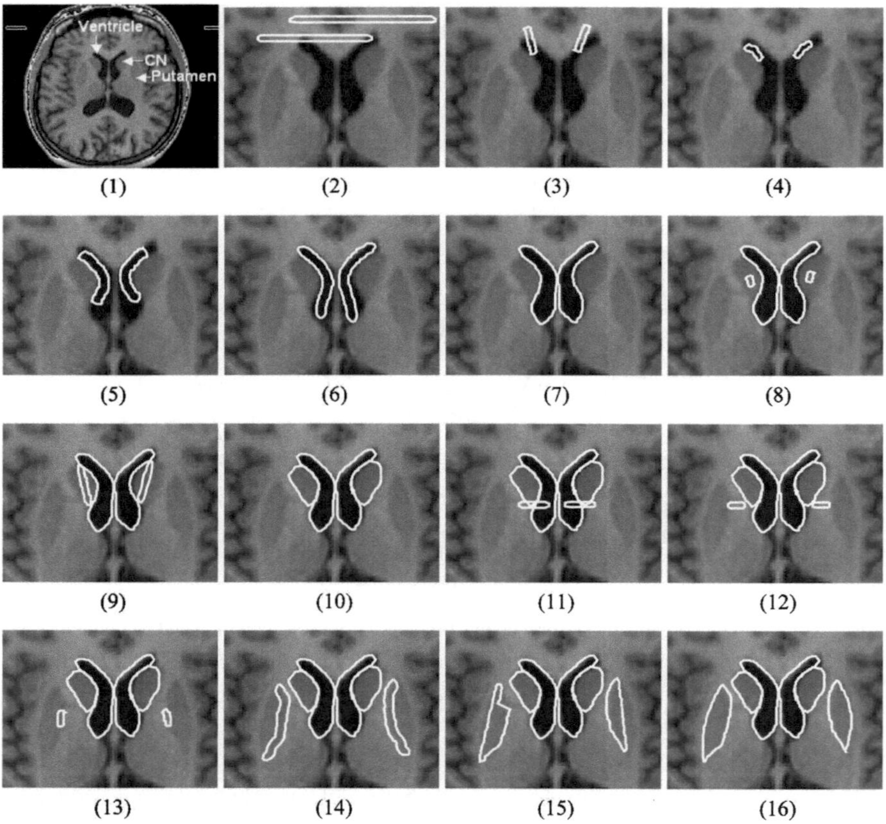

Fig. 6 Automatic brain MR image segmentation by multiple deformable organisms (from [9]). The sequence of images illustrates the temporal progression of the segmentation process. Deformable lateral ventricle (**1–7**), caudate nucleus (**8–10**), and putamen (**11–16**) organisms are spawned in succession and progress through a series of behaviors to detect, localize, and segment the corresponding structures in the MR image

3 Functional Models

Complementary to the physics-based deformable models discussed thus far are *functional models*, which emulate physics with enough accuracy that they may be used for the purposes of visually realistic simulation. For over two decades, we have been developing functional deformable models for use in computer graphics and animation [2, 15, 19–21]. Our most recent research on functional models focuses on the biomechanical simulation of humans. The ensuing sections briefly review the biomechanical models that we have developed of the human face, neck-head-face complex, and entire body.

3.1 Facial Simulation

Biomechanically simulating the human face presents deep challenges, and we started working on this problem approximately 20 years ago [8, 23]. Conceptually, our face models are organized hierarchically into several levels of abstraction related to the behavioral control of facial expression, the anatomy of facial muscle structures, the histology and biomechanics of facial tissues, as well as facial geometry and appearance. The face model is muscle-actuated. Its 44 contractile muscles of facial expression are arranged in an anatomically consistent manner within the bottom layer of a synthetic facial soft tissue. The tissue is modeled as a lattice of uniaxial viscoelastic units assembled into multilayered prismatic elements with epidermal, dermal, sub-cutaneous fatty tissue, fascia, and muscle layers. The elements enforce volume preservation constraints and model contact response against the skull substrate. Expressive facial tissue deformations result from numerically simulating the physical response of the element assembly to the stresses induced by appropriately coordinated facial muscle contractions. The face simulation runs at real-time, interactive rates on a PC.

3.2 Biomechanically Simulating and Controlling the Neck-Head-Face Complex

The neck has a complex anatomical structure and it plays an important role in supporting the head atop the cervical spine, while generating the controlled head movements that are essential to so many aspects of human behavior. We have developed a biomechanical model of the human head-neck system that emulates the relevant anatomy [7] (Fig. 7). Characterized by appropriate kinematic redundancy (seven cervical vertebrae coupled by three-DOF joints) and muscle actuator redundancy (72 neck muscles arranged in three muscle layers), our model presents a challenging motor control problem, even for the relatively simple task of balancing the mass of the head atop the cervical column in gravity.

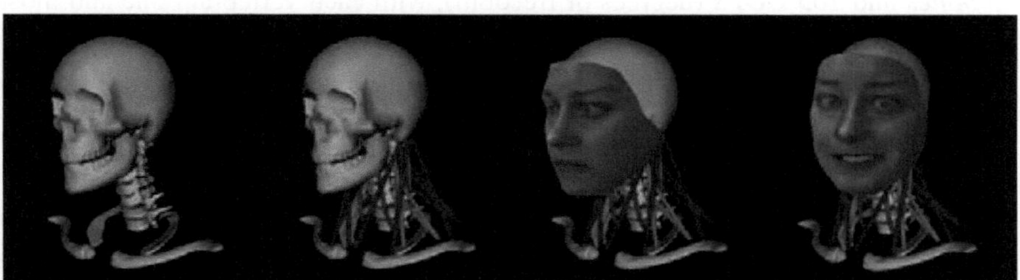

Fig. 7 Biomechanical, musculoskeletal neck-head-face model with 72 Hill-type neck muscle actuators, animated in gravity by a neuromuscular controller. The biomechanical face model incorporates a soft tissue simulation with 44 embedded muscles of facial expression

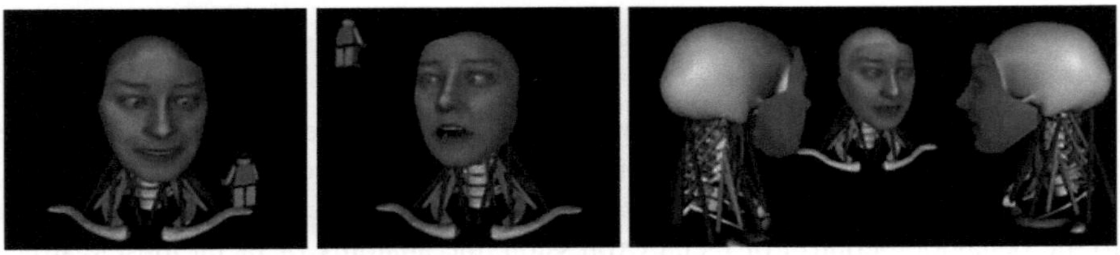

Fig. 8 Head-Eye gaze behavior (*left*); the model gazing at a visual target in different directions. Autonomous behavior-based interaction between three face-head-neck systems (*right*)

We have developed a neuromuscular control model for the neck that emulates the relevant biological motor control mechanisms. Incorporating low-level reflex and high-level voluntary sub-controllers, our hierarchical controller provides input motor signals to the numerous muscle actuators. In addition to head pose and movement, it controls the coactivation of mutually opposed neck muscles to regulate the stiffness of the head-neck multibody system. Taking a machine learning approach, the neural networks within our neuromuscular controller are trained offline to efficiently generate the online pose and tone control signals necessary to synthesize a variety of autonomous movements for the behavioral animation of the human head and face (Fig. 8), with the latter also simulated biomechanically as described in the previous section.

3.3 Comprehensive Biomechanical Simulation of the Human Body

Extending the above work, we have recently been developing a comprehensive biomechanical model of the human body [6], confronting the combined challenge of modeling and controlling more or less all of the relevant articular bones and skeletal muscles, as well as simulating the physics-based deformations of the soft tissues, including muscle bulging (Fig. 9).

In particular, we have created a physics-based skeletal model that consists of *75 bones* and *165 DOFs* (degrees of freedom), with each vertebral bone and most ribs having independent DOFs. To be properly actuated and controlled, our detailed bone model requires a comparable level of detail with respect to muscle modeling. We incorporate a staggering *846 muscles*, which are modeled as piecewise line segment Hill-type force actuators. We have also developed an associated physics-based animation controller that computes accelerations to drive the musculoskeletal system toward a sequence of preset target key poses, and then computes the required activation signal for each muscle through inverse dynamics.

Our volumetric human body model incorporates detailed skin geometry, as well as the active muscle tissues, passive soft tissues, and skeletal substructure. Driven by the muscle activation inputs and resulting skeletal motion, a companion simulation

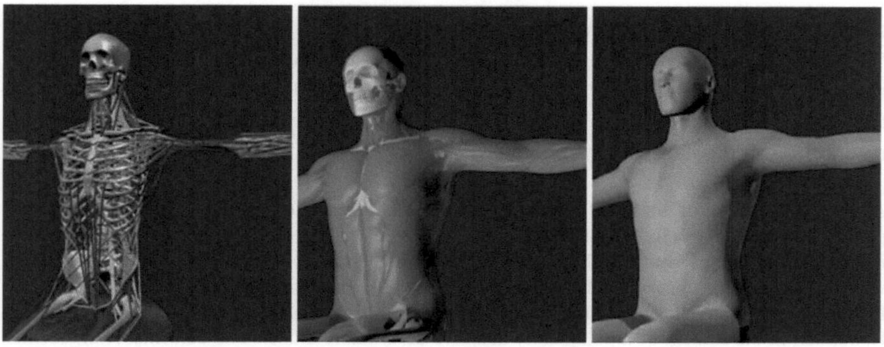

Fig. 9 Our comprehensive human body simulation is characterized by the biomechanical modeling of the relevant musculoskeletal tissues. The skeleton with 75 bones is actuated by 846 muscles (*left*). The motion of the skeleton and the activation level of each muscle deforms the inner soft tissue (*center*) and, hence, the outer skin (*right*)

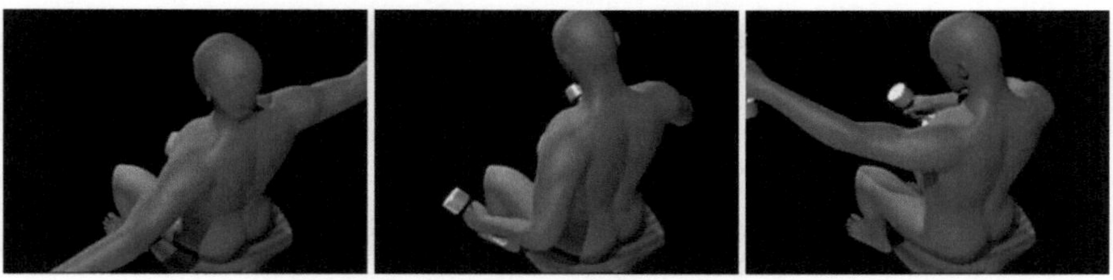

Fig. 10 An inverse dynamics motor controller drives the musculoskeletal system to track a sequence of target poses

of a volumetric, finite element model of the soft tissue introduces the visual richness of more detailed three-dimensional models of the musculature. Specifically, we achieve robust and efficient simulation of soft tissue deformation by decoupling the visualization geometry from the simulation geometry within the finite element framework. The flesh is modeled as an isotropic, quasi-incompressible Mooney–Rivlin material. A total of *354,000 Body-Centered-Cubic (BCC) tetrahedral finite elements* are simulated to create detailed deformation of the embedded high-resolution surfaces of the skin and each of the muscles.

Figure 10 demonstrates biomechanically simulated flexing motions of the arms carrying dumbbell loads in gravity.

4 Conclusion

I have reviewed our work on deformable and functional models for use in image analysis, particularly in medical imaging, and in the biomechanical simulation of the human body. Within the overarching physics-based framework, deformable models and functional models are complementary inasmuch as the former exploits physics to analyze visual data, whereas the latter exploits physics to synthesize visually realistic simulations. Both model categories have attracted intense interest from the target research communities and they will continue to pose intellectually provocative research problems in the foreseeable future.

Acknowledgements I am grateful to João Tavares and Renato Jorge for inviting me to deliver a plenary lecture at the VIPIMAGE 2009 Conference and for encouraging me, and patiently waiting for me, to prepare this article. I am grateful to the many colleagues who have collaborated with me in the development of the work surveyed, whose names appear in the list of references. I would especially like to acknowledge the invaluable contributions of Tim McInerney and Ghassan Hamarneh in the context of topologically adaptive deformable models and deformable organisms, as well as Sung-Hee Lee and Eftychios Sifakis in the context of human modeling and simulation.

References

1. Carlbom, I., Terzopoulos, D., Harris, K.: Computer-assisted registration, segmentation, and 3D reconstruction from images of neuronal tissue sections. IEEE Trans. Med. Imag. **13**(2), 351–362 (1994)
2. Faloutsos, P., van de Panne, M., Terzopoulos, D.: Dynamic free-form deformations for animation synthesis. IEEE Trans. Visual. Comput. Graph. **3**(3), 201–214 (1997)
3. Hamarneh, G., McInerney, T., Terzopoulos, D.: Deformable organisms for automatic medical image analysis. In: Proceedings of the 3rd International Conference on Medical Image Computing and Computer Assisted Interventions (MICCAI'01), Utrecht, The Netherlands, pp. 66–75, Berlin, Germany, Springer (2001)
4. Hamarneh, G., McIntosh, C., McInerney, T., Terzopoulos, D.: Deformable orgnisms: An artificial life framework for automated medical image analysis. In: Schaefer, G., Hassanien, A., Jiang, J. (eds.) Computational Intelligence in Medical Imaging: Techniques and Applications, Chap. 15, pp. 435–474. CRC Press, Boca Raton, FL (2008)
5. Kass, M., Witkin, A., Terzopoulos, D.: Snakes: Active contour models. Int. J. Comput. Vis. **1**(4), 321–331 (1988)
6. Lee, S.-H., Sifakis, E., Terzopoulos, D.: Comprehensive biomechanical modeling and simulation of the upper body. ACM Trans. Graph. (Proc. ACM SIGGRAPH'09) **28**(4), 99:1–17 (2009)
7. Lee, S.-H., Terzopoulos, D.: Heads up! Biomechanical modeling and neuromuscular control of the neck. ACM Trans. Graph. **25**(3), 1188–1198 (2006)
8. Lee, Y., Terzopoulos, D., Waters, K.: Realistic modeling for facial animation. In: Computer Graphics Proceedings, Annual Conference Series, Proc. ACM SIGGRAPH'95, pp. 55–62. August 1995
9. McInerney, T., Hamarneh, G., Shenton, M., Terzopoulos, D.: Deformable organisms for automatic medical image analysis. Med. Image Anal. **6**(3), 251–266 (2002)
10. McInerney, T., Terzopoulos, D.: A dynamic finite element surface model for segmentation and tracking in multidimensional medical images with application to cardiac 4D image analysis. Comput. Med. Imag. Graph. **19**(1), 69–83 (1995)
11. McInerney, T., Terzopoulos, D.: Topologically adaptable snakes. In: Proceedings of 5th International Conference on Computer Vision (ICCV'95), pp. 840–845, Cambridge, MA, June 1995
12. McInerney, T., Terzopoulos, D.: Deformable models in medical image analysis: A survey. Med. Image Anal. **1**(2), 91–108 (1996)
13. McInerney, T., Terzopoulos, D.: Topology adaptive deformable surfaces for medical image volume segmentation. IEEE Trans. Med. Imag. **18**(10), 840–850 (1999)

14. McInerney, T., Terzopoulos, D.: T-snakes: Topology adaptive snakes. Med. Image Anal. **4**(2), 73–91 (2000)
15. Metaxas, D., Terzopoulos, D.: Dynamic deformation of solid primitives with constraints. Comput. Grap. (Proc. ACM SIGGRAPH'92) **26**(2), 309–312 (1992)
16. Terzopoulos, D.: On matching deformable models to images. Technical Report 60, Schlumberger Palo Alto Research (1986) Reprinted in *Topical Meeting on Machine Vision,* Technical Digest Series, vol. 12 (Optical Society of America, Washington, DC) 1987, pp. 160–167
17. Terzopoulos, D.: The computation of visible-surface representations. IEEE Trans. Pattern Anal. Mach. Intell. **PAMI-10**(4), 417–438 (1988)
18. Terzopoulos, D.: Deformable models: Classic, topology-adaptive and generalized formulations. In: Osher, S., Paragios, N. (eds.) Geometric Level Set Methods in Imaging, Vision, and Graphics, Chap. 2, pp. 21–40. Springer, New York (2003)
19. Terzopoulos, D., Fleischer, K.: Deformable models. Vis. Comput. **4**(6), 306–331 (1988)
20. Terzopoulos, D., Fleischer, K.: Modeling inelastic deformation: Viscoelasticity, plasticity, fracture. Comput. Graph. (Proc. ACM SIGGRAPH'88) **22**(4), 269–278 (1988)
21. Terzopoulos, D., Platt, J., Barr, A., Fleischer, K.: Elastically deformable models. Comput. Graph. (Proc. SIGGRAPH'87) **21**(4), 205–214 (1987)
22. Terzopoulos, D., Szeliski, R.: Tracking with Kalman snakes. In: Active Vision, pp. 3–20. MIT Press, Cambridge, MA (1992)
23. Terzopoulos, D., Waters, K.: Physically-based facial modelling, analysis, and animation. J. Visual. Comp. Animat. **1**(2), 73–80 (1990)
24. Terzopoulos, D., Witkin, A., Kass, M.: Constraints on deformable models: Recovering 3D shape and nonrigid motion. Artif. Intel. **36**(1), 91–123 (1988)

Medical-GiD: From Medical Images to Simulations, 4D MRI Flow Analysis

Eduardo Soudah, Julien Pennecot, Jorge S. Pérez, Maurizio Bordone, and Eugenio Oñate

Abstract Medical imaging techniques, such as MRI and CT scanning, are valuable tools for getting a lot of information non-invasively and it is useful for reconstructing the geometry of complex objects about the patients. Medical-GiD is a medical image platform that incorporates a module to read directly the blood velocity profile from the MR scan, in particular for deformable registration of 4D MRI images, Electrocardiography (ECG)-synchronized and respiration controlled 3D magnetic resonance (MR) velocity mapping (flow-sensitive 4D MRI), 3D morphologic and three-directional blood flow data. Furthermore, Medical-GiD is focus in the medical image processing in the biomechanical research field to generating meshes from the medical images, to apply in Computational Fluid Dynamics (CFD) or structural mechanics (stress analysis). To date, these techniques have largely been applied to compute meshes for numerical simulations, but with Medical-GiD, we will have the integration between the real data and numerical simulations.

Keywords Computational Fluid Dynamics · Mesh generation · Blood flow · Aorta · Magnetic resonance

1 Introduction

According to World Health Organization estimates, 17 million people around the globe die of cardiovascular disease (CVD) each year. About 600 million people with high blood pressure are at risk of heart attack, stroke and cardiac failure. Low and middle-income countries contributed to 78% of CVD deaths. By 2010 CVD is estimated to be the major cause of death in developed countries. This huge impact has motivated the development of new non-invasively techniques in order

E. Soudah (✉), J. Pennecot, J.S. Pérez, M. Bordone, and E. Oñate
International Center for Numerical Methods in Engineering, Technical University of Catalonia, Barcelona, Spain
e-mail: esoudah@cimne.upc.edu; ronda@cimne.upc.edu; mbordone@cimne.upc.edu; onate@cimne.upc.edu

J.M.R.S. Tavares and R.M.N. Jorge (eds.), *Computational Vision and Medical Image Processing: Recent Trends*, Computational Methods in Applied Sciences 19,
DOI 10.1007/978-94-007-0011-6_8,

to understand cardiovascular pathologies and interventions. The effect of blood flow on arterial wall remodeling in the investigation of vascular hemodynamics within the vascular vessels is of great interest, for example in the aorta coarctation. The identification of patients with aortic disease requires a detailed understanding of the link between vascular malformation and altered hemodynamics, and how is the relationship between the blood flow and the aortic wall; it has the potential to greatly enhance the understanding of the pathogenesis and progression of vascular diseases and to aid in the decision of whether treatment is warranted. In this perspective, 4D Phase-Contrast non-invasive magnetic resonance imaging (MRI), with its intrinsic sensitivity to blood flow, offers the unique possibility to simultaneously acquire morphology and spatially co-registered hemodynamic information non-invasively.

2 Methodology

2.1 Medical-GiD

Medical-GiD is a homemade software development in CIMNE, designed for qualitative evaluation of medical images, in particular for deformable registration of 4D MRI images. Medical-GiD is written in the Tcl interpreted language so that it is integrated as a module of the Personal Pre and Post Processor GiD [4]. GiD is a universal, adaptive and user-friendly graphical user interface for geometrical modeling, data input and visualization of results for all types of numerical simulation programs. The object oriented structure has been implemented using Snit in order to be integrated Medical-GiD as a module of GiD or other programs. Medical-GiD is based on several open source libraries able to read and write different images formats using Insight Segmentation and Registration Toolkit library (ITK) [6]. For the image processing tasks, Medical-GiD uses ITK libraries and an inner development filters for noise filtering and eddy current correction in MR phase velocity data. The program GUI is based on VTK [23, 25] (Visualization toolkit) which is an open source toolkit which can be integrated freely in commercial software as well ITK.

2.2 Architecture Design

In Fig. 1, the architecture structure of Medical-GiD is shown. The architecture is based on two different modules communicated by ITK-VTK filter. The whole visualization process is programmed using the VTK toolkit and the glue used to cement the code and create the GUI is Tcl/Tk [22]. Using the visualization the user can change some of the parameters used during the image processing. Those parameters are passed back to ITK and the image processing is updated for a new visualization. Although the user guide of ITK says that ITK has been wrapped

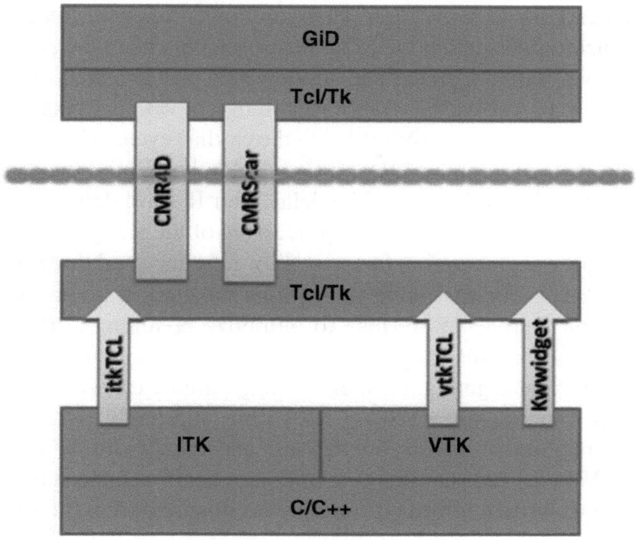

Fig. 1 Medical-GiD Structure. CMR4D and CMRScar are the vertical applications. To add new vertical applications in Medical-GiD is really easy because is application oriented to the problem

using many scripting languages, such as Tcl, Java and Python, there are almost no documentation available online or off the shelves on how to use the wrapped functions. Therefore, we have not been able to use libraries using Tcl, and we have developed our own wrappers in C++. Although this seems (and was) a hard task, it allowed us to implement our own C++ classes to interact with the image and provide to implement easier our filters. A special care has been taken to use programming languages as well as libraries compatible with the actual form of GiD. The Tcl/Tk language is used for the GUI and as cement for the code. Snit has been used to develop an object oriented code in Tcl. And the two toolkits used (ITK and VTK) are open source code which are freely implementable into a commercial code.

2.3 Magnetic Resonance

Measurements were carried out using a 3 T MR system (Magnetom TRIO; Siemens, Erlangen, Germany) time-resolved, 3D MR velocity mapping based on an RF-spoiled, gradient-echo sequence with interleaved three-directional velocity encoding (predefined fixed velocity sensitivity = 150 cm/s for all measurements). Data were acquired in a sagittal-oblique, 3D volume that included the entire thoracic aorta and the proximal parts of the supra aortic branches. Each 3D volume was carefully planned and adapted to the individual anatomy (spatial resolution, $2.1 \times 3.2 - 3.5 \times 3.5 - 5\,\text{mm}^3$). In the in vivo situation, measurements may be compromised by the active cyclic motion of the heart (cardiac contraction and dilation) and the passive motion of the heart due to respiration. These motion components may lead to image artifacts and uncertainties about the exact measurement site in the aorta. Only if the breathing state was within a predefined window data was accepted for the geometrical reconstruction. To resolve the temporal evolution of vascular geometry and blood flow, measurements were synchronized with the cardiac cycle. The velocity data was recorder in intervals of Temporal Resolution (TeR) throughout the cardiac starting after the R-wave of the ECG. The initial delay after R-wave detection was required for execution of the navigator pulse and processing of the navigator signal. Twofold acquisition (k-space segmentation factor = 2) of reference and three-directional velocity sensitive scans for each cine time frame resulted in a temporal resolution of eight repetition time = 45–49 ms. To minimize breathing artifacts and image blurring, respiration control was performed based on combined adaptive k-space reordering and navigator gating. Further imaging parameters were as follows: rectangular field of view = $400 \times (267 - 300)\,\text{mm}^2$, flip angle $= 15°$, time to echo = 3.5–3.7 ms, repetition time = 5.6–6.1 ms, and bandwidth = 480–650 Hz per pixel [10–12]. Velocity measurements a voluntary healthy, male subject underwent MR examinations; written informed consent was obtained from the subject.

2.4 Segmentation and Meshing for Computational Simulations

The development of computational simulations in medicine, molecular biology and engineering has increased the need for quality finite element meshes. For the segmentation procedure Medical-GiD includes a variety of ITK filters, which are used interactively by the clinicians to determinate the volume of interest of the problem. After segmenting the medical image we end with a file with the image data and the value of the isosurface value defining the boundary of the volume of interest. The imaging data V is given in the form of sampled function values on rectilinear grids,

$$V = F(x_i, y_j, z_k)|0 \leq i \leq n_x, 0 \leq j \leq n_y, 0 \leq k \leq n_z; \tag{1}$$

We assume a continuous function F is constructed through the trilinear interpolation of sampled values for each cubic cell in the volume. The format used to read the medical data is VTK structured point as it is agreed in [9]. The description of this format can be found in [9]. The image in this format can also be rendered as a volume and manipulated with ITK. Given an isosurface value defining the boundary of the volume of interest we can extract a geometric model of it. We are interested in creating a distcretization of the volume suitable for finite element computation. The following methods are able to generate a finite element meshes that can be used in the computational analysis: (1) Dual contouring, (2) Marching Cubes, (3) Advancing front, and (4) Isosurface stuffing. All of them has been integrated into Medical-GiD.

In order to generate in Medical-GiD a volume mesh valid for the computational simulation from the voxels, the Fig. 2 shows two different procedures to reach it.

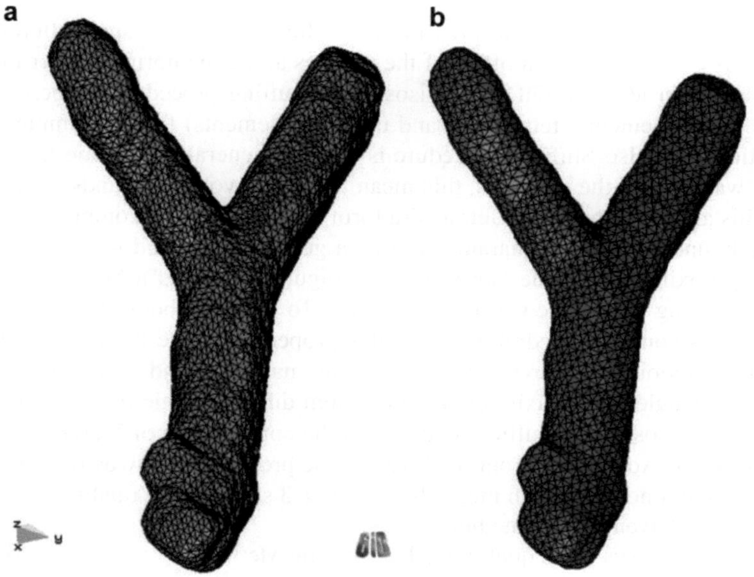

Bifucartion generated using Marching Cube, smoothing and advanting front methods.

Bifurcation generated using Isosurface stuffing directly from the image.

Fig. 2 Meshes generated using the IsoStuffing and Marching Cubes methods

Figure 2a shows the boundary mesh generated using this combination of methods. We combine the Marching Cubes method to generate first the boundary mesh first and then, after a smoothing, an Advancing Front [8] method to fill the interior with tetrahedral. The Marching Cubes [9] algorithm visits each cell in the volume and performs local triangulation based on the sign configuration of the eight vertices. If one or more vertex of a cube have values less than the user-specified isovalue, and one or more have values greater than this value, we know the voxel must contribute some component of the isosurface. By determining which edges of the cube are intersected by the isosurface, we can create triangular patches which divide the cube between regions within the iso-surface and regions outside. By connecting the patches from all cubes on the isosurface boundary, we get a surface representation. The Advancing Front [8] is an unstructured grid generation method. Grids are generated by marching from boundaries (front) towards the interior. Tetrahedral elements are generated based on the initial front. As tetrahedral elements are generated, the "initial front" is updated until the entire domain is covered with tetrahedral elements, and the front is emptied. Figure 2a shows tetrahedral mesh generated using Marching Cubes, smoothing and Advancing Front methods. Some of the triangles generated by the Marching Cubes method do not exhibit good quality to be used in finite element computation. In order to improve the quality of those elements we apply a Laplacian smooth technique which is volume preserving. The smoothing algorithm implemented tries to preserve the volume after each application of the laplace operator by doing an offset of the vertices along the normal. Other method implemented in Medical-GiD is the isosurface stuffing procedure to increase the quality of the elements (tetrahedral and triangles elements) for the computational simulations. The Iso-Stuffing procedure is ideal to generate a volume mesh with quality warranty of the elements, this mean angle and volume bounds are guaranteed. This algorithm generates tetrahedra form a small set of precomputed stencils, and the boundary mesh is guaranteed to be a geometrically and topologically accurate approximation of the isosurface [7]. Figure 2b shows a bifurcation mesh generated using Isosurface stuffing procedure. To compare both procedures, next figure shows some tetrahedral and triangles properties of the bifurcation meshes generated previously. Figures 3 and 4 show the maximum and minimum angle to boundary triangles and maximum and minimum dihedral angle to tetrahedral elements for the Isosurface Stuffing method and the combination of Marching Cubes, smoothing and Advancing Front methods. These properties show us the quality of our meshes attained with both methods. Next Fig. 3 shows mesh quality for Marching Cubes + Advance front methods

Next Fig. 4 shows mesh quality for Iso-Stuffing Method.

We notice that the mesh quality attained with the isosurface stuffing method (Fig. 4) is higher quality than the mesh generated with the combination of the

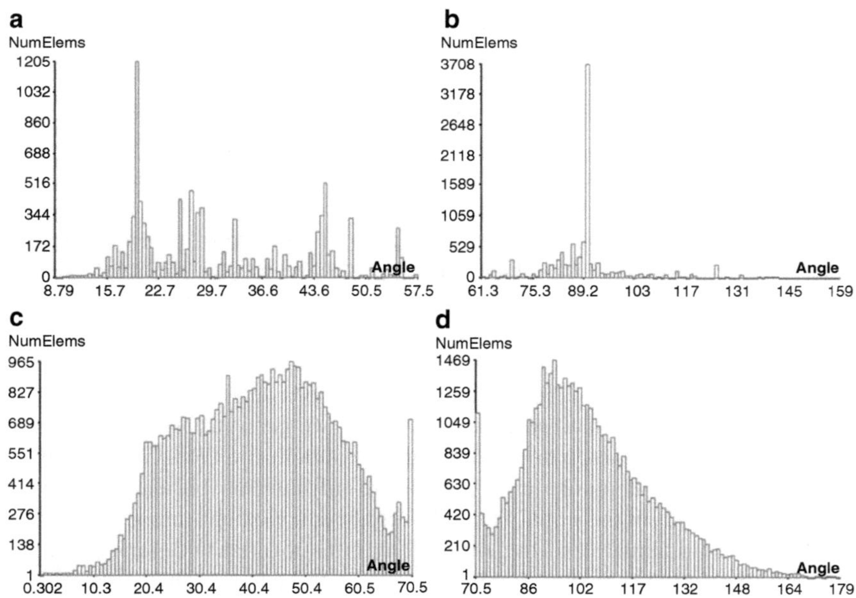

Fig. 3 Mesh quality for Marching Cubes + Advance Frontal methods. (**a**) histogram for the minimum angle of the boundary triangles elements, (**b**) histogram for the maximum angle of the boundary triangles elements, (**c**) histogram for the minimum dihedral angle of the Tetrahedral elements, and (**d**) histogram for the maximum dihedral angle of the Tetrahedral elements

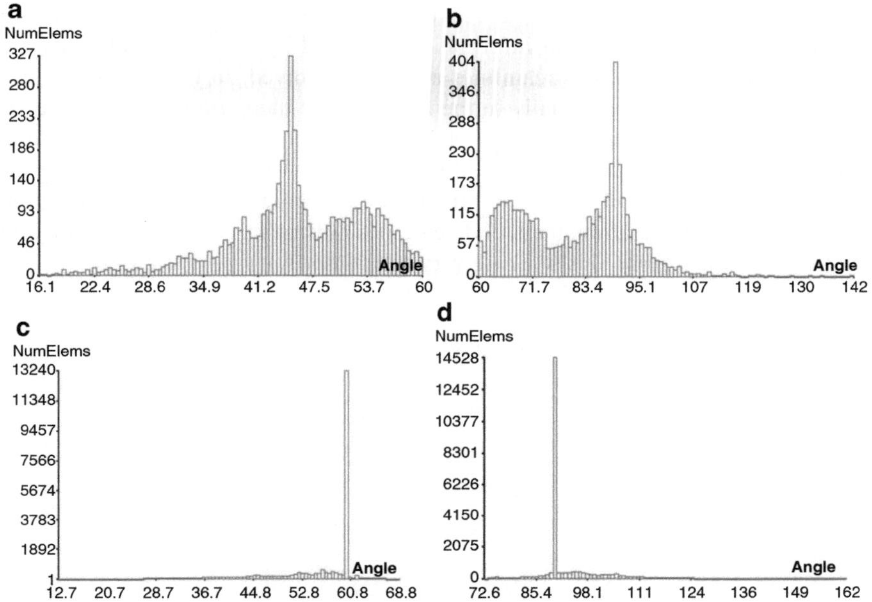

Fig. 4 Mesh quality for Iso-stuffing method. (**a**) histogram for the minimum angle of the boundary triangles, (**b**) histogram for the maximum angle of the boundary triangles, (**c**) histogram for the minimum dihedral angle of the tetrahedral elements, and (**d**) histogram for the maximum dihedral angle of the tetrahedral elements

Marching Cubes, Smoothing and Advancing front methods (Fig. 3), furthermore, using Isosurface method it is possible to generate the mesh directly from the image data.

3 Results

In order to assess the performance of the image and geometry processing (geometrical 3D reconstruction and mesh generation) and the mathematical models, we have compared the MRI velocity measurements with the CFD simulations in the aorta.

3.1 Aortic Blood Flow Analysis

The obtained ECG-synchronized time series of 3D data sets were read in Medical-GiD and underwent fully automated noise filtering, segmentation, meshing and visualization inside Medical-GiD, which offered different data visualization options to illustrate the dynamics of 3D blood flow encoded in the velocity data.

Visualization of the patterns and dynamics of 3D blood flow was spatially registered with the anatomical information provided by the magnitude data and included vector graphs, 3D streamlines and time-resolved. In the original images there are a lot of noise, especially in the zones where there are no tissues (the velocity seems to have a random value where there is air). Figure 5 shows the three components of the velocity in the third iteration (Vx, Vy, Vz) and magnitude image. The third iteration of the whole MRI data has been used for the segmentation, because during this iteration, the blood velocities pulsing through the aorta are high and therefore the threshold is working very satisfactorily.

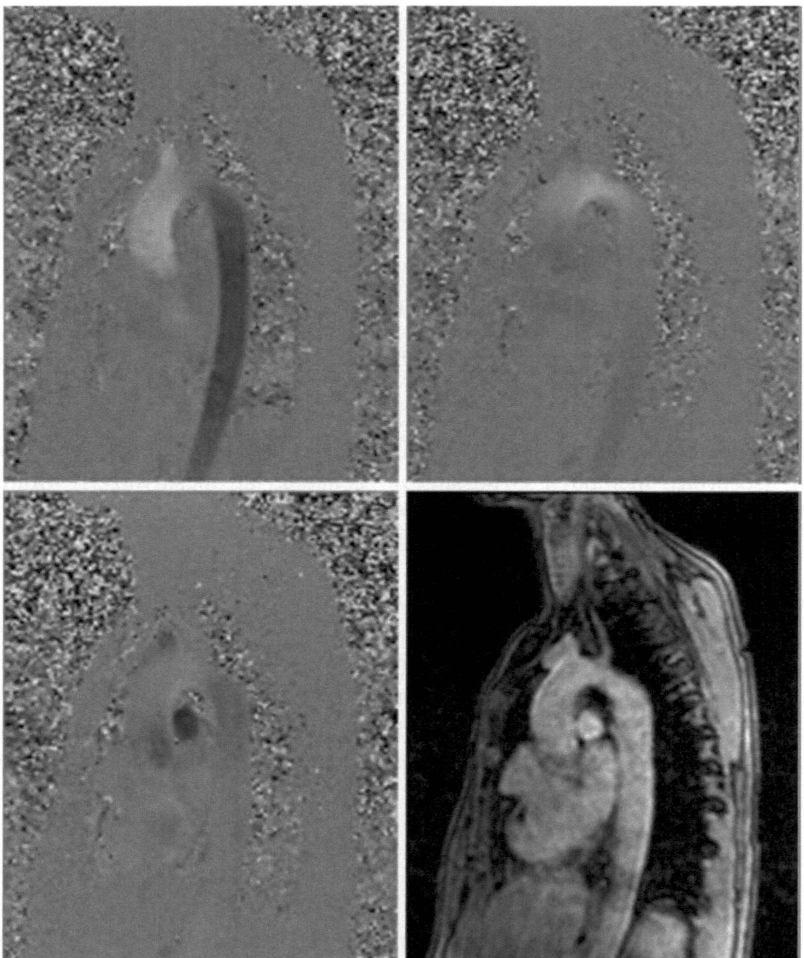

Fig. 5 Phase contrast image (through plane velocity encoding) in Vx, Vy, Vz and magnitude image at the third iteration

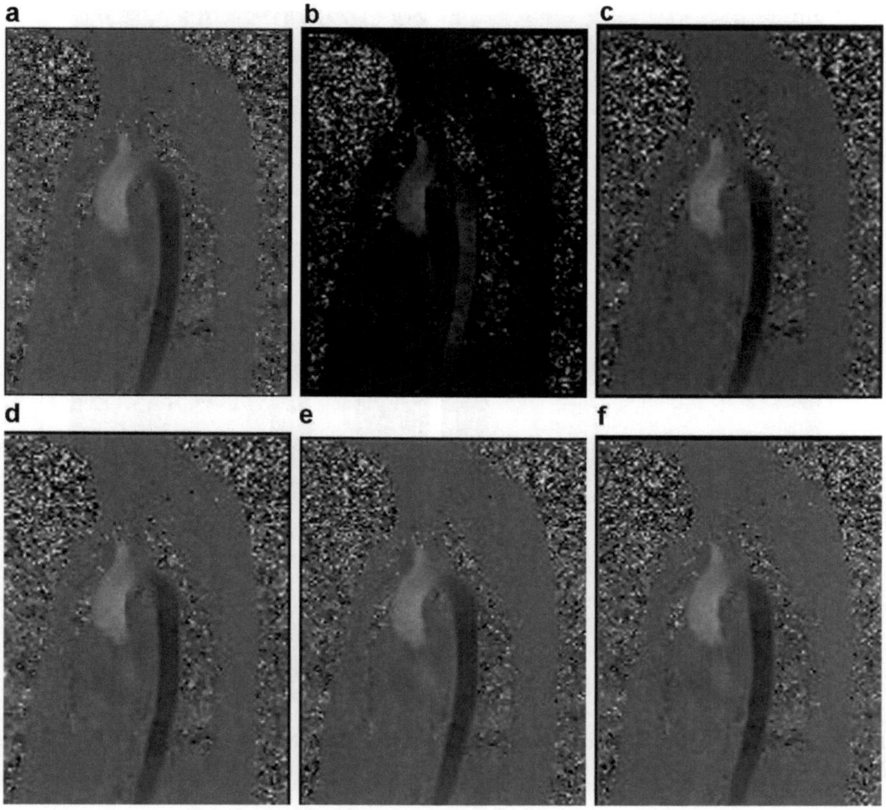

Fig. 6 Results obtained applying different noise filters. (**a**) Original image with noise, (**b**) with media filter, (**c**) with standard deviation filter, (**d**) with entropy filter, (**e**) with asymmetric filter, and (**f**) with homogeneity filter

To eliminate the noise of the original image. Different algorithms have been applied (Media, Standard deviation, entropy, asymmetric filter and homogeneity filter), Fig. 6 shows the results obtained afterwards the filters have been applied. We obtained segmentation of the aorta by applying a standard deviation filter and threshold filter to the velocity magnitude of blood in the vector data. In order to select only the region of interest and not only the zones of high velocity magnitude which would include the air surroundings (noise), we applied a standard deviation filter to compute the velocity magnitude and then we used a connected threshold to choose points inside the aorta. We chose to use a neighborhood connected threshold image filter, this means that a voxel is accepted if itself and all its neighbors have a velocity magnitude above a defined threshold. Furthermore all voxels selected need to be connected with at least one seed point. The results almost exactly math the aorta, but it looks like an eroded (thinner) version of the aorta. Indeed voxels located close to the edge of the aorta have their neighborhood crossing over outside of

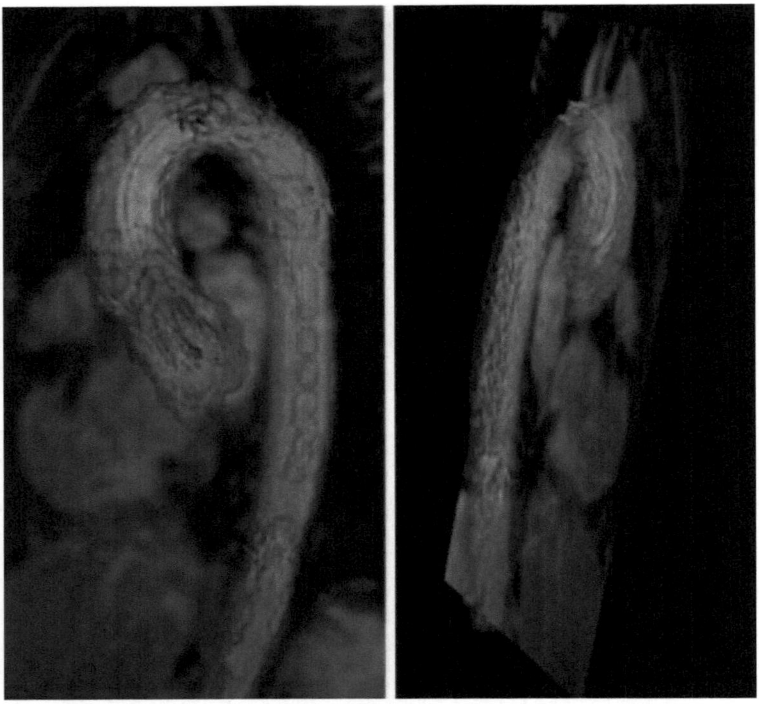

Fig. 7 Visualization of the velocity vector field getting from MRI within the aorta using for Medical-GiD

the aorta. Those points are really noisy and may have a value of velocity magnitude below the threshold and therefore the voxel is not selected as part of the aorta. It is then necessary to "dilate" the aorta by one or two pixels to capture exactly the aorta. The following image shows 3D blood velocity field in the descendent aorta obtained directly from the MRI. The segmentation is then used as a mask for the velocity image and is superimposed on a slice of the scalar data. Figure 7 shows respectively the longitudinal section and detail of the aorta. The color lines represent the blood velocity field inside the aorta. Concerning the calibration of the magnetic resonance machine, a special procedure has been developed to obtain the blood velocity field: this special algorithm has to be properly adjusted to the velocity encoding parameters of the MRI.

Furthermore, vector graphs representing the pixel wise, three-directional blood flow velocities could be superimposed on selected cut planes and animated over the cardiac cycle. For an overview over 3D blood flow patterns at a single time frame within the cardiac cycle, paths originating from the predefined emitter planes and tangent to all measured velocity vectors (3D streamline) were calculated. Temporal information could be added by generating traces within the 3D volume representing the path of imaginary massless particles within the measured time-resolved velocity vector fields starting at a specified time within the cardiac cycle (time-resolved, 3D particle traces).

3.2 Blood Flow Velocity Decoding

Blood flow velocity in each voxel depends on acquisition velocity sensitivity and gray scale. In general the velocities are encoded in the phase difference images such that there is a linear relationship between the gray scale value and the underlying velocity. Velocity in cm/s = ((PixelValue − GrayScale)/GrayScale) × Venc; where venc is the velocity sensitivity in cm/s (in our case venc = 150 cm/s), GrayScale depends of the DICOM (in our case 2,048) and PixelValue is the value of the gray color of the phase contrast image (see Sect. 2.3).

3.3 Numerical Simulation

In this work, blood is assumed as 3D, steady, incompressible, homogeneous, Newtonian fluid with no external forces applied on it, while the arterial wall is comprised from non-elastic and impermeable material. The newtonian approximation is acceptable in large arteries how it have been explained previously. Mathematically a newtonian fluid can be expressed as symmetric stress tensor by the follow constitutive equation:

$$\rho = -p\mathbf{I} + 2\mu\varepsilon(\mathbf{u}) \tag{2a}$$

$$\varepsilon(\mathbf{u}) = \frac{1}{2}\left(\nabla\mathbf{u} + \nabla\mathbf{u}^T\right) \tag{2b}$$

where p is the fluid pressure, **I** is the unit tensor, μ denotes the apparent fluid viscosity and $\varepsilon(u)$ is the rate-of-strain tensor (2b). Therefore, according to this, blood flow is simulated with average blood properties: fluid viscosity $\mu = 0.0035$ Pa·s and density $\rho = 1{,}050\,\text{kg/m}^3$. Considering a fluid domain(large artery) Ω based on the arbitrary Lagrangian method [3] and adopting the following notation: $\Omega(0,t)$ is a 3D arterial region, and x = (x_1, x_2, x_3) is an arbitrary point of Ω. For x ε Ω and t > 0 the conservation of momentum and continuity in the compact form are described by the following equations:

$$\rho\cdot\left(\frac{\partial\mathbf{u}}{\partial\mathbf{t}} + (\mathbf{u}\cdot\nabla\mathbf{u})\right) + \nabla\,\mathbf{p} - \nabla\cdot(\mu\,\triangle\,\mathbf{u}) = \rho\cdot\mathbf{f} \tag{3a}$$

$$\nabla u = 0 \tag{3b}$$

where **u** = **u** (x, t) denotes the velocity vector, **p** = **p** (x, t) the pressure field, ρ density, μ the dynamic viscosity of the fluid and f the volumetric acceleration. It is now possible to recast the Navier–Stokes equations that are used to describe the pulsatile blood flow in large arteries on the time-dependent domain Ω with appropriate boundary conditions. The boundary conditions of system (3) are prescribed velocities on the walls and inflow boundaries, as well as prescribed pressure p on the outflow boundary. The volumetric forces ($\rho \cdot \mathbf{f}$) are not taken in to account in the present analysis.

The solution of system (3) requires considerable computational effort. It is impossible to advance in time using the momentum equation unless we know the pressure, but we cannot know the pressure unless we know the velocity. It is possible, however, to proceed as in a full Stokes problem which at every time step solves for $\mathbf{u}$ and $\mathbf{p}$ simultaneously but this turns out to introduce more problems than it is worth, including being a very slow numerical procedure. Instead, we may note that the pressure field $\mathbf{p}$ is essentially determined by the incompressibility constraint, and it is this idea which Chorin [1] used to invent the popular projection method or fractional step-method. The projection method is based on the Helmholtz decomposition principle, which states that any sufficiently regular vector function can be split into a divergence free and a rotation-free vector field. In [5] and [20] was shown that this decomposition can be applied to the weak formulation of the Navier–Stokes equations in appropriate spaces. The technique splits the problem (3a), (3b) in the sequence of an advection diffusion problem for an auxiliary non-divergence-free velocity field and a projection of the intermediate velocity field onto the divergence-free functional space. The first step is to compute an intermediate velocity field, $\mathbf{u}^*$, using the momentum equation but using an approximation to $\nabla \mathbf{p}$. Thus, because this is only an approximation, $\mathbf{u}^*$ will not necessarily be divergence free. The second step is to project $\mathbf{u}^*$ onto the space of divergence-free vector fields, which incidentally will calculate the pressure $\mathbf{p}$ at the next time step for us. For an excellent overview of various projection methods, including convergence properties and the derivation of formulae see [1]. In [17–19, 21] this technique have been applied in cardiovascular research.

Due to the highly convective flow in the ascending aorta and in the general in the cardiovascular system, the numerical scheme requires a stabilization technique in order to avoid oscillations in the numerical solution. In this study an innovative stabilization method based on the Finite Increment Calculus(FIC) concept [14–16] is applied that preserves the consistency of the scheme. Convergence was achieved when all mass, velocity component and energy changes, from iteration to iteration, were less than 10^8. The stabilized Navier–Stokes equations are solved numerically by means of a finite-element method, and its implementation was done in Tdyn [2, 13] a fluid dynamics and multi-physics simulation environment.

The geometry used for the numerical simulation has been obtained using the isostuffing procedure (Fig. 8).

For the validation of the blood flow a good qualitative agreement of 3D blood velocities predicted by CFD with the MRI velocity measurements, we can see the 3D blood velocity profile predicted by CFD (Fig. 9) compared with the data measured by MRI (Fig. 7). However, each technique has limitations that introduce differences between the corresponding blood flow velocity fields. It is important to understand these differences in order to better interpret the results obtained with each technique, and to be aware of the regions along the arteries where each technique is expected to over simplify the velocity patterns or yield under or over estimations of the velocity.

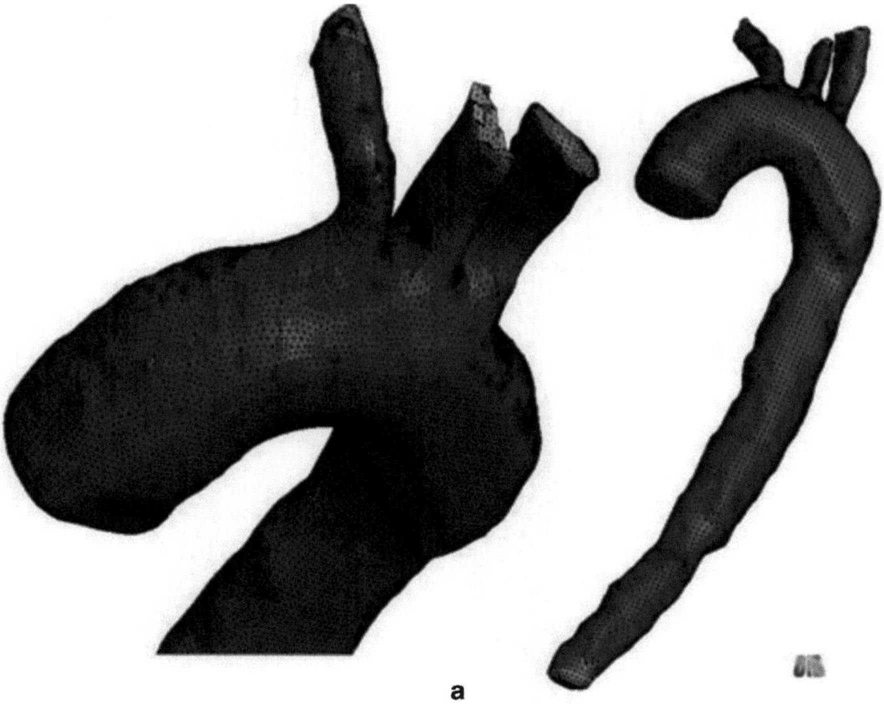

Fig. 8 Aorta mesh getting by Iso stuffing procedure

In Fig. 10 shows the velocity profile in fourth different sections of the aorta (ascendent aorta, aortic arch I, aortic arch II and descendent aorta). We have compared the numerical results obtained with the CFD simulation with the real values obtained with the MRI (Sect. 3.1) notice that the different between both is negligible.

4 Conclusion

Mean aortic flow velocity is probably of greater use as a trend indicator of cardiovascular diseases, aorta coarctation and atherosclerosis plaque as a result of the recirculating flow, the wall shear stresses at the inner wall are low and oscillating, predisposing to the development of atherosclerosis. In Figs. 6 and 7 we observe how in the internal part of the arch aortic, Brachiocephalic, Left Subclavian and Left.Ext Carotid a change of the flow direction and flow recirculating is produced due the complex geometry of the vessels and the high velocity profile. These changes of the direction in these parts are directly related with the atheroma plaque formation, as in the carotid. We have compared these results with experimental results and other medical studies and the common area of grow up of the atheroma

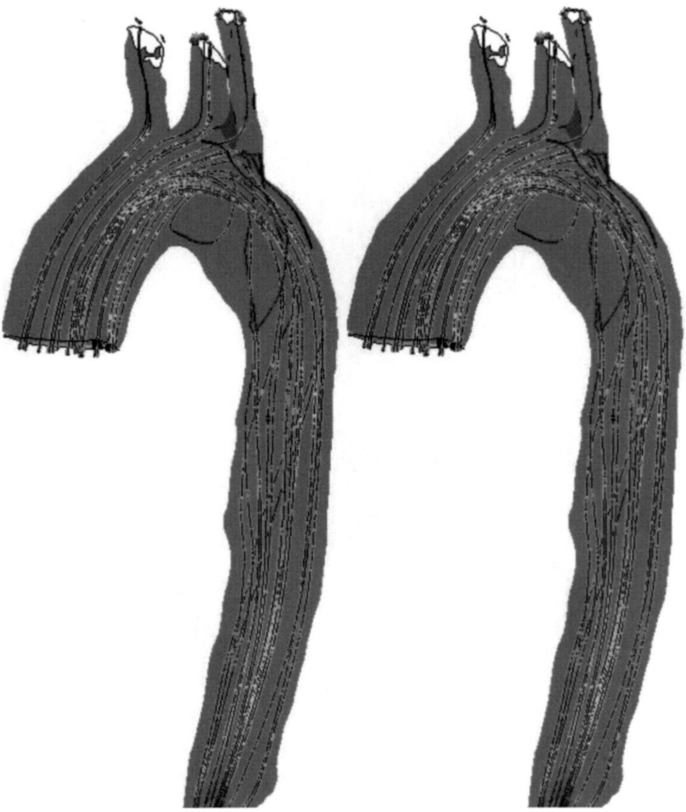

Fig. 9 Streamlines inside the Aorta

plaque fit in with the numerical recirculation areas [24]. This model shows that transient fluid flow in the aorta can be simulated, in particular in the aortic arch, and also are useful for studies of the arch branched graft in the treatment of aortic aneurysm or aortic dissection. Medical-GiD is a development environment of medical images treatment and computational simulation that can help us to understand these phenomena. One of the main applications of Medical-GiD is working directly from the data of 4D-MRI images, allowing in a unique user-interface: filtering, segmented, meshing and visualizes a real blood flood profiles. Medical-GiD is designed to be integrated easily in other programs, as GiD. Other visualization and segmentation tools will be implemented according to the clinician's requirements. Medical-GiD is based on ITK, VTK, TCL-TK libraries and C++ applications for visualize, segmentation and meshing of 3D and 4D images in Linux and Windows. Future works will include advanced techniques in image processing, meshing and also improvements in the fitting techniques of the velocity encoding parameters.

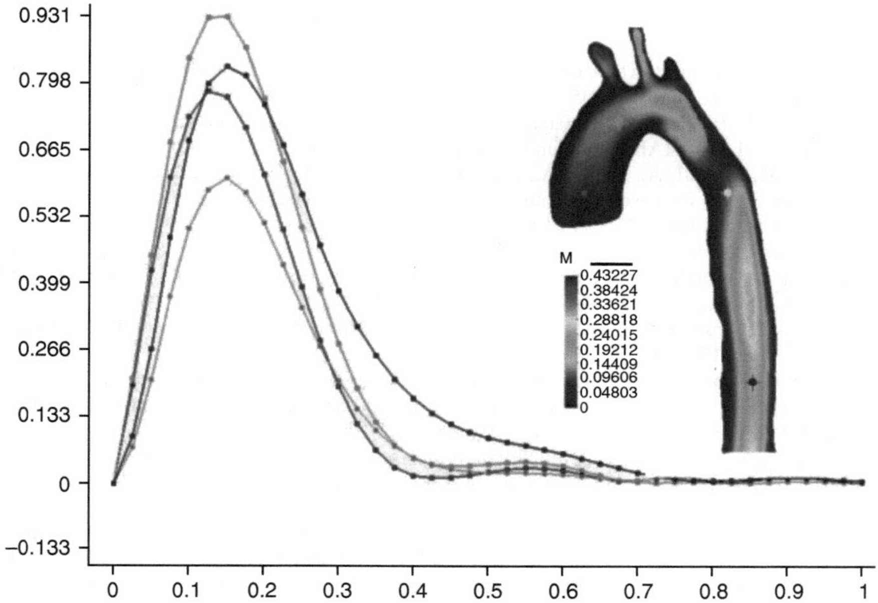

Fig. 10 Numerical results in the ascendent aorta, aortic arch I, aortic arch II and descendent aorta

Acknowledgements The authors would like to acknowledge Dr. Frances Carreras (from Hospital de la Santa Creu i Sant Pau) and Michael Markl (from the Departments of Diagnostic Radiology and Medical Physics, Freiburg, Germany) for their contributions and the support give us to do this work. The medical images used during this work are from the Departments of Diagnostic Radiology, Medical Physics; Neurology and Clinical Neurophysiology; and Cardiovascular Surgery, University Hospital Freiburg, Freiburg, Germany.

References

1. Chorin, A.J.: Numerical solution of the Navier Stokes Equations. Math. Comput. **22**, 745–762 (1968)
2. COMPASS Ingeniera y Sistemas SA.Tdyn. Environment for Fluid Dynamics (Navier Stokes equations), Turbulence, Heat Transfer, Advection of Species and Free surface simulation. Theoretical background and Tdyn 3D tutorial, March 2002
3. Formaggia, L., Nobile, F., Quarteroni, A., Veneziani, A.: Multiscale modelling of the circulatory system: a preliminary analysis. Comput. Visual. Sci. **2**, 75–83 (1999)
4. GiD Reference Manual. The personal pre and postprocessor. Ribó, R., de Riera Pasenau, M.A., Escolano, E., Suit, J., Colls, A., May 2010, CIMNE. (ftp://www.gidhome.com/pub/GiD_Documentation/Docs/GiD_Reference_Manual.pdf)
5. Girault, V., Raviart, P.-A.: Finite Element Methods for Navier-Stokes Equations, p. 374 Springer, Berlin/Heidelberg/New York/Tokyo: (1986)
6. The ITK Software Guide Second Edition. Ibáñez, L., Schroeder, W., Ng, L., Cates, J., and the Insight Software Consortium, August 30, 2005, Kitware Inc.

7. Labelle, F., Shewchuk, J.R.: Isosurface Stuffing: fast tetrahedral meshes with good dihedral angles. ACM Transactions on Graphics, **26**(3), Article 57, July 2007
8. Lohner, R., Parikh, P.: Three dimensional grid generation by the advancing-front method. Int. J. Numer. Meth. Fluid. **8**, 1135–1149 (1988)
9. Lorensen, W.E., Cline, H.E.: Marching cubes: A high resolution 3D surface construction algorithm. ACM SIGGRAPH Computer Graphic, **21**(4), 163–169, July 1987
10. Markl, M., Harloff, A., Bley, T.A., Frydrychiwicz, A., et al.: Time-resolved 3D MR velocity mapping at 3T: improved navigator-gated assessment of vascular anatomy and blood flow. J. Magn. Reson. Imag. Art: 06-0195, 25:000–000 (2007)
11. Markl, M., Draney, M.T., Hope, M.D., et al.: Time-resolved 3D velocity mapping in the thoracic aorta: visualization of three-directional blood flow patterns in healthy volunteers and patients. J. Comput. Assist. Tomogr. **28**, 459–468 (2004)
12. Markl, M., Chan, F.P., Alley, M.T., et al.: Time-resolved 3D phase-contrast MRI. J. Magn. Reson. Imag. **17**, 499–506 (2003)
13. Oñate, E., García, J., Idelsohn, S.R., del Pin, F.: Finite calculus formulation for finite element analysis of incompressible flows. Eulerian, ALE and Lagrangian approaches. Comput. Meth. Appl. Mech. Eng. Elsevier, Laussane (Switzerland) (2006). ISSN 0045-7825
14. Oñate, E., Valls, A., García, J.: FIC/FEM formulation with matrix stabilizing terms for incompressible flows at low and high Reynolds numbers. Comput. Mech. Springer, Berlin (2006). ISSN: 0178-7675 (Paper) 1432-0924 (Online)
15. Oñate, E., Valls, A., García, J.: Computation of turbulent flows using a Finite calculus – finite element formulation. Int. J. Numer. Meth. Fluid. Wiley, London (GB) (2007). ISSN 0271-2091
16. Oñate, E., Valls, A., García, J.: Modeling incompressible flow at low and high reynolds numbers via a Finite calculus–Finite element approach. J. Comput. Phys. Elsevier, New York (USA) (2007). ISSN 0021-9991
17. Perktold, K., et al.: Pulsatile non-Newtonian blood flow in three-dimensional carotid bifurcation models: a numerical study of flow phenomena under different bifurcation angles. J. Biomed. Eng. **13**, 507–515 (1991)
18. Perktold, K., Rappitsch, G.: Mathematical modeling of local arterial flow and vessel mechanics. In: Crolet, J., Ohayon, R. (eds.) Computational Methods for Fluid Structure Interaction, pp. 230–245. Wiley, New York (1994)
19. Schroeder, W., Martin, K., Lorensen, B.: Visualization toolkit. An Object-Oriented approach to 3D graphics, 4th edn. Kitware Inc. (2006)
20. Quartapelle, L.: Numerical solution of the incompressible Navier–Stokes equations. Birkhäuser Verlag, Basel (1993)
21. Taylor, C.A.: A Computation Framework for Investigating Hemodynamic Factors in Vascular Adaptation and Disease, Thesis. Stanford University, California, USA (1996)
22. Welch, B., Jones, K., Hobbs, J.: Practical programming in Tcl and Tk, 4th edn. Published by Prentice Hall, PTR (2003)
23. Schroeder, W., Martin, K., Lorensen, B.: The visualization toolkit. An Object-Oriented approach to 3D graphics, 4th edn. Kitware Inc. (2006)
24. van Steenhoven, A.A., van de Vossea, F.N., Rindt, C.C.M., Janssenu, J.D., Renemanb, R.S.: Experimental and numerical analysis of carotid arterv blood flow. Liepsch, D.W. (ed.) Blood Flow in Large Arteries: Applications to Atherogenesis and Clinical Medicine. Monogr Atheroscler, vol. 15, pp. 250–260. Basel, Karger (1990)
25. VTK User's Guide, Install, use and extent the visualization toolkit. Version 5, Kitware Inc. March 2010

KM and KHM Clustering Techniques for Colour Image Quantisation

Mariusz Frackiewicz and Henryk Palus

Abstract This paper deals with the comparison of two clustering techniques k-means (*KM*) and k-harmonic means (*KHM*) in the case of their use in colour image quantisation. The classical *KM* technique establishes good background for this comparison. Authors proposed two original heuristic initialisation methods, one arbitrary(*DC*) and one adaptive (*SD*), that were used in both techniques. Apart from specific validity indices for clustering, the results were also evaluated by means of average colour differences in RGB (*PSNR*) and CIELAB colour spaces (ΔE) and additionally difference of colourfulness (ΔM). Experimental tests realised on benchmark colour images show the superiority of *KHM* over *KM*. Other problems with both clustering techniques (e.g., empty clusters) have also been highlighted.

Keywords Colour image quantisation · k-means · k-harmonic means

1 Introduction

There is not a problem to observe that in each digital colour image we appear only a small subset of all possible 16.7 millions colours, limited by the number of pixels and the content of image. Colour image quantisation is the process of transformation of a true colour image (typically eight bit onto each colour component) into an image consisting of a small number of specially selected colours (colour palette). Colour quantisation is widely presented in colour image processing handbooks [5, 9].

New colours in quantisation process are selected by minimizing the colour difference between the original image and the quantised image. Low value of colour difference (quantisation error) needs a palette designed for the particular image, i.e. adaptive palette. The quantisation error depends on the number of unique colours in the original image, the number of colours in the palette (e.g., 8, 16, 32, 64, 128 or 256 colours), the method of choice of colours for the palette and the pixel classifying technique.

M. Frackiewicz (✉) and H. Palus
Silesian University of Technology, ul. Akademicka 16, 44-100 Gliwice, Poland
e-mail: Mariusz.Frackiewicz@polsl.pl; Henryk.Palus@polsl.pl

J.M.R.S. Tavares and R.M.N. Jorge (eds.), *Computational Vision and Medical Image Processing: Recent Trends*, Computational Methods in Applied Sciences 19,
DOI 10.1007/978-94-007-0011-6_9, © Springer Science+Business Media B.V. 2011

The colour quantisation is a kind of lossy compression technique. Colour quantisation is also very often used as an auxiliary operation in computer vision, computer graphics and multimedia. It can be helpful in image segmentation process as presegmentation stage [8] and applied in colour image watermarking [26]. Colour quantisation is also an important step in content-based image retrieval (CBIR) systems based on colour histograms with reduced dimensions [28]. Algorithms of colour quantisation are still used to present the true colour images on devices with limited number of colours. A good example of such case can be the display on a mobile phone.

The paper will be organized as follows. In Sect. 2, we will introduce both clustering techniques used in colour quantisation. In Sect. 3, will be presented three criteria used for the evaluation of quantisation. The experimental results, mainly comparison tests, will be described in Sect. 4. The hints for solving problems of initialisation and avoiding empty clusters will be contained in Sects. 5 and 6. Finally, we will conclude this chapter in Sect. 7.

2 Clustering Techniques

Clustering is the process of partitioning a set of objects (pattern vectors) into subsets of similar objects called clusters. Pixel clustering in three-dimensional colour space on the basis of their colour similarity is one of approaches in the field of colour quantisation. Clustering is often seen as an unsupervised classification of pixels on the base of its colours similarity. Colours, dominated in the image and corresponding to objects, create dense clusters in the colour space in a natural way.

2.1 KM Technique

One of the most popular and fastest clustering techniques is the k-means (*KM*) technique. *KM* has been developed in the sixties [19] and has been described in classical Anderberg's handbook [1]. During the first step of *KM* algorithm a fixed number of clusters and initial cluster centres in the colour space are chosen. The main idea is to modify the positions of cluster centres so long as the sum of distances between all points of clusters and their cluster centres will be minimal. During these modifications all points are allocated to closest cluster centres using a predefined e.g. Euclidean metric. After each allocation a new positions of cluster centres are computed as arithmetical means of cluster points. The algorithm usually stops if the difference between new and old positions of cluster centres is less than the previously defined value of threshold.

In general *KM* converges to a locally optimal solution. The results of *KM* depend on different factors such as method of determination of initial cluster centres, used colour space, applied metric etc. Such sensitivity to initialisation is an important disadvantage of *KM* technique. On the other hand there is one of the fastest methods to perform clustering.

2.2 KHM Technique

Bin Zhang [30, 31] has proposed a few years ago a new improved version of *KM* based on harmonic means, instead of arithmetic means, and named k-harmonic means (*KHM*). We assumed that a colour image contains n pixels and is treated as clustering data set $X = \{x_1, \ldots, x_n\}$. During the initialisation step the number of clusters k and values of starting cluster centres $C = \{c_1, \ldots, c_k\}$ are determined. Additionally, the *KHM* technique needs an input parameter p, that should be equal or larger than two. The membership function $m(c_j|x_i)$ defines the degree of membership of x_i pixel in the cluster with the centre c_j [16]. This function has following basic properties:

$$\begin{cases} m(c_j|x_i) \geq 0 \\ \sum_{j=1}^{k} m(c_j|x_i) = 1 \end{cases} \tag{1}$$

In the case of *KM* technique a "hard membership" is applied:

$$m(c_j|x_i) \in \{0, 1\} \tag{2}$$

$$m(c_j|x_i) = \begin{cases} 1 \text{ } if \text{ } l = arg \underbrace{min}_{j} \|x_i - c_j\|^2 \\ 0 \text{ } otherwise \end{cases} \tag{3}$$

In the case of *KHM* technique a "soft membership" is applied:

$$0 \leq m(c_j|x_i) \leq 1 \tag{4}$$

$$m(c_j|x_i) = \frac{\|x_i - c_j\|^{-p-2}}{\sum_{j=1}^{k} \|x_i - c_j\|^{-p-2}} \tag{5}$$

The weight function $w(x_i)$ defines an influence of pixel x_i on computing new components of cluster centre c_k. This function has following basic properties:

$$w(x_i) > 0 \tag{6}$$

but in the case of *KM* we have:

$$w(x_i) = 1 \tag{7}$$

In the case of *KHM* technique following variable weights are applied:

$$w(x_i) = \frac{\sum_{j=1}^{k} \|x_i - c_j\|^{-p-2}}{\left(\sum_{j=1}^{k} \|x_i - c_j\|^{-p}\right)^2} \tag{8}$$

We calculate new cluster centres using a formula that is common for both *KM* and *KHM* techniques:

$$C_j = \frac{\sum_{i=1}^{n} m(c_j|x_i)w(x_i)x_i}{\sum_{i=1}^{n} m(c_j|x_i)w(x_i)} \tag{9}$$

The *KM* technique minimizes following objective function:

$$KM(X,C) = \sum_{i=1}^{n} \min_{j\in\{1\ldots k\}} \left\| x_i - c_j \right\|^2 \tag{10}$$

The *KHM* technique minimizes following objective function:

$$KHM(X,C) = \sum_{i=1}^{n} \frac{k}{\sum_{j=1}^{k} \frac{1}{\left\| x_i - c_j \right\|^p}} \tag{11}$$

The clustering process can be organized in different colour spaces. Among colour spaces a special role plays the CIELAB colour space [29]. The Euclidean distance in this space is approximately equal to the perceptual difference between colours. Therefore we investigated colour quantisation using both spaces: basic RGB and perceptually uniform CIELAB space.

The *KHM* technique has recently attracted much attention in the field of image segmentation, e.g. colour images [15], MR images [10] and multispectral images [18]. This algorithm has been applied also to telecommunication systems [2], economical models [11] and flexible manufacturing systems [14]. Nowadays, the results from *KHM* are additionally improved by using such modern optimization techniques as simulated annealing (SA) [12], tabu search (TS) [13] and particle swarm optimization (PSO) [27].

3 Tools for Evaluation of Quantisers

Both *KM* and *KHM* techniques were tested in RGB and CIELAB colour spaces. Objective image quality measures are very important in the evaluation process of different colour quantisers. Commonly used measures are Mean Squared Error (*MSE*) and average colour difference in CIELAB colour space (ΔE). The *MSE* for colour image is defined by:

$$MSE = \frac{1}{MN} \sum_{i=1}^{M} \sum_{j=1}^{N} \left[(R_{ij} - R_{ij}^*)^2 + (G_{ij} - G_{ij}^*)^2 + (B_{ij} - B_{ij}^*)^2 \right] \tag{12}$$

where M and N are the image dimensions in pixels, R_{ij}, G_{ij}, B_{ij} are colour components of the pixel of location (i, j) in original image and R_{ij}^*, G_{ij}^*, B_{ij}^* are colour components of the pixel in quantised image. The smaller the *MSE* value, the better is the quantised image. Unfortunately, this measure sometimes bad correlates with subjective visual quality of image. Other common error measure applied to evaluation of quantisation is Peak Signal-to-Noise Ratio (*PSNR*), related with *MSE* directly.

Next quality measure ΔE, which takes the colorimetric aspects into account, can be expressed as:

$$\Delta E = \frac{1}{MN}\sum_{i=1}^{M}\sum_{j=1}^{N}\sqrt{(L_{ij} - L_{ij}^{*})^2 + (a_{ij} - a_{ij}^{*})^2 + (b_{ij} - b_{ij}^{*})^2} \tag{13}$$

where L_{ij}, a_{ij}, b_{ij} denote the colour components of the pixel of location (i, j) in original image and L_{ij}^{*}, a_{ij}^{*}, b_{ij}^{*} are CIELAB colour components of the pixel in quantised image.

Additional third measure of quantisation error is based on the idea of colourfulness of the image. If we assume that the colourfulness of image calculated after colour quantisation should be equal to the colourfulness of original image, then we can use following difference of colourfulness as a tool for evaluation of quantisation [22]:

$$\Delta M = \left| M_{orig} - M_{quant} \right| \tag{14}$$

where M_{orig} is the colourfulness of original image and M_{quant} is the colourfulness of quantised image. Above formula became with success applied also to colour image filtering [23].

According to [17] the colourfulness of image can be computed using following formula:

$$M = \sqrt{\sigma_{rg}^2 + \sigma_{yb}^2} + 0.3\sqrt{\mu_{rg}^2 + \mu_{yb}^2} \tag{15}$$

where σ_{rg}, σ_{yb} are the standard deviations and μ_{rg}, μ_{yb} are the mean values of opponent colour components of the image pixels. The opponent components are approximated by following simplified equation:

$$rg = R - G \tag{16}$$

$$yb = 0.5(R + G) - B \tag{17}$$

where rg – red-green opponency, yb – yellow-blue opponency.

Formulae for computing of colourfulness are simple and good correlate with the perceptual colourfulness of the image, which was confirmed experimentally in [17].

4 KM versus KHM: Comparison Tests

The first comparison tests have been performed with the use of colour rendition chart named ColorChecker Chart (X-Rite, USA). This chart, proposed more than thirty years ago for colour investigations in such branches of colour imaging technology as photography, television and graphic arts [21], includes 24 specially prepared colour patches that have strictly defined colorimetric coordinates in the standard colour systems. The digital image Chart (640 × 480 pixels) has been acquired in good illumination conditions. This image was quantised into 25 colours (all 24 patches and background).

Figures 1 and 2 present quantisations results in RGB and CIELAB spaces for both investigated techniques with the use of DC and SD initialisations (see the Sect. 5). We visually evaluated results: all colour patches with perceived colour errors have been marked by multiplication signs (X). The number of these signs in case of KHM is much smaller than in case of KM technique (5 versus 29).

The quantitative evaluation needs clustering validity indexes or measures of quantisation quality. Basic indexes of cluster validity can be defined as [24]:

$$VM_1 = 10\,000\,\frac{Intra}{Inter_1} \tag{18}$$

$$VM_2 = 10\,000\,\frac{Intra}{Inter_2} \tag{19}$$

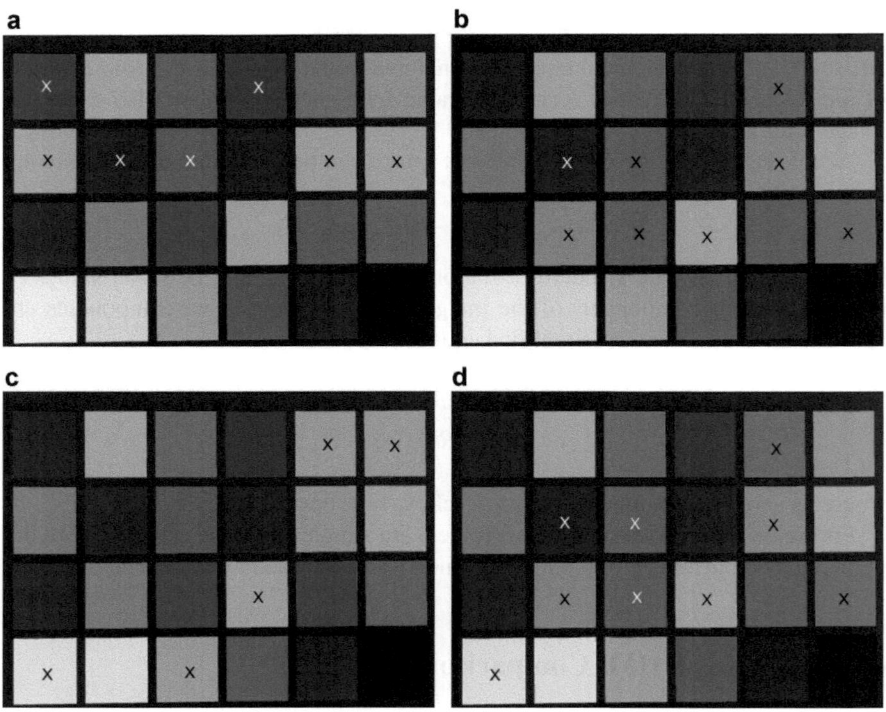

Fig. 1 *KM* quantisation results for the Chart image ($k = 25$): (**a**) RGB space, DC initialisation, (**b**) LAB space, DC initialisation, (**c**) RGB space, SD initialisation, (**d**) LAB space, SD initialisation

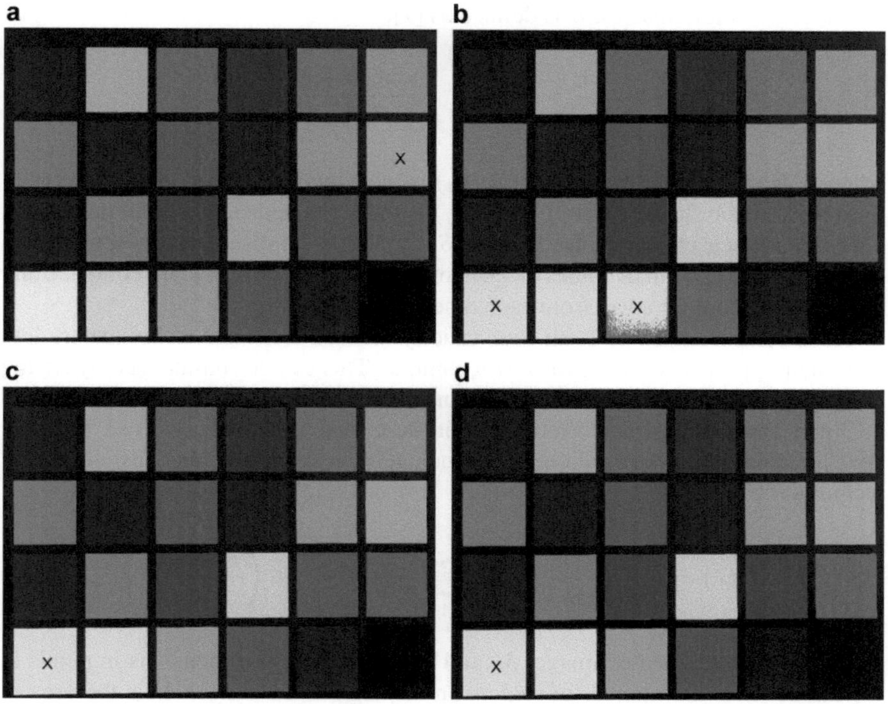

Fig. 2 *KHM* quantisation results for the Chart image ($k = 25$): (**a**) RGB space, *DC* initialisation, (**b**) LAB space, *DC* initialisation, (**c**) RGB space, *SD* initialisation, (**d**) LAB space, *SD* initialisation

where *Intra* and $Inter_1$, $Inter_2$ are average intra-cluster and inter-cluster distances. The intra-cluster distance measures the within cluster variability (cluster compactness):

$$Intra = \frac{1}{MN} \sum_{j=1}^{k} \sum_{x \in K_j} \|x - C_j\|^2 \tag{20}$$

where M and N are the image dimensions, k is the number of clusters and C_j is the cluster centre of the cluster K_j. The inter-cluster distance, complimentary to the intra-cluster distance, is a measure of separation between cluster centres:

$$Inter_1 = \sum_{i=1}^{k-1} \sum_{j=i+1}^{k} \left(\|C_i - C_j\|\right)^2 \tag{21}$$

$$Inter_2 = \min\left(\|C_i - C_j\|\right)^2 \tag{22}$$

where $i = 1, 2, \ldots, k - 1$ and $j = i + 1, \ldots, k$.

Davies–Bouldin index *DB* is defined as [7]:

$$DB = \frac{1}{k}\sum_{i=1}^{n} \max_{i=1, i \neq j} \left\{ \frac{S_n(C_i) + S_n(C_j)}{S(C_i, C_j)} \right\} \tag{23}$$

where k is the number of clusters, $S_n(C_i)$ is the average distance of all patterns in cluster i to their cluster centre C_i, $S_n(C_j)$ is the average distance of all patterns in cluster j to their cluster centre C_j, and $S(C_i, C_j)$ is the distance between clusters centres C_i and C_j. Small values of *DB* correspond to clusters that are compact, and whose centers are far away from each other.

As is clear from Table 1, all four validity indexes for *KHM* technique are less than their appropriate values for *KM* technique. This can be summarised by saying that the *KHM* generates for image Chart much better structure of pixel clusters.

Apart from three quantisation criteria described in Sect. 3, we can also use special function for evaluation of segmentation results generated by clustering techniques [3]:

$$Q(I) = \frac{1}{10\,000MN}\sqrt{R}\sum_{i=1}^{R}\left[\frac{e_i^2}{1+\log A_i} + \left(\frac{R(A_i)}{A_i}\right)^2\right] \tag{24}$$

where I is the segmented image, M and N are the image dimensions in pixels in the image, R is the number of regions in the segmented image, A_i is the area of the region i, $R(A_i)$ is the number of regions having an area equal to A_i and e_i is the colour error of region i. The colour error in RGB space is calculated as the sum of the Euclidean distances between colour components of pixels of region and components of average colour, which is an attribute of this region in the segmented image. The colour errors in different colour spaces are not comparable and therefore are transformed back to the RGB space. First term of (24) is a normalization factor, the second term penalizes results with too many regions (oversegmentation), and the third term penalizes results with non-homogeneous regions. Last term is scaled by the area factor because the colour error is higher for large regions. The main idea of using this kind of function can be formulated as follows: the lower the value of $Q(I)$, the better is the segmentation result.

Table 1 Validity indexes for the image chart

	Intra		VM_1		VM_2		*DB*	
KM	RGB	LAB	RGB	LAB	RGB	LAB	RGB	LAB
Chart_DC	564	688	0.538	0.738	34 789	28 822	0.592	0.900
Chart_SD	270	710	0.321	0.909	18 324	30 230	0.568	1.046
	Intra		VM_1		VM_2		*DB*	
KHM	RGB	LAB	RGB	LAB	RGB	LAB	RGB	LAB
Chart_ DC	100	300	0.110	0.343	1 841	12 352	0.398	0.696
Chart_SD	94	132	0.106	0.152	1 686	1 706	0.431	0.475

Table 2 Quantisation errors for the image chart

	PSNR		ΔE		ΔM		$Q(I)$	
KM	RGB	LAB	RGB	LAB	RGB	LAB	RGB	LAB
Chart_DC	25.35	24.51	8.43	3.99	3.73	5.76	5 952	7 275
Chart_SD	28.57	24.37	5.26	2.03	3.77	6.02	2 646	6 858
	PSNR		ΔE		ΔM		$Q(I)$	
KHM	RGB	LAB	RGB	LAB	RGB	LAB	RGB	LAB
Chart_DC	32.96	28.13	3.19	0.57	0.99	3.17	795	2 108
Chart_SD	33.25	31.72	2.76	0.56	0.66	2.81	752	1 179

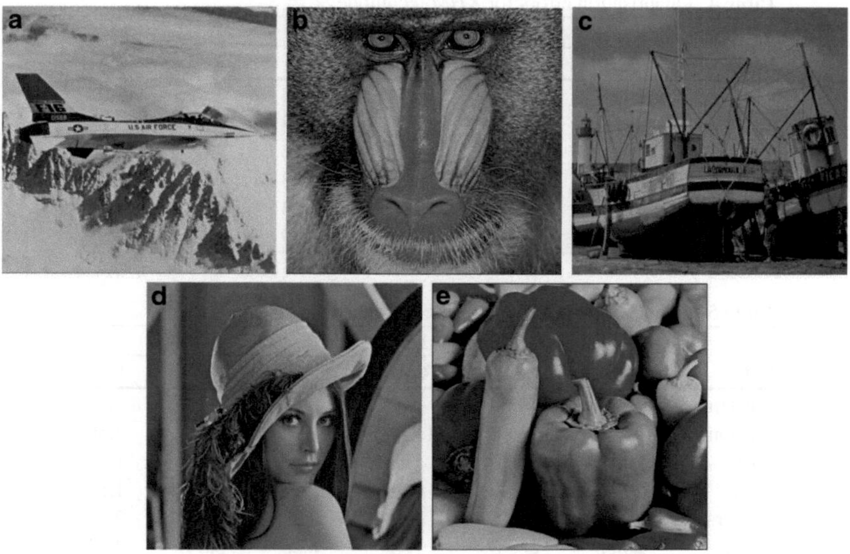

Fig. 3 Test images used in the experiment: (**a**) Airplane, (**b**) Baboon, (**c**) Boats, (**d**) Lena, (**e**) Peppers

As is clear from Table 2, all four measures give better results for *KHM* technique than for *KM* technique. This can be summarised by saying that the *KHM* generates for image Chart much better quantised and segmented images.

For further experiments a representative set of five test images has been chosen. All images are commonly used in the community of colour image processing. These images have the same spatial resolution (512 × 512 pixels) and are presented in Fig. 3. During tests the images were quantised into 8 and 16 colours.

Tables 3–6 show the results of comparison different measures of quantisation errors. The colour quantisation is better if $PSNR$ value is higher and errors ΔE and ΔM are smaller. During analysis of experimental results we can observe some ambivalence: if we use for evaluation $PSNR$ values (based on RGB space) then we achieve that quantisations in the case of RGB-based *KM* and *KHM* techniques are

Table 3 Quantisation errors for *KM* technique, $k = 8$

	PSNR		ΔE		ΔM	
KM	RGB	LAB	RGB	LAB	RGB	LAB
Airplane	27.86	27.00	5.01	4.66	8.29	5.39
Baboon	22.42	20.24	14.50	12.97	7.51	5.68
Boats	26.85	25.76	7.26	6.56	8.19	3.45
Lena	26.87	25.75	8.39	7.24	5.26	3.06
Peppers	24.62	22.96	10.59	9.59	4.65	3.84
Overall	**25.72**	**24.34**	**9.15**	**8.20**	**6.78**	**4.28**

Table 4 Quantisation errors for *KHM* technique, $k = 8$

	PSNR		ΔE		ΔM	
KHM	RGB	LAB	RGB	LAB	RGB	LAB
Airplane	29.69	28.84	4.57	4.35	4.49	3.84
Baboon	22.32	20.33	14.72	12.88	6.55	5.08
Boats	26.74	25.56	7.28	6.73	8.05	3.23
Lena	26.44	25.70	8.45	7.33	6.38	2.70
Peppers	24.59	22.93	10.62	9.64	4.19	4.38
Overall	**25.96**	**24.67**	**9.13**	**8.19**	**5.93**	**3.85**

Table 5 Quantisation errors for *KM* technique, $k = 16$

	PSNR		ΔE		ΔM	
KM	RGB	LAB	RGB	LAB	RGB	LAB
Airplane	31.34	30.09	3.87	3.46	3.46	3.37
Baboon	24.84	23.18	11.60	10.01	4.33	3.56
Boats	29.88	28.20	5.53	4.95	3.77	1.90
Lena	29.49	27.80	6.30	5.51	2.71	1.57
Peppers	27.11	25.46	8.32	7.33	2.45	2.27
Overall	**28.53**	**26.95**	**7.12**	**6.25**	**3.34**	**2.53**

Table 6 Quantisation errors for *KHM* technique, $k = 16$

	PSNR		ΔE		ΔM	
KHM	RGB	LAB	RGB	LAB	RGB	LAB
Airplane	32.36	31.25	3.72	3.31	3.43	3.14
Baboon	24.76	22.58	11.61	10.20	4.40	3.47
Boats	29.74	28.43	5.39	4.86	3.92	1.81
Lena	29.32	27.87	6.34	5.42	2.97	1.77
Peppers	27.10	25.07	8.25	7.23	2.62	2.06
Overall	**28.66**	**27.04**	**7.06**	**6.20**	**3.47**	**2.45**

better than in the case of CIELAB-based techniques. But if we use for evaluation ΔE values (based on CIELAB space) then we achieve that quantisations are better in the case of CIELAB-based techniques. The use of additional criterion ΔM solves this contradiction. The change of colourfulness is smaller if we use CIELAB space for both *KM* and *KHM* techniques. Therefore our final choice of colour space is CIELAB space. If we compare *KHM* to the *KM*, both realized in CIELAB space, we observe that all three average values of criterion are better in the case of *KHM*.

Clustering techniques, used in described experiments, needed to define some parameters. We established, that the number of iterations was equal to 15 and, in the case of *KHM*, we chose the value of parameter $p = 2.7$. It is compliant with the authors of KHM proposal [31]. We applied to both cases (*KM*, *KHM*) the same adaptive method of initialisation named SD, that is described in the next section.

5 Choice of Initialisation Method

Some clustering techniques, also *KM* and *KHM*, need a priori information about initial cluster centres, i.e. starting points of algorithm. Classical version of *KM* uses random initialisation methods. Sometimes these methods generate empty clusters. From point of view of optimisation theory we should consider that no single method of initialisation will guarantee the achievement of global minimum for objective function. Both clustering techniques need automatic initialisation methods which lead to good local minimum. Efficient initialisation methods are still active field of research [6].

We have tested two deterministic initialisation methods: one arbitrary and one adaptive method. The first method is based on uniform partitioning of diagonal of RGB cube (DC) and in the second is used the size of pixel cloud of colour image and it is marked as SD.

First, the mean values and standard deviations (SD) for each RGB component of all image pixels are calculated. Next, each standard deviation determines surroundings of corresponding mean values, which are then uniformly splitted into k equal intervals. The centres of these intervals are colour components of initial cluster centres.

Tables 7 and 8 present the results of comparison both initialisation methods for *KM* and *KHM* techniques. We can observe that SD adaptive initialisation is a bit better than DC initialisation. The *KHM* technique is less sensitive to initialisation and needs computationally faster variants similarly to recently realized fast FCM clustering techniques, which were described in work [25].

Table 7 Quantisation errors for tested initialisations of *KM*

	PSNR		ΔE		ΔM	
KM	DC	SD	DC	SD	DC	SD
Airplane	30.81	30.09	3.42	3.46	2.84	3.37
Baboon	23.22	23.18	10.16	10.01	3.85	3.56
Boats	27.82	28.20	5.16	4.95	2.19	1.90
Lena	27.50	27.80	5.77	5.51	1.98	1.57
Peppers	25.37	25.46	7.21	7.33	2.57	2.27
Overall	**26.94**	**26.95**	**6.34**	**6.25**	**2.69**	**2.53**

Table 8 Quantisation errors for tested initialisations of *KHM*

	PSNR		ΔE		ΔM	
KHM	*DC*	*SD*	*DC*	*SD*	*DC*	*SD*
Airplane	31.12	31.25	3.47	3.31	3.30	3.14
Baboon	22.78	22.58	10.37	10.20	2.96	3.47
Boats	28.28	28.43	4.91	4.86	2.03	1.81
Lena	27.78	27.87	5.43	5.42	1.53	1.77
Peppers	25.21	25.07	7.22	7.23	2.55	2.06
Overall	**27.03**	**27.04**	**6.28**	**6.20**	**2.47**	**2.45**

Table 9 The number of empty clusters (*KM* technique)

	$DC,\ k = 25$		$SD,\ k = 25$	
KM	RGB	LAB	RGB	LAB
Chart	1	0	0	0

Table 10 The number of empty clusters (*KM* technique)

	$DC,\ k = 8$		$SD,\ k = 8$		$DC,\ k = 16$		$SD,\ k = 16$		$DC,\ k = 32$		$SD,\ k = 32$	
KM	RGB	LAB	RGB	LAB	RGB	LAB	RGB	LAB	RGB	LAB	RGB	LAB
Airplane	2	1	0	0	2	1	0	0	6	3	0	0
Baboon	0	0	0	0	1	0	0	0	1	0	0	0
Boats	0	0	0	0	1	2	0	0	5	4	0	0
Lena	1	1	0	0	2	2	0	0	5	3	0	0
Peppers	0	0	0	0	0	0	0	0	0	0	0	0

6 Empty Clusters

KM and *KHM* techniques need "good" initialisations what means high quality clustering achieved by small number of iterations. "Good" initialisation should not lead to formation of empty clusters during clustering process, i.e. any centre of cluster should not remain empty. If a cluster becomes empty then the unique number of colours in quantised image will be smaller than k. In such case the quantisation technique needs an additional repairing procedure of solve the problem of empty clusters by changing their centres or splitting a newly created cluster. Therefore sometimes are developed clustering methods that, during clustering process, limit a minimum size of each cluster [4].

It was checked how many empty clusters comes into being during pixel clustering by *KM* and *KHM* techniques with different initialisations. First for the image Chart quantised into 25 clusters. Table 9 shows that KM might produce empty clusters. The KHM technique in this case, in contrast to KM, returns only non-empty clusters. In the following Table 10 are presented the numbers of empty clusters for five benchmark images quantised by *KM* technique.

This research confirms that DC initialisation in *KM* technique for some images generates empty clusters. If k is increased then the number of empty clusters is increased too. Therefore we can see the sense of applying the SD method of initialisation. Results for SD initialisation presented in both tables are encouraging. During tests of 300 colour images from image data base accessible on the University of Berkeley (USA) webpage [20] we have find for SD only few cases of empty clusters. The *KHM* technique always creates non-empty clusters.

7 Conclusions

We proposed a new approach to colour image quantisation, based on *KHM* clustering. This approach reduces the quantisation errors expressed as $PSNR$, ΔE and ΔM and is less sensitive to initialisation than *KM* technique. *KHM* technique does not generate empty clusters. The general drawback of *KM* and *KHM* techniques in comparison with non-iterative algorithms of colour quantisation is its longer execution time. The further research will be focused on using the new perceptual colour metric (CIEDE 2000) and accelerating computations for clustering processes by parallel programming and using GPU card.

Acknowledgements This work has been supported by the Polish Ministry of Science and Higher Education under RD grant no. N N516 374736 from the Science Budget 2009–2011.

References

1. Anderberg, M.: Cluster Analysis for Applications. Academic Press, New York, USA (1973)
2. Boppana, D., Rao, S.: Clustering-based blind maximum likelihood sequence detection for GSM and TDMA systems. In: Proceedings of the 45th Midwest Symposium on Circuits and Systems, vol. 1, pp. 427–430. Tulsa, OK, USA (2002)
3. Borsotti, M., Campadelli, P., Schettini, R.: Quantitative evaluation of color image segmentation results. Pattern Recogn. Lett. **19**(8), 741–747 (1998)
4. Bradley, P.S., Bennett, K.P., Demiriz, A.: Constrained k-means clustering. Tech. Rep. MSR-TR-2000-65, Microsoft Research, Redmond, WA, USA (2000)
5. Brun, L., Tremeau, A.: Digital color imaging handbook, chapter Color quantization, pp. 589–637. CRC Press, Boca Raton, FA, USA (2003)
6. Celebi, M.: Effective initialization of k-means for color quantization. In: Proceedings of the IEEE International Conference on Image Processing (ICIP2009), Cairo, Egypt (2009)
7. Davies, D., Bouldin, D.: A cluster separation measure. IEEE Trans. Pattern Anal. Mach. Intell. **1**(4), 224–227 (1979)
8. Deng, Y., Manjunath, B.: Unsupervised segmentation of color-texture regions in images and video. IEEE Trans. Pattern Anal. Mach. Intell. **23**(8), 800–810 (2001)
9. Domański, M., Bartkowiak, M.: The colour image processing handbook, chapter Compression, pp. 242–304. Chapman and Hall, London, UK (1998)
10. Ekin, A., Jasinschi, R.: A robust thresholding method with applications to brain MR image segmentation. In: Proceedings of EUSIPCO, Florence, Italy (2006)
11. Giordani, P., Kohn, R.: Adaptive independent Metropolis-Hastings by fast estimation of mixture of normals. http://www.riksbank.com/upload/research/conferences/bayes2006/aimh_august1.pdf

12. Güngör, Z., Ünler, A.: K-harmonic means data clustering with simulated annealing heuristic. Appl. Math. Comput. **184**(2), 199–209 (2007)
13. Güngör, Z., Ünler, A.: K-harmonic means data clustering with tabu-search method. Appl. Math. Model. **32**(2), 1115–1125 (2008)
14. Güngör, Z., Ünler, A.: Applying k-harmonic means clustering to the part-machine classification problem. Expet. Syst. Appl. **36**(2), 1179–1194 (2009)
15. Hamerly, G., Elkan, C.: Alternatives to the k-means algorithm that find better clusterings. In: Proceedings of the 11th ACM Conference on Information and Knowledge Management (CIKM2002), McLean, VA, USA, pp. 600–607 (2002)
16. Hamerly, G.J.: Learning structure and concepts in data through data clustering. Ph.D. Thesis, University of California, San Diego (2003)
17. Hasler, D., Suesstrunk, S.: Measuring colourfulness for natural images. In: Electronic Imaging 2003: Human Vision and Electronic Imaging VIII, Proceedings of SPIE, vol. 5007, pp. 87–95 (2003)
18. Li, Q., Mitianoudis, N., Stathaki, T.: Spatial kernel k-harmonic means clustering for multi-spectral image thresholding. IET Image Process. **1**(2), 156–167 (2007)
19. Mac Queen, J.: Some methods for classification and analysis of multivariate observations. In: Proceedings of the 5th Berkeley Symposium on Mathematics, Statistics, and Probabilities, vol. I, pp. 281–297. Berkeley and Los Angeles, CA, USA (1967)
20. Martin, D., Fowlkes, C., Tal, D., Malik, J.: A database of human segmented natural images and its application to evaluating segmentation algorithms and measuring ecological statistics. In: Proceedings of the 8th International Conference on Computer Vision, pp. 416–423. Vancouver, BC, Canada (2001)
21. McCamy, C., Marcus, H., Davidson, J.: A color rendition chart. J. Appl. Photogr. Eng. **2**(3), 95–99 (1976)
22. Palus, H.: On color image quantization by the k-means algorithm. In: Droege, D., Paulus, D. (eds.) Proceedings of 10. Workshop Farbbildverarbeitung, pp. 58–65. Toenning, Germany (2004)
23. Palus, H.: Colourfulness of the image and its application in image filtering. In: Proceedings of 5th IEEE International Symposium on Signal Processing and Information Technology (ISSPIT 2005), pp. 884–889. Athens, Greece (2005)
24. Ray, S., Turi, R.: Determination of number of clusters in k-means clustering and application in colour image segmentation. In: Proceedings of the 4th International Conference on Advances in Pattern Recognition and Digital Techniques, pp. 137–143. Calcutta, India (1999)
25. Schaefer, R., Zhou, H.: Fuzzy clustering for colour reduction in images. Telecommun. Syst. **40**, 17–25 (2009)
26. Tsai, P., Hu, Y., Chang, C.: A color image watermarking scheme based on color quantization. Signal Process. **84**(1), 95–106 (2004)
27. Ünler, A., Güngör, Z.: Particle swarm optimization based k-harmonic means data clustering. In: Proceedings of the 38th International Conference on Computers and Industrial Engineering, vol. 1, pp. 379–387. Beijing, China (2008)
28. Wang, M., Yang, W., Acharya, R.: Color clustering techniques for color content-based image retrieval from image databases. In: Proceedings of IEEE International Conference on Multimedia Computing and Systems, pp. 442–449. Ottawa, Canada (1997)
29. Wyszecki, G., Stiles, W.: Color Science: Concepts and Methods, Quantitative Data and Formulae. Wiley, New York, USA (1982)
30. Zhang, B.: Generalized k-harmonic means – boosting in unsupervised learning. Tech. Rep. TR HPL-2000-137, Hewlett Packard Labs, Palo Alto, CA, USA (2000)
31. Zhang, B., Hsu, M., Dayal, U.: K-harmonic means – data clustering algorithm. Tech. Rep. TR HPL-1999-124, Hewlett Packard Labs, Palo Alto, CA, USA (1999)

Caries Detection in Panoramic Dental X-ray Images

João Oliveira and Hugo Proença

Abstract Dental Caries, also known as dental decay or tooth decay, is defined as a disease of the hard tissues of the teeth caused by the action of microorganisms found in plaque on fermentable carbohydrates (principally sugars). Therefore, the detection of dental caries in a preliminary stage is an important task. This chapter has two major purposes: firstly to announce the availability of a new data set of panoramic dental X-ray images. This data set contains 1,392 images with varying types of noise, usually inherent to this kind of images. Second, to present a complete case study for the detection of dental caries in panoramic dental X-ray images.

Keywords Caries Detection · Medical Diagnosis · Image Classification

1 Introduction

Dental Caries, also know as tooth decay, are a preventable disease. Given its dynamic nature, once established, they can be treated or reversed prior to significant cavitation takes place. Primary diagnosis involves visual inspection of all the visible tooth surfaces. Dental radiographs (X-rays) may show dental caries before they are visible, particularly caries between the teeth. Large dental caries are usually apparent to the human observer, but smaller lesions can be difficult to detect. Visual and tactile inspections along with radiographs are therefore employed frequently among dentists.

1.1 Dental X-ray

Dental X-rays are pictures of the teeth, bones, and soft tissues around them that help find problems within the teeth, mouth, and jaws. X-ray pictures reveal

J. Oliveira (✉) and H. Proença
Department of Computer Science, IT - Instituto de Telecomunicações, University of Beira Interior, Covilhã, Portugal
e-mail: joaopoli@gmail.com

J.M.R.S. Tavares and R.M.N. Jorge (eds.), *Computational Vision and Medical Image Processing: Recent Trends*, Computational Methods in Applied Sciences 19,
DOI 10.1007/978-94-007-0011-6_10,

cavities, hidden dental structures, and bone loss that cannot be seen during a visual examination. Dental X-rays may also be done as follow-up after dental treatment. There are three main different types of dental X-ray: bitewing, periapical and panoramic. A full-mouth series of periapical X-rays are most often done during a person's first visit to the dentist. Bitewing X-rays are used during checkups to look for tooth decay. Panoramic X-rays may be used occasionally, depending on the expert opinion.

1.2 Main Applications

Automated image analysis processes have been achieving higher relevance for many purposes and the results can be considered satisfactory. In the specific area of medical image processing, the detection of health situations as earliest as possible increases the role of such automated systems.

1.3 Clinical Environments

Dental X-ray images are also used in clinical environments, in the detection and prediction of Bone Mineral Density (BMD) for the diagnosis of osteoporosis. In [11] authors assessed the trabecular pattern of dental X-rays to predict BMD.

In [12] authors proposed a framework to segment dental X-ray images. The segmentation contains two phases: training, in which they manually selected images representative of the whole. These images are segmented based on a hierarchy of regions of detectable "level set". Further features are extracted by Principal Component Analysis (PCA) [10], and feed a Support Vector Machine (SVM) classifier scheme [5, 13]. In the segmentation of new data the SVM provides the initial contours corresponding to the possible lesion region.

1.4 Biometrics

Dental X-ray are also used for the identification of deceased individuals [9]. This process is based on the comparison of the Ante-Mortem (AM) and Post-Mortem (PM) dental X-rays. In [4] the tooth contour is extracted for matching purposes of dental radiographs, which is done by the directional snake process [15]. Three main stages are performed: initialization, convergence to the gradient and an adjustment at the end of the process. In the first stage authors initialize the snake, for that the gumline detection is performed. The gumline is the "visual line" that separates the root area from the crown area. The method takes advantage of the fact that there is an intensity increase at the gum lines from the crow area to the root area. The Gradient

Vector Flow (GVF) field of the edges detected by the Canny operator is used as the external energy for the convergence gradient stage. In the final stage the fine adjustments are based on the fact that true pixels boundaries always had in their neighbor pixels of lower intensities. The external energy is defined by (1), where $E_{ext,1}$ is the external energy of the teeth boundaries, $E_{ext,2}$ corresponds to the image intensity and ω controls the trade-off between the gradient and the intensity. The results of this paper are quite interesting, but it should be noted that authors simply applied the method to bitewing dental X-ray images, that are much more easier to handle, due to the limited amount of available information.

$$E_{ext} = E_{ext,1} + \omega E_{ext,2} \tag{1}$$

In [3] the matching of dental X-ray images for human identification, is based on the gap valley detection, tooth isolation, contour extraction (crown and root) and in the contours matching edge. This method is manually initialized, where the user is asked to mark a point between jaws. Further, the horizontal projection of the intensities is calculated, being expected that near this point will be a gap intensity valley. Based on this, using the probability function:

$$p_{v_i}(D_i, y_i) = p_{v_i}(D_i) p_{v_i}(y_i), \tag{2}$$

where

$$p_{v_i}(D_i) = c\left(1 - \frac{D_i}{\max_k D_k}\right), \tag{3}$$

and

$$p_{v_i}(y_i) = \frac{1}{\sqrt{2\Pi}\sigma} e^{-(y_i - y)^2 \div \sigma^2}. \tag{4}$$

A set of points were extracted and connected with a spline function into a smooth curve. Hereinafter the teeth gap valley detection is based on the sum of intensities of the perpendicular lines to the boundary. The tooth isolation is obtained through the previous step, i.e., each pair of consecutive perpendicular lines contain a single tooth between them. The contour extraction is based in the probability of each pixel in the Region of Interest (ROI), which in this case corresponds to the isolated tooth, belonging to the ROI, starting from the center of the region targeted in the previous steps. Finally, the contour comparison is performed in order to obtain human identification. Despite the good results obtained by the authors, this method is very dependent on the users input as a wrong initialization point has the consequence of not yielding any segmented tooth.

1.5 Teeth Segmentation

Segmentation is known to be one of the most difficult image processing tasks and it plays an important role in most subsequent image analysis stages, namely in pattern recognition and matching. Segmentation consists in the partitioning of an image into its constituent regions and in the extraction of the objects of interest. However, there is no image segmentation technique that performs well in all problems. In addition, the performance of a segmentation technique is greatly affected by images noise.

In [16], authors performed the teeth segmentation in digitalized dental X-ray films using mathematical morphology, proposing new approach to the problem of identification of the PM through dental X-rays. Mathematical morphological method are used in the segmentation of teeth and a decrease in processing of contrast in grayscale to improve the segmentation problem. The ROI is a rectangular area in the original image containing a tooth. The three main rules for the extraction are, firstly the retrieving of the largest possible number of teeth, secondly only operate in bitewing and periapical X-rays and finally in the worst case extract at least one tooth per image. To perform the segmentation authors divided the grayscale range into three regions: brightest areas that corresponds to teeth, middle areas that correspond to the bones and finally the darkest areas concerning the background.

The segmentation process is divided into four main stages, firstly the internal noise filtering that consists in the teeth gap valley detection and in the partitioning of the jaws. This step uses both horizontal and vertical projection of the sum intensities for the detection of the gap valley between the upper and the lower jaw. Secondly is the threshold operation, where the main goal is to divide the teeth from the background and the dental bones. Due to the shading effect present in the images, the extraction of only one threshold is not advisable. Therefore, the extraction of three thresholds was performed, based on the cumulative histogram of the filtered images. Next we perform labeling of the connected components [6, 8], in this case, four different types of connected components: (a) the teeth, considered as ROI, (b) more than one tooth due to overlap, (c) connected components corresponding to the background or bones, and (d) corresponding to parts of the teeth, such as root or crowns. Finally, the refinement where the selection of the best candidates of the connected components is carried out.

1.6 Active Contours Without Edges

Based on techniques of curve evolution, Mumford–Shah functional and level sets, the active contour without edges model [2] can detect objects whose boundaries are not necessarily defined by the gradient. In the level set formulation, the problem becomes a "mean-curvature flow" evolving the active contour, which will stop on the desired boundary. However, the stopping term does not depend on the image gradient, as in the classical active contour models, but is instead related to a particular image property. Assuming that a image ω_0 is composed by two related regions of approximately constant intensities, ω_0^i and ω_0^j. The object that we want to segment is represented by the values of ω_0^i and the boundary is denoted by C_0. Therefore, inside the object we have $\omega_0 \approx \omega_0^i$ and $\omega_0 \approx \omega_0^j$ outside the object boundary. Defining the fitting term, given by (5):

$$F_1(C) + F_2(C) = \int_{inside(C)} |\omega_0(x, y) - c_1|^2 dxdy$$

$$+ \int_{outside(C)} |\omega_0(x, y) - c_2|^2 dxdy \qquad (5)$$

where C is the variable curve, and the constants c_1, c_2, depending on C, are the intensities averages of ω_0 inside and outside C. In this case the fitting term is given by the boundary of the object C_0, as shown in (6):

$$\inf_C \{F_1(C) + F_1(C)\} \approx 0 \approx F_1(C_0) + F_1(C_0). \qquad (6)$$

For example, if the curve C is outside the object, then $F_1(C) > 0$ and $F_2(C) \approx 0$. If the curve C is inside the object, then $F_1(C) \approx 0$ but $F_2(C) > 0$. If the curve C is both inside and outside the object, then $F_1(C) > 0$ and $F_2(C) > 0$. Finally, the fitting energy is minimized if $C = C_0$ i.e., if the curve C is on the boundary of the object. Authors [2] minimized the fitting term and they also added some regularizing terms, such as the length of the curve C and the area of the region inside C, making the energy functional defined by $F(c_1, c_2, C)$, as shown in (7):

$$F(c_1, c_2, C) = \mu * Length(C) + \nu * Area(inside(C))$$

$$+\lambda_1 \int_{inside(C)} |\omega_0(x, y) - c_1|^2 dxdy$$

$$+\lambda_2 \int_{outside(C)} |\omega_0(x, y) - c_2|^2 dxdy \qquad (7)$$

where $\mu, \nu \geq 0$, $\lambda_1, \lambda_2 > 0$ are fixed parameters.

This technique of active contours is used in our work in two different stages: in the teeth gap valley detection and in the tooth segmentation.

2 Main Goal/Motivation

The main goal of this work, is to detect dental caries in panoramic dental X-ray images, by signalling the infected teeth in the image. To the best of our knowledge, there is a lack of a complete case study in the literature, as only methods that describe parts of the whole process can be found. This work should interest the scientific community, as it can constitute a comparison term for other methods concerned with the detection of dental caries in panoramic X-ray images.

3 Data-Set

Images of our data-set were captured by an Orthoralix 9,200 DDE X-ray camera. There are a total of 1,392 grayscale images in the data set, with varying types of dental structures, mouth sizes and number of teeth per image, as can be seen in Fig. 1. Another major point of interest of this data set are maps that localize dental cavities acting as ground truth of automated methods. Also, we believe that this set of images is useful to evaluate the current teeth segmentation methods.

3.1 Morphological Properties

When compared to other types of stomatology images, radiographic images are highly challenging, due to several reasons:

- Different levels of noise, due to the moving imaging device that captures a global perspective of the patient's mouth.
- Low contrast, either global or on local regions of the images, dictated by the mouth topology and morphologic properties, which are very complex.
- Blurring that makes difficult the straightforward detection of edges.
- Noise originated by the spinal-column that covers the frontal teeth in some images, as shown in Fig. 1.

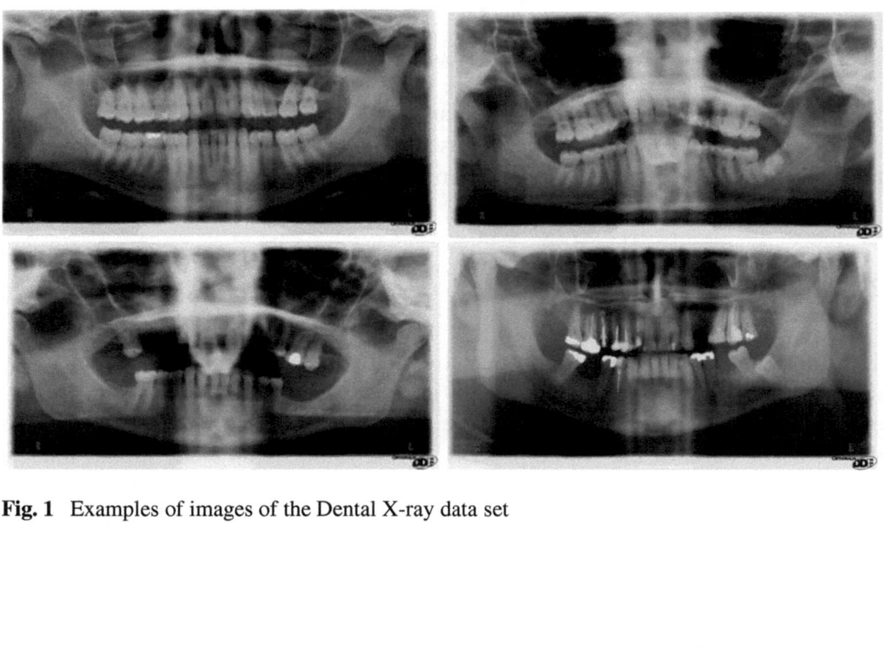

Fig. 1 Examples of images of the Dental X-ray data set

4 Method

As show in Fig. 2, our work comprises four different stages. The first stage is based in a statistical analysis of the images morphology, in order to define a preliminary ROI that takes out the nasal and chin bones. Next, we detect the upper and the lower jaws, based on the extraction of primitive points between jaws and in a polynomial fitting process that connects all the primitive points. The second stage is the teeth gap valley detection, where first we detect the gap valleys based in active contours techniques [2]. This process is applied in each jaw represented in the polar coordinate system. Secondly, we divide each tooth by extracting the points that are minimums in their contour neighborhood. The third stage consists in the accurate segmentation of each tooth. Here, we also used the active contours technique. Finally, we extracted the dental features and classified dental caries. A large variety of features were used to feed our binary classifier: statistical, image characteristics, region based features, texture based features and features based on the tooth border.

4.1 ROI Definition

Our method starts by the detection of a ROI, that should contain the mouth and teeth and discard non-useful information, as the nasal and chin bones. This stage is based in a statistics of the sizes and positions of each component in each image. For each image of a training set we measured four distances (R_1, R_2, R_3, R_4),

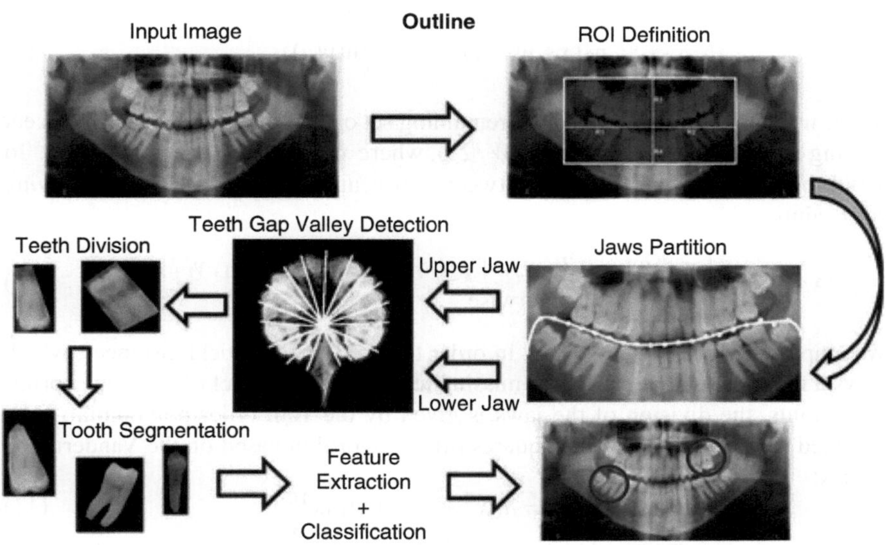

Fig. 2 The Outline of our developed work

defined by $R_i = \sqrt{(x_c - x_{R_i})^2 + (y_c - y_{R_i})^2}$, where $(x_c, \ y_c)$ corresponds to the image center $(x_c, \ y_c) = (w/2 = 1408, \ h/2 = 770)$ and $(x_{R_i}, \ y_{R_i})$ corresponds to four points extracted from the left, right, upper and lower side of the mouth. The histograms of R_i enabled us to fit corresponding Gaussian distributions for each one, defined by their mean and standard deviation: $(\mu, \ \sigma)$. Based on these distributions, we obtained the minimum value for each R_i that would appropriately crop the data with 95% certainty. Furthermore, a margin guarantees that slightly different images will be appropriately cropped, even at the expresses of a small increment of useless regions. The values obtained were $R_1 \approx 897.77$, $R2 \approx 863.36$, $R3 \approx 406.31$, and $R4 \approx 471.27$.

4.2 *Jaws Partition*

This stage concerns about the partition of the jaws. Firstly, the extraction of points between the jaws and then connecting those points by a polynomial least squares fitting scheme, a derivation of the least squares fitting procedure [7]. The set of points is obtained based on the horizontal projection $v(u)$ of the images, given by (8), where $I(x, i)$ denotes the intensity value at line x and column i:

$$v(u) = \sum_{i=0}^{w} I(x, i) \tag{8}$$

The initial point $p_0(x_0, w - 1)$ is defined at the far right of the image and at the line that has minimum $v(u)$ value:

$$p_0(x_0, w - 1) = \arg\min_x(v(u)) \tag{9}$$

where w is the image width and the remaining set of points p_i are regularly spaced, starting from $p_0 : p_i(x_i, (w - 1) - W/21)$, where x_i is obtained similarly to x_0. To avoid too high vertical distances between consecutive p_i, we added the following constraints:

$$p_i(x_i, y_i) = \begin{cases} p_i(x_{i+1} + T, y_i), & \mid p_i(x_i, y_i) - p_{i+1}(x_{i+1}, y_{i+1}) \mid > T \\ p_i(x_i, y_i), & \text{otherwise} \end{cases} \tag{10}$$

We empirically obtained $T = 20$, in order to avoid huge vertical distances, which plays a major role in dealing with missing teeth. Having the set of $p_i(x_i, y_i)$ primitive points, the division of the jaws is given by the 10th order polynomial, (11), obtained by a polynomial least squares fitting algorithm based on the Vandermond matrix:

$$p(x) = a_0 x^0 + \ldots + a_{10} x^{10} \tag{11}$$

The performance of this stage depends on the number of the missing teeth present in the input image, specially when more than one consecutive tooth is missing.

4.3 Teeth Gap Valley Detection

Having jaws divided, the next goal is to detect the teeth gap valley. These valleys tend to be darker than the teeth themselves, although exceptions are due to teeth overlap. We started by the transformation of the data from cartesian coordinates to polar coordinates, used to easy the division between teeth radial lines. The next step is the contour segmentation, regarded always as a typical active contours problem. The object of interest is in the center of the image, therefore, the contour can be initialized as the image border. In the third step we calculate for each contour point the distance between the image center and extracted the minimum points, which correspond to the teeth gap valleys. Finally, we crop the selected regions.

Morphological operators In order to increase the contrast of the input images, we applied a pre-processing filter (top and bottom hat transform):

$$\begin{aligned} I_{output} &= (I_{Original} + TH_{Original}) - BH_{Original} \\ I_{outputFinal} &= (I_{output} + TH_{output}) - BH_{output} \end{aligned} \tag{12}$$

where $I_{Original}$ corresponds to the input image, $TH_{Original}$ is the output of the top hat transform $BH_{Original}$ is the output bottom hat transform. The resulting image of the pre-processing filter is $I_{outputFinal}$. We used a rectangular structuring element with dimensions $[w/4, h/2]$, where w and h are the width and height of the image, respectively. This choice was based in a training set of 500 images, selected from the whole data set. As can be seen in the left column of Fig. 3, pre-processing increased the contrast of the image. A less successful example can be seen in the right column of the Fig. 3, where pre-processing contributed for the disappearance of the frontal teeth. This occurs only in these because they are thinner and can't reflect as much radiation as do pre molars and molars. Other cases are due to the poor quality of the image. Jaws were divided simply by a horizontal linear partition of the image. The upper jaw was cropped in the lower value of the polynomial found in the previous stage. The lower jaw was cropped in the higher value that the polynomial takes.

Polar Coordinates In the polar coordinate system each point is defined by a distance to a fixed point and the angle from a fixed direction. The polar coordinates r (the radial coordinate) and θ (the angular coordinate, often called the polar angle). Equation (13) gives the method used to transform an (x, y) point in polar coordinates [1]:

$$\begin{aligned} r &= \sqrt{x^2 + y^2} \\ \theta &= \tanh \frac{y}{x} \end{aligned} \tag{13}$$

where $\tanh \frac{y}{x}$ corresponds to a two argument inverse tangent which takes the signs of x and y into account to determine in which quadrant θ lies. The resulting images

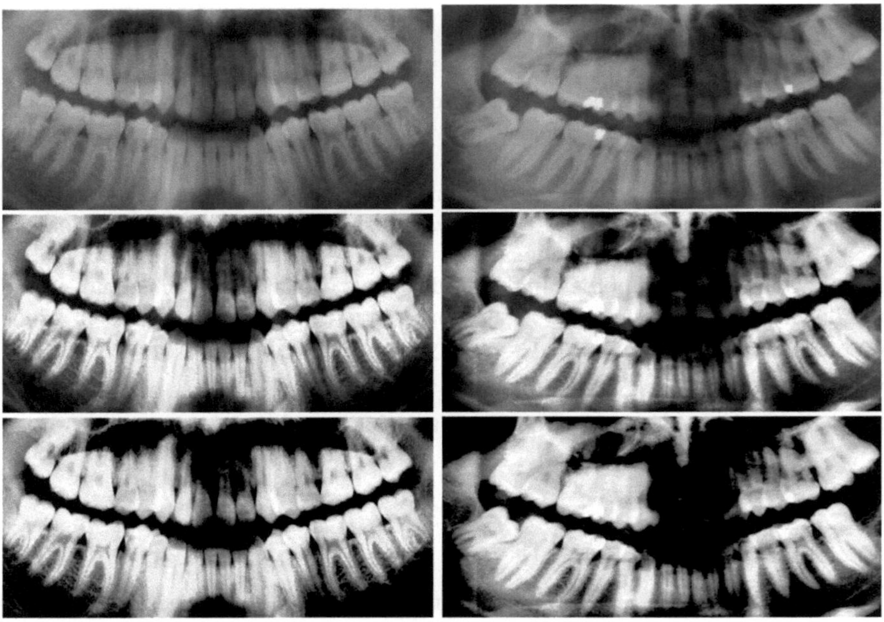

Fig. 3 Examples of a successful (*left* column) and failure (*right* column) cases of the preprocessing module

in polar coordinates had dimensions $[h * 2; h * 2]$, where h corresponds to the height of the original input image. With this step, we transformed our problem in a typical active contours problem.

Active Contours Without Edges This segmentation method seeks for the minimization of an energy model, given by (7) and requires proper initialization of the contour mask. After the analysis of a training set composed by 200 images we defined the initial mask corresponding to four independent elements in each image quadrant:

$$I_{mask}(x, y) = \begin{cases} ([w * 0.10...(w/2) * 0.90], [h * 0.10...(h/2) * 0.90]) = 255 \\ ([(w/2) + (w/2) * 0.10...w * 0.90], \\ \quad [h * 0.10...(h/2) * 0.90]) = 255 \\ ([(w/2) + (w/2) * 0.10...w * 0.90], \\ \quad [(h/2) + (h/2) * 0.10...h * 0.90]) = 255 \\ ([w * 0.10...(w/2) * 0.90], \\ \quad [(h/2) + (h/2) * 0.10...h * 0.90]) = 255 \end{cases} \tag{14}$$

where w and h correspond to the image width and height, respectively. Data was resized to $1/4$, due to computational concerns, obtaining final sizes of $\frac{w}{4}, \frac{h}{4}$.

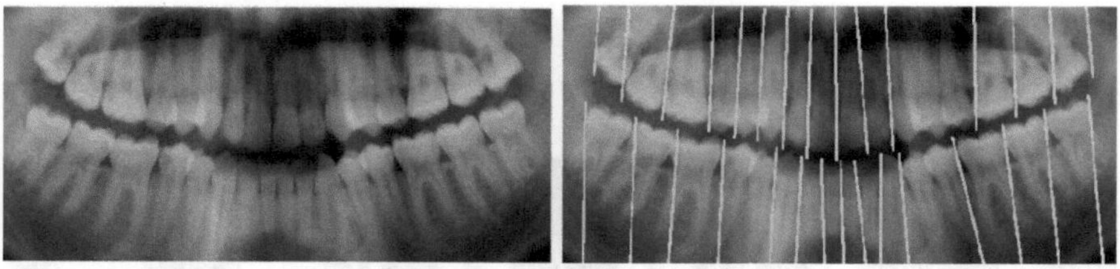

Fig. 4 An example of our method for the teeth gap valley detection

4.4 Teeth Division

This step is based on the minimum values extracted in the previous step:

- Let $c_1, ..., c_n$ be the set of contour points, where $c_i = (x_i, y_i)$. Let (x_c, y_c) be the image center. Let d_i be the distances between the center and the contour, i.e., $d_i = \sqrt{(x_i - x_c)^2 + (y_i - y_c)^2}$.
- Let $D_i = \{d_i, ..., d_n\}$ correspond to the distances vector. We eliminated all distances based on $d_i^2 = D_i \cap (A_1^{-1})$ where $A_1 = [D_i < 0.10 * h]$.
- A Gaussian filter was used to smooth the distance values. Let $d_i^3 = d_i^2 \otimes G_{\sigma,r}$ where $G_{\sigma,r}$ is a Gaussian Kernel [14, 17] of sigma $\sigma = 10$ and radius $r = 100$.
- Defining d_i^m as the local minimums extracted from d_i^3, i.e., $d_i^m = (((d_i^3(x-3) > d_i^3(x-2) > d_i^3(x-1)) > d_i^3(x))\ \&\&\ (d_i^3(x) < d_i^3(x+1)))$.

As shown in the Fig. 4 the extraction of the minimum values is very dependent on the coordinates transitions, because it is inherent a loss of information in such transitions. This leads to the cutting of some teeth.

4.5 Tooth Segmentation

This process is quite similar to the teeth gap valley detection stage. The input images contain only one tooth and the problem is to distinguish between teeth and background corespondent to the gum line and the gum itself. The pre-processing was similar to the one applied earlier. As shown in Fig. 5 the use of the active contours technique appears to have been a very good option. It should be stressed that all segmented regions actually contain the tooth, i.e., the region corresponding to the tooth is always inside the resulting region, although sometimes together with some background noise. In other cases, overlap teeth leaded to the inclusion of multiples teeth in the segmented region, as shown in Fig. 5.

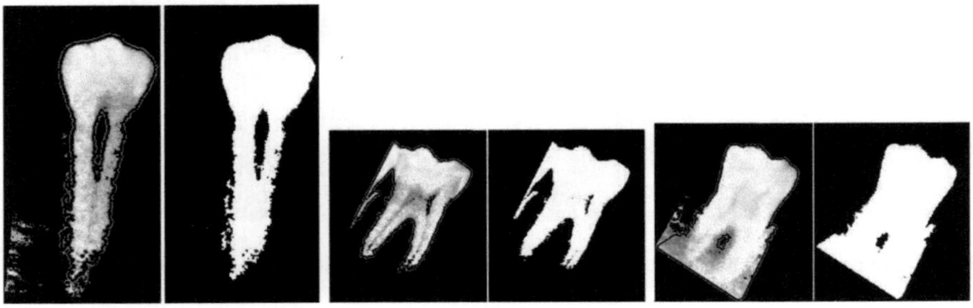

Fig. 5 Examples of the active contours method applied to our input images

4.6 Dental Caries Classification

This stage starts by the extraction of features that apriority could carry relevant information to the problem. To do this we created a training set of 1,098 images, with 549 images with dental caries and 549 images of healthy teeth. This training set contains all types of teeth, but with pre molars and molars in majority due to a similar proportion in the complete data set. We used large heterogeneous types of features, hence the importance of using algorithms for selecting the best ones, which was carried out by the PCA algorithm. Features have five main categories:

1. Features based on simple pixel statistics; such as pixel intensity and maximum pixel intensity.
2. Statistic features as the entropy, mean-value and variance.
3. Region based features such as the Hu moments, the Zernike moments, area and perimeter.
4. Features based on the segmented boundary, as chain codes, Fourier descriptors, signature and angular function.
5. Features based on the image texture, as the energy and third moment.

Table 1 shows the types of features that contain 95 and 99% of the total variance in the training set, according to each of the above defined types. The "Variance" column gives the percentage of features of the corresponding type that were selected by the PCA. "Number Features" gives the total number of features selected. It can be seen that the features based on the region boundary and the region itself had a significant preponderance when compared to other types of features. In turn, features based on the image properties do not add too much information to the feature set. Note that the statistical features based on the boundary and in the region correspond to a significant portion of the selected feature set by the PCA algorithm.

Table 1 Results from applying the PCA in our initial feature set

	Variance	Number features	Variance	Number features
Features based on	95%	65	99%	128
Image properties	6.1	4	3.1	4
Region	97	63	93.75	120
Boundary	100	65	100	128
Texture	46.2	30	39	50
Statistical	93	60	92.2	118

5 Results

5.1 Segmentation

In this section we discuss the results of all the stages of our work. Starting by a few observations regarding the way these results were obtained as well as the sets we defined. For the ROI definition, jaws partition, teeth gap valley detection and tooth segmentation stages ground truth was given by visual inspection, with a two-folder cross validation. It should be stressed that all results were based on an error-free inputs from previous stages. This was performed in order to avoid that errors in the earliest stages corrupt the results obtained by the final ones. Table 2 shows the results obtained by the first three stages of our method.

Results of the ROI definition and of the jaws partition are quite satisfactory, obtaining an accuracy above 90%. For these two steps and concerning the visual inspection we considered as *correct* the presence of all teeth in the output image resulting of the ROI definition. Regarding the jaws partition we considered *correct* any polynomial that divides each jaw without cutting any tooth.

5.2 Classification

Feature normalization is a necessary step because feature values lie within different dynamic ranges. A straightforward technique is the normalization to same mean and variance. Other linear techniques limit the features value in the range of [0, 1] by proper scaling. We empirically evaluated each of the above described strategies.

Artificial Neural Network A feed-forward artificial Neural Network (NN) was used for classification proposes. Table 3 contains the best result obtained for the test set using the PCA features with the covered variance of 99%. Figure 6 shows the correspondent Receiver Operating Characteristic (ROC) curve. As we can observe, the results can be considered satisfactory. Also, there is an increase of the accuracy rating after the appliance of the PCA for a 99% variance coverage, which denotes the importance of the attributes selection performed by the PCA.

Table 2 Results of our method stages up to the dental caries detection

Stages	Results (% of correct)	Number of Images
ROI definition	95.7	700
Jaws partition	92.6	700
Teeth gap valley	87.5	700
Tooth segmentation	71.91	1,098

Table 3 Confusion matrix for the ANN classifier for the normalized test set between [0, 1] after the appliance of the PCA for a 99% variance coverage

Class	No dental caries	Dental caries	Total
No dental caries	548	1	549
Dental caries	13	536	549
Total	561	537	1,084
Accuracy	98,70%		

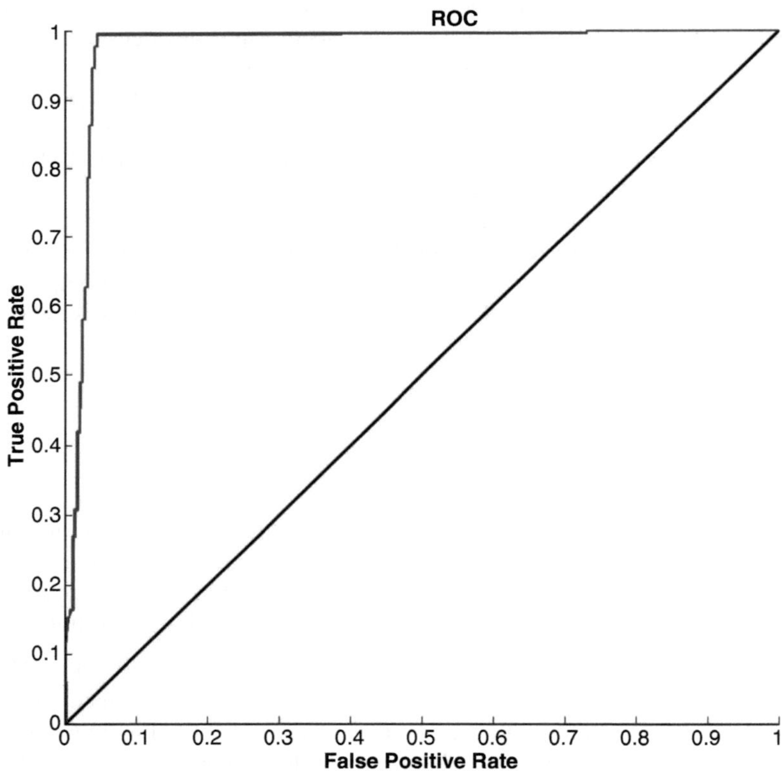

Fig. 6 ROC for the ANN classifier for the normalized test set between [0, 1] after the appliance of the PCA for a 99% variance coverage

Another conclusion drawn from these results is that extracted features have enough discriminating capacity to decide with high confidence whether a tooth contains or not a dental cavity.

6 Conclusion and Further Work

The main contribution of this work is the development of a complete case study for the dental caries detection in dental panoramic X-ray. Also we announced the availability of a new data set of panoramic dental X-ray images, which can constitute a tool for the research community in the development of stomatologic-related applications. This data set has varying morphologic properties that make it valuable to the scientific community. These include the number of teeth per image, the shape of the mouth and teeth as well as the levels of noise. Concerning the first two stages of the proposed method, results were considered satisfactory, obtaining in the ROI definition a accuracy of 95.7% and in the jaws partition a result of 92.6%. The other three stages had the accuracy rating of 87.5% (teeth gap valleys detection) and 71.91% (tooth segmentation). Finally, the accuracy of the classification module was 98.70%. These results regard each stage independently, which enabled us to perceive the actual merits of each module without corruption of the results due to errors in previous stages. Regarding further work the jaws partition, it is very important to detect missing teeth because in these situations our method tends to fail. Finally, our main goal is to start the detection of other types of dental diseases, using the described dental X-ray data set.

References

1. Anton, H.A., Bivens, I., Davis, S.: Calculus, 7th edn. Wiley, New York, USA, ISBN 978-0471381570 (2001)
2. Chan, T.F., Vese, L.A.: Active contours without edges. IEEE Trans. Image Process. **10**, 266–277 (2001)
3. Chen, H., Jain, A.K.: Matching of dental x-ray images for human identification. Pattern Recogn. **37**, 1519–1532 (2004)
4. Chen, H., Jain, A.K.: Tooth contour extraction for matching dental radiographs. In proceedings of the 17th International Conference on Pattern Recognition (ICPR'04), vol. III, 522–525, Cambridge, United Kingdom (2004)
5. Cristianini, N., Shawe-Taylor, J.: An Introduction to Support Vector Machines and Other Kernel-based Learning Methods, 1st edn. Cambridge University Press (2002)
6. Davies, E.R.: Machine Vision: Theory, Algorithms, Practicalities, 3rd edn. Morgan Kaufmann, Publishers Inc, San Diego, USA, ISBN 978-0122060939 (2005)
7. Dyer, S.A., He, X.: Least-squares fitting of data by polynomials. IEEE Instru. Meas. Mag. **3**, 46–51 (2001)
8. Gonzalez, R.C., Woods, R.E.: Digital Image Processing, 3rd edn. Prentice-Hall (2008)
9. Jain, A., Hong, L., Pankanti, S.: Biometrics: promising frontiers for emerging identification market. Comm. ACM, **43**, 91–98 (2000)

10. Jollie, I.T.: Principal component analysis, 2nd edn. Springer Series in Statistics, New York (2002)
11. Li, S., Fevens, T., Krzyzak, A., Li, S.: An automatic variational level set segmentation framework for computer aided dental x-rays analysis in clinical environments. Comput. Med. Imag. Graph. **30**, 65–74 (2006)
12. Li, S., Fevens, T., Krzyak, A., Jin, C., Li, S.: Semi-automatic computer aided lesion detection in dental x-rays using variational level set. Pattern Recogn. **40**, 2861–2873 (2007)
13. Meyer, D., Leisch, F., Hornik, K.: The support vector machine under test. IEEE Trans. Image Process. **55**, 169–186 (2003)
14. Nixon, M.S., Aguado, A.S.: Feature Extraction and Image Processing, 1st edn. Newnes (2002)
15. Park, H., Schoepflin, Y., Kim, T.: Active contour model with gradient directional information: directional snake. IEEE Trans. Circ. Syst. Video Tech. **11**, 252–256 (2001)
16. Said, E.H., Nassar, D.E.M., Fahmy, G., Ammar, H.H.: Teeth segmentation in digitized dental x-ray films using mathematical morphology. IEEE Trans. Inf. Foren. Sec. **1**, 178–189 (2006)
17. Shapiro, L.G., Stockman, G.C.: Computer Vision, 1st edn. Prentice-Hall (2001)

Noisy Medical Image Edge Detection Algorithm Based on a Morphological Gradient Using Uninorms

Manuel González-Hidalgo, Arnau Mir Torres, Daniel Ruiz Aguilera, and Joan Torrens Sastre

Abstract Medical images edge detection is one of the most important pre-processing steps in medical image segmentation and 3D reconstruction. In this paper, an edge detection algorithm using an uninorm-based fuzzy morphology is proposed. It is shown that this algorithm is robust when it is applied to different types of noisy images. It improves the results of other well-known algorithms including classical algorithms of edge detection, as well as fuzzy-morphology based ones using the Łukasiewicz t-norm and umbra approach. It detects detailed edge features and thin edges of medical images corrupted by impulse or gaussian noise. Moreover, some different objective measures have been used to evaluate the filtered results obtaining for our approach better values than for other approaches.

Keywords Noise reduction · Edge detection · Mathematical morphology · Uninorms · Representable uninorm · Idempotent uninorm

1 Introduction

Edge detection is a fundamental pre-processing step in applications such as image segmentation and computer vision, and its performance is relevant for the final results of the image processing. Over years, many efforts have been devoted in the literature, and also are currently devoted, to propose approaches to extract contour features. These different approaches vary from the classical approaches [19] based on a set of convolution masks, to the new techniques based on fuzzy sets [2]. Nevertheless, many of them fail or diminish their effectiveness in presence of noise.

M. González-Hidalgo (✉)
Computer Graphics, Vision and Artificial Intelligence Group, Mathematics and Computer Science Department, University of the Balearic Islands, Spain
e-mail: manuel.gonzalez@uib.es

A.M. Torres, D.R. Aguilera, and J.T. Sastre
Fuzzy Logic and Information Fusion Group, Mathematics and Computer Science Department, University of the Balearic Islands, Spain
e-mail: arnau.mir@uib.es; daniel.ruiz@uib.es; dmijts0@uib.es

J.M.R.S. Tavares and R.M.N. Jorge (eds.), *Computational Vision and Medical Image Processing: Recent Trends*, Computational Methods in Applied Sciences 19,
DOI 10.1007/978-94-007-0011-6_11, © Springer Science+Business Media B.V. 2011

The fuzzy mathematical morphology is a generalization of binary morphology [21] using techniques of fuzzy sets [1, 5, 7, 17]. The basic tools of mathematical morphology are the so-called morphological operations that are applied to an image A, which is modified through the so called structural element B, whose size and shape are chosen in order to study the structure of the image A. The basic morphological operations are: erosion, dilation, opening and closing. Mathematical morphology, either crisp or fuzzy, provides an alternative approach to image processing based on the shape concept represented by the structural element (see for instance [21]).

The fuzzy operators used to build a fuzzy morphology are conjunctors and implications. Among them, the most commonly used are the t-norms and their residual implications. Recently conjunctive uninorms, as a particular case of conjunctors, have also been used in this area [8, 10–14]. In the two recent works [10, 12] the authors use two kinds of left-continuous conjunctive uninorms in order to obtain a mathematical morphology with "good" properties, including duality between the morphological operators.

This work can be seen as a continuation of [12] and [13] where the authors made a comparative study of the results obtained using the morphology based on uninorms with those obtained using t-norms and using the classical umbra approach. In these works, it is checked out that uninorms detect the edges of the images better than other approaches. Also, in [12], properties of idempotence and generalized idempotence for opening and closing operators based on uninorms are shown and in [13] (see also [14]) the authors study the feasibility of alternate filters (alternate compositions of openings and closings), from opening and closing of the fuzzy morphology based on uninorms, in order to use them in the elimination and reduction of noise. Thus, the aim of this paper is to extend this study to a residual operator based on alternate filters using uninorms. The alternate filters are used in elimination and reduction of noise, while the residual operator is used to highlight certain components of the image.

The residuals and morphological gradients are still under study and they have applications in image analysis. See, by example [12, 13] and references therein. Thus, in [15], it is proposed a directional transition detection algorithm based on morphological residues, considering linear structurant elements. In 2002, T. Chen et al. in [4], design on the basis of mathematical morphology, a new detector of soft edges in dark regions called "Pseudo Top-Hat" which provides, in the case of the classical image of the video cameraman, a better performance than those achieved by other edge detection methods used to compare the results. In [23], morphological gradients based on openings and closings were used to detect edges in CT medical images altered by noise. The results were compared with other contours detectors, improving the obtained edge images. More recently, in [16, 18] gradient operators are applied again to edge detection and image segmentation, respectively. Thus, in [16], an edge detector is developed for obtaining thin edges in regions or images with low-contrast. Tested with multiple images, even some of them corrupted by noise type salt and pepper and Gaussian noise of mean zero and variance 0.02, the method performs very well in comparison with the other four methods with which they work. In [18] operators were designed based on multiscale morphological gradients, addressing the segmentation problem of images to Computed Axial Tomography (CAT). All these works show that the morphological gradients remain relevant and useful in the analysis and image processing. In this work the feasibility of alternate filters will be studied, from opening and closing of the fuzzy morphology based on uninorms (studied in detail in [10, 12]). Following the ideas in [13], where the authors used the alternate filters in the reduction of noise, we will use them in the design of an edge detection algorithm for medical images reaching a compromise between elimination and smoothing of noise and the detection of the features in medical images. A preliminary work in this direction is [11] where the proposed algorithm was already introduced. In this work, we study the performance of this algorithm in presence of different types of noise, impulse and Gaussian. Moreover, the behaviour of this algorithm is investigated depending on the amount of noise in the images. Some different objective measures are used to evaluate the filtered results, the Mean Square Error (MSE) and the Signal to Noise Ratio (SNR) (see [19]), and the recently defined Structural Similarity Index Measurement (SSIM) (see [22], Sect. III-B, pp. 603–605). It can be noticed that we obtain better results when we use uninorms that when we use other detectors considered in this work.

This work is organized as follows. In the next section we introduce the fuzzy morphological operators dilation, erosion, opening and closing based on a conjuntor and an implicator. We also recall the two types of left-continuous conjunctive uninorms, jointly with their residual implicators, used in our morphological approach. For these kinds of fuzzy operators, the majority of the good algebraic and morphological properties are guaranteed and we recall the most important ones in this section. Section 3 describes the proposed edge detector algorithm. This algorithm has three steps: first, we preprocess the image by an alternate filter in order to filter the noise and smooth the image; second, we apply a Beucher gradient by dilation and last, we apply a global threshold to transform the edge image into a binary image. Section 4 is devoted to the comparison experiments between our proposed algorithm and other classical edge detectors as Canny, Prewitt and LoG, and classical fuzzy algorithms as Łukasiewicz t-norm and umbra approach. The interpretation of the results is also included. In Sect. 5, conclusions and future work are pointed out.

2 Fuzzy Morphological Operators and Its Properties

We assume as known the basics facts on uninorms used in this work which, in any case, can be found in [6, 9, 20]. We will use the following notation: $\mathcal{I}$ is an implication, $\mathcal{C}$ a conjunctor, $\mathcal{N}$ a strong negation, and finally A is a gray-scale image and B is a gray-scale structural element.

We recall the definitions of fuzzy morphological operators following the ideas of De Baets in [5]. The method consists in fuzzify the logical operations, i.e. the Boolean conjunction and the Boolean implication, to obtain fuzzy operators. An n-dimensional gray-scale image is modeled as an $\mathbb{R}^n \longrightarrow [0, 1]$ function. The values of an image must be in [0, 1] in order to consider it as a fuzzy set. Then, we will proceed to explain this method from the following definitions and propositions.

Definition 1. The *fuzzy dilation* $D_{\mathcal{C}}(A, B)$ and *fuzzy erosion* $E_{\mathcal{I}}(A, B)$ of A by B are the gray-scale images defined by

$$D_{\mathcal{C}}(A, B)(y) = \sup_x \mathcal{C}(B(x-y), A(x)) \tag{1}$$

$$E_{\mathcal{I}}(A, B)(y) = \inf_x \mathcal{I}(B(x-y), A(x)). \tag{2}$$

Note that the reflection of a gray-scale image B denoted by $-B$, and defined by $-B(y) = B(-y)$, for all $y \in \mathbb{R}^n$. Given two images B_1, B_2, we will say that $B_1 \subseteq B_2$ when $B_1(y) \leq B_2(y)$ for all $y \in R^n$.

Definition 2. The *fuzzy closing* $C_{\mathcal{C},\mathcal{I}}(A, B)$ and *fuzzy opening* $O_{\mathcal{C},\mathcal{I}}(A, B)$ of A by B are the gray-scale images defined by

$$C_{\mathcal{C},\mathcal{I}}(A, B)(y) = E_{\mathcal{I}}(D_{\mathcal{C}}(A, B), -B)(y) \tag{3}$$

$$O_{\mathcal{C},\mathcal{I}}(A, B)(y) = D_{\mathcal{C}}(E_{\mathcal{I}}(A, B), -B)(y). \tag{4}$$

The conjunctors and implications used in this paper are two types of left-continuous conjunctive uninorms and their residual implications. Specifically these two types of uninorms are the following:

- The representable uninorms: Let $e \in]0, 1[$ and let $h : [0, 1] \longrightarrow [-\infty, \infty]$ be a strictly increasing, continuous function with $h(0) = -\infty$, $h(e) = 0$ and $h(1) = +\infty$. Then

$$U_h(x, y) = \begin{cases} h^{-1}(h(x) + h(y)), & \text{if } (x, y) \notin \{(1, 0), (0, 1)\}, \\ 0, & \text{in other case,} \end{cases}$$

  is a conjunctive representable uninorm with neutral element e, see [9], and its residual implication $\mathcal{I}_{U_h}$ is given by

$$\mathcal{I}_{U_h}(x, y) = \begin{cases} h^{-1}(h(y) - h(x)), & \text{if } (x, y) \notin \{(0, 0), (1, 1)\}, \\ 1, & \text{in other case.} \end{cases}$$

  Moreover, U_h satisfies self duality (except at the points (0,1) and (1,0)) with respect to the strong negation $\mathcal{N}(x) = h^{-1}(-h(x))$, see [6].
- A specific type of idempotent uninorms: Let $\mathcal{N}$ be a strong negation. The function given by

$$U^{\mathcal{N}}(x, y) = \begin{cases} \min(x, y), & \text{if } y \leq \mathcal{N}(x), \\ \max(x, y), & \text{in other case,} \end{cases}$$

is a conjunctive idempotent uninorm. Its residual implication is given by (see [20])

$$\mathcal{I}_{U^{\mathcal{N}}}(x, y) = \begin{cases} \min(\mathcal{N}(x), y), & \text{if } y < x, \\ \max(\mathcal{N}(x), y), & \text{if } y \geq x. \end{cases}$$

These two types of left-continuous conjunctive uninorms guarantee most of the good algebraic and morphological properties associated with the morphological operators obtained from them ([6, 10, 12, 20]). Among these properties, we highlight those described below. In all properties, U is a left-continuous conjunctive uninorm with neutral element $e \in]0, 1[$, $\mathcal{I}_U$ its residual implication, A is a gray-level image and B a gray-scale structural element:

- The fuzzy dilation $D_{\mathcal{U}}$ is increasing in both arguments, the fuzzy erosion $E_{\mathcal{I}}$ is increasing in their first argument and decreasing in their second one, the fuzzy closing $C_{U,\mathcal{I}_U}$ and the fuzzy opening $O_{U,\mathcal{I}_U}$ are both increasing in their first argument.
- If $B(0) = e$ the fuzzy dilation is extensive and the fuzzy erosion is anti-extensive

$$E_{\mathcal{I}_U}(A, B) \subseteq A \subseteq D_U(A, B).$$

- Moreover, the fuzzy closing is extensive and the fuzzy opening is anti-extensive:

$$O_{U,\mathcal{I}_U} \subseteq A \subseteq C_{U,\mathcal{I}_U}(A, B).$$

- The fuzzy closing and the fuzzy opening are idempotent, i.e.:

$$C_{U,\mathcal{I}_U}(C_{U,\mathcal{I}_U}(A, B), B) = C_{U,\mathcal{I}_U}(A, B),$$
$$O_{U,\mathcal{I}_U}(O_{U,\mathcal{I}_U}(A, B), B) = O_{U,\mathcal{I}_U}(A, B).$$

- If $B(0) = e$, then

$$E_{\mathcal{I}_U}(A, B) \subseteq O_{U,\mathcal{I}_U}(A, B) \subseteq A \subseteq C_{U,\mathcal{I}_U}(A, B) \subseteq D_U(A, B).$$

- For the two previous conjunctives uninorms of type U_h and $U^{\mathcal{N}}$, the duality between fuzzy morphological operators is guaranteed.

3 The Proposed Edge Detector Algorithm

The main goal of this work is to develop an algorithm which can detect and preserve, in presence of noise, edge features in the low-contrast regions of medical images. In this work, we make use of a residual operator from fuzzy opening and closing operations in order to detect edge images and, at the same time, denoise the image. Recall that a residual operator of two morphological operations or transformations is their difference. In previous works, [12] and [13], we present the performance of fuzzy gradients and top-hat transformations based on uninorms in order to detect edges in natural images. In these works the displayed experiments show that the uninorms outperform the results obtained using t-norms and the classical umbra approach.

From the operation properties of the fuzzy morphology based on uninorms, it is satisfied that

$$O_{U,\mathcal{I}_U}(C_{U,\mathcal{I}_U}(A, B), B) \subseteq C_{U,\mathcal{I}_U}(A, B).$$

Let B be such that $B(0) = e$ and consider $F = O_{U,\mathcal{I}_U}(C_{U,\mathcal{I}_U}(A, B), B)$. So we have, using the properties stated in the previous section (see also [12]), the following chain of inclusions

$$E_{\mathcal{I}_U}(C_{U,\mathcal{I}_U}(F, B), B) \subseteq C_{U,\mathcal{I}_U}(F, B) \subseteq D_U(C_{U,\mathcal{I}_U}(F, B), B).$$

Then we can compute the next residual operator

$$\delta^{1+}_{U,\mathcal{I}_U}(A, B) = D_U(C_{U,\mathcal{I}_U}(F, B), B) \setminus C_{U,\mathcal{I}_U}(F, B). \tag{5}$$

In (5), the so called *alternate filters*, alternate composition of opening and closing, are involved. These alternate filters are used to remove and to smooth noise in [13, 14]. So, the proposed algorithm is the following: Firstly, we preprocess the image by an alternate filter in order to filter the noise and smooth the image, and then we apply a Beucher gradient by dilation. Once the residual image (5) is obtained, a global threshold experimentally obtained is then applied to transform the edge image into a binary image.

The previous filtering of the image allows us to minimize the effect of the noise on the image without altering or slightly altering the outer edge of the regions that compose the image and maintaining the edge features of the image. To binarize the obtained image in (5), a value threshold between 0.85 and 0.98 of the maximum value of the histogram is taken. In the next section we present some experimental results obtained using the previous algorithm.

4 Experimental Results and Analysis

In the following experiments, the idempotent uninorm $U^{\mathcal{N}}$ with $\mathcal{N}(x) = 1 - x$ and the representable uninorm U_h with $h(x) = \ln\left(\frac{x}{1-x}\right)$ have been used. The obtained results are compared with the Łukasiewicz t-norm and the classic development based on *umbra approach* (see [17]). In particular, the structural element used by the morphological operators is given by a 3×3 matrix:

$$\begin{pmatrix} 0 & 1 & 0 \\ 1 & 1 & 1 \\ 0 & 1 & 0 \end{pmatrix} \cdot e \tag{6}$$

where e is the neutral element of the uninorm. When we select the Łukasiewicz t-norm as conjunctor the structural element is represented by the matrix

$$\begin{pmatrix} 0.86 & 0.86 & 0.86 \\ 0.86 & 1.00 & 0.86 \\ 0.86 & 0.86 & 0.86 \end{pmatrix},$$

except in the experiments shown in Fig. 8. This structural element has been used by Nachtegael and Kerre in [17] and by the authors in [12–14]. In the case of the classical umbra approach the structural element is given by the matrix

$$\begin{pmatrix} 219 & 219 & 219 \\ 219 & 255 & 219 \\ 219 & 219 & 219 \end{pmatrix}.$$

The performance of the proposed fuzzy mathematical morphology based on edge detection algorithm is evaluated in this section, and experimental results compared with other existing methods are also presented. The method has been applied to medical images and salt and pepper noise corrupted medical images. The noise in the images has been added using the standard functions of Matlab R2008a Also, the edge images processed by the Canny, Prewitt, LoG (Laplacian of Gaussian operator), Zero-Cross and Roberts edge detectors have been obtained using default parameters of Matlab. Except in Fig. 1c where we have used a sensitivity threshold for the Prewitt method equal to 0.05 because, in this case, we got an almost empty edge image using the default setting. In all cases, various sets of parameters have been tested and only those providing more adequate results are shown in the figures.

The MRI head image shown in Fig. 1a of size 256×228 contain dark regions and many features of brain wrinkles and head cavities. The contrast in these dark regions is so low that edge features in these regions are very difficult to detect. Canny [3] an many others establish the unavoidable trade-off between localization and signal strength. The Canny, Prewitt, LoG edge detectors are applied to the image and the experimental results are displayed in Fig. 1b–d.

The results obtained with the proposed algorithm using the Łukasiewicz t-norm as conjunction and its residual implication, and using the classical umbra approach are displayed in (Fig. 1e–f). It can be seen that the performance of the proposed edge detector algorithm using uninorms (Fig. 1g–h) is better than those of the previous ones. Using uninorms and the proposed algorithm, many thin features in the MRI head image are detected and have a strong intensity. In [12] we can see as the edge images obtained by a pure morphological approach (morphological gradient) produce a good edge detection performance, but many really thin edges are still unable to be detected.

In the following experiments, noise type salt and pepper was added to the test images in order to study the robustness of the proposed algorithm. To remove noise

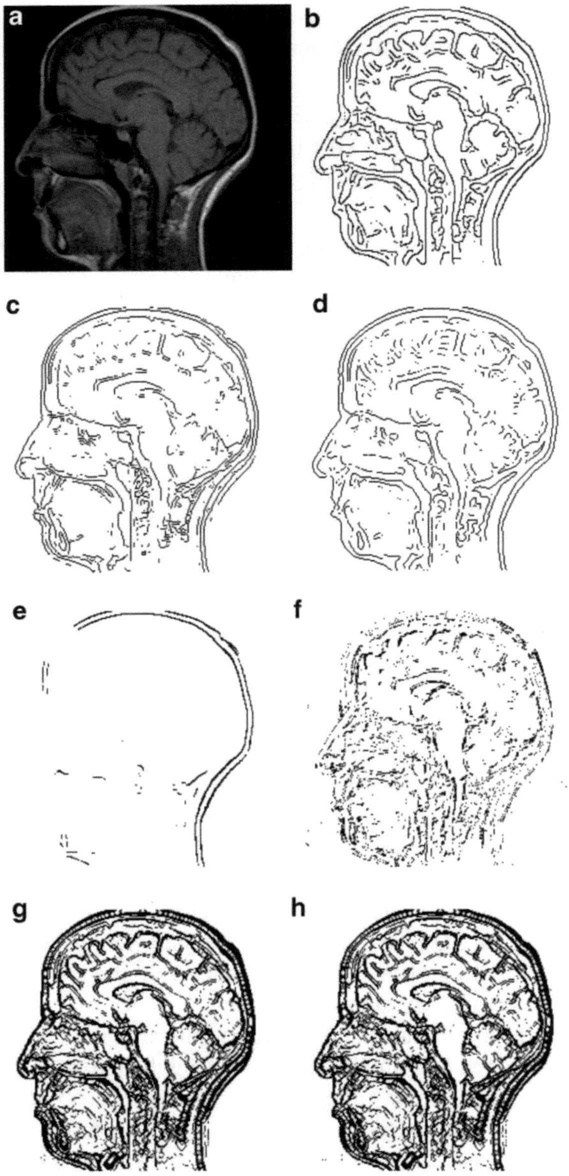

Fig. 1 (**a**) Original MRI image. (**b–d**) Edge detection obtained by Canny, Prewitt and LoG edge detectors, respectively. (**e, f**) Using the proposed algorithm with Łukasiewicz t-norm and umbra approach, respectively. (**g, h**) Results obtained by the proposed approach using the representable and idempotent uninorm, respectively

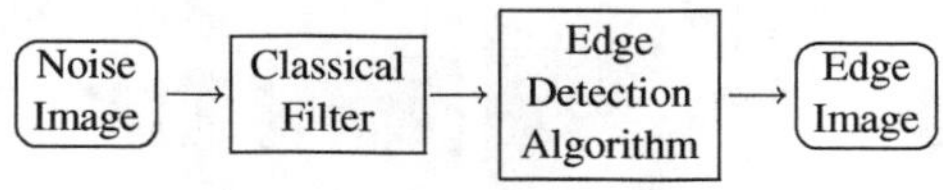

Fig. 2 Block diagram for edge detection using a classical detector

in the image, a classical filter of $n \times n$ mask was applied to the noisy image before applying a classical edge detector algorithm. In particular a median filter with $n = 3$ was applied to remove salt and pepper noise and a Wiener filter with $n = 5$ was applied in presence of Gaussian noise. The block diagram of the process is illustrated in Fig. 2. With this set of experiments we show that the proposed edge detection algorithm can adequately extract edge features even when the image is noisy.

The original lungs CT image of size 430×338 displayed in Fig. 3a contains many interesting features. A salt and pepper noise function with parameter 0.02 was added to the image (Fig. 3b). In this case, the Canny and zero-cross were also applied to the image after a median filter was used to remove noise. The proposed algorithm using representable and idempotent uninorms can successfully extract the boundaries of the lungs and the main edge features of the image. Compare with the so one obtained using t-norms and the umbra approach. Note that, the Canny edge detector fails to detect the outer edge of body, and the two classical edge detectors fail to separate the boundaries of the lungs, showing some gaps in the obtained boundary. Something similar happens with the detected edges of osseous structures.

In Fig. 4 we display the results obtained by the proposed fuzzy edge detection algorithm when four different salt and pepper noise functions, of parameter 0.04, 0.06, 0.08 and 0.1 respectively, were added to the image shown in Fig. 3a. Our goal is to study the performance of the proposed algorithm when we increase the amount of noise present in the image. The results obtained with the proposed algorithm are shown in Fig. 4a–d. Comparing these results with those shown in Fig. 3h, we can see as the edges image are little affected with the increase of noise and many features remain detected.

A number of different objective measures can be utilized to evaluate the previous filtering step in our fuzzy approach providing a quantitative evaluation of the filtering results. Among them, the MSE, the SNR, and the SSIM (see [22]). Let O_1 and F_2 be two images of dimensions $M \times N$. We suppose that O_1 is the original noise-free image and F_2 is the restored image for which some filter has been applied. The MSE, SNR, and SSIM values defined in (7)–(9) are used to evaluate the filtering performance.

$$MSE(F_2, O_1) = \frac{1}{MN} \sum_{i=1}^{M} \sum_{j=1}^{N} (O_1(i,j) - F_2(i,j))^2. \tag{7}$$

$$SNR(F_2, O_1) = 10 \cdot \log_{10} \left(\frac{\sigma_1^2}{MSE} \right), \tag{8}$$

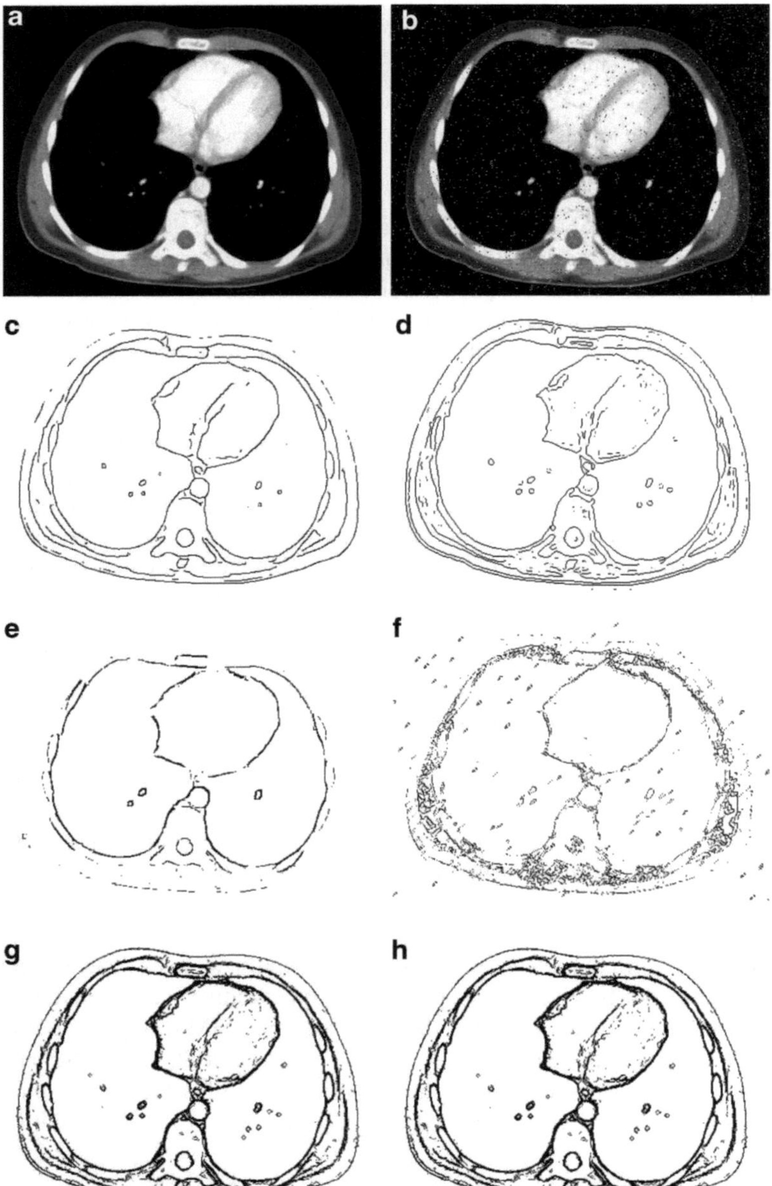

Fig. 3 (**a**) Original lungs CT image. (**b**) Corrupted with 0.02 salt and pepper noise. (**c, d**) Results by Canny and zero-cross edge detectors, respectively. (**e, f**) Results obtained by the proposed algorithm using the Łukasiewicz t-norm and umbra approach, respectively. (**g, h**) Results obtained by the proposed algorithm using a representable and an idempotent uninorm, respectively

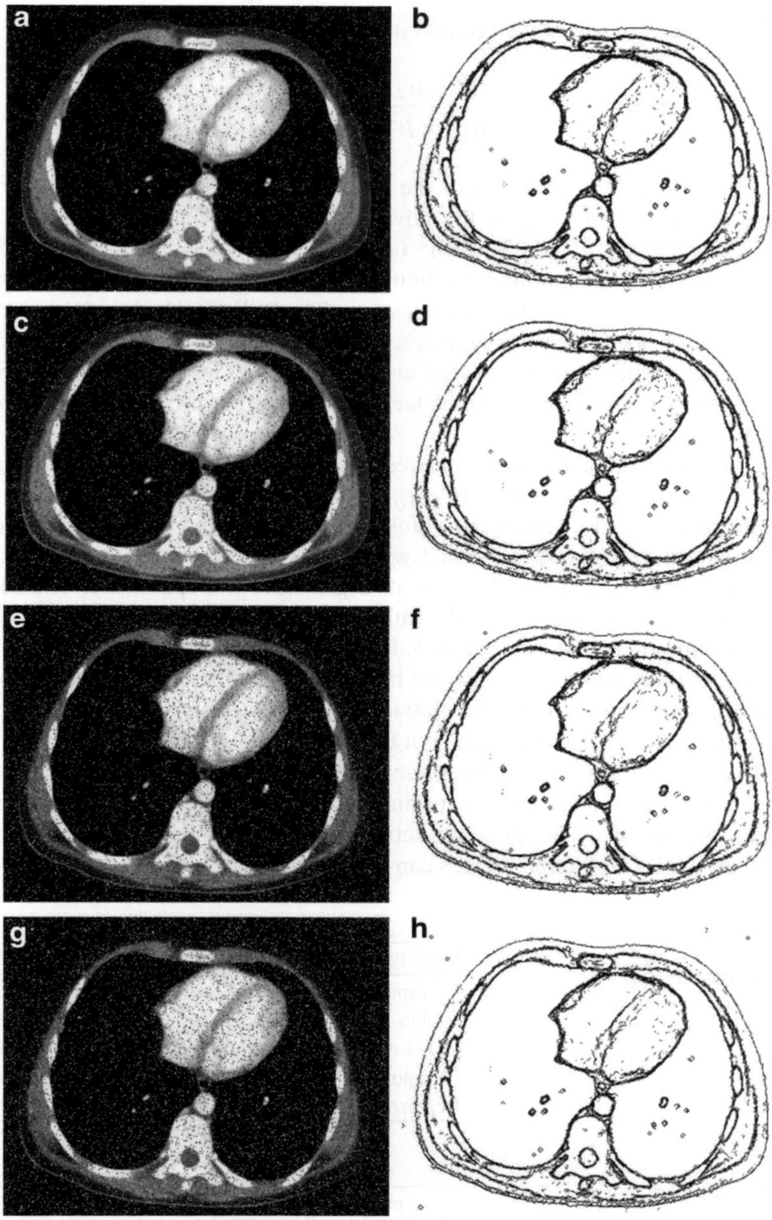

Fig. 4 From *top* to *bottom*, corrupted original image (*left*) and results (*right*) obtained by the proposed algorithm using the same idempotent uninorm and structural element than in Fig. 3h, when we corrupted the original image with 0.04, 0.06, 0.08 and 0.1 salt and pepper noise, respectively

where σ_1^2 is the variance of the original image O_1,

$$SSIM(F_2, O_1) = \frac{(2\mu_1\mu_2 + C_1)}{(\mu_1^2 + \mu_2^2 + C_1)} \cdot \frac{(2\sigma_{12} + C_2)}{(\sigma_1^2 + \sigma_2^2 + C_2)}, \tag{9}$$

where μ_k, $k = 1, 2$ is the mean of the image O_1 and F_2 respectively, σ_k^2 is the variance of each image, σ_{12} is the covariance between the two images, $C_1 = (0.01 \cdot 255)^2$ and $C_2 = (0.03 \cdot 255)^2$ (see [22] for details). Recently, SSIM was introduced under the assumption that human visual perception is highly adapted for extracting structural information from a scene. The SSIM is an alternative complementary framework for quality assessment based on the degradation of structural information. Smaller values of MSE and larger values of both SNR and SSIM ($0 \leq SSIM \leq 1$) are indicators of better capabilities for noise reduction and image recovery.

The values of these measures between the original image and filtered image $C_{U,\mathcal{I}_U}(F, B)$, where $F = O_{U,\mathcal{I}_U}(C_{U,\mathcal{I}_U}(A, B), B)$, associated to the experiments displayed in Fig. 3, are depicted in Table 1. It can be noticed that when we use uninorms the measures are improved with respect to the other cases. The original and corrupted image can be seen in Fig. 3a and b respectively. The filtered images using the umbra approach, the Łukasiewicz t-norm, the idempotent and representable uninorms are shown in Fig. 5. It can be seen in this figure, that the filtered images using the uninorm approach are more similar to the original image than the filtered images obtained using the classical or t-norm approach, in the sense that more noise is removed, as is pointed out in Table 1.

Table 2 shows the values of these measures in function of the amount of noise added to the original image in the experiments of Fig. 4. Notice that, when the noise increases, the values of the measures remain acceptable and SSIM values are still higher than 0.99. The filtered images can be seen in Fig. 6.

Table 1 MSE, SNR and SSIM for filtered images shown in Fig. 5 associated to the experiments displayed in Fig. 3

Filter type	MSE	SNR	SSIM
Corrupted Img.	578.826	11.0088	0.96108
Umbra App.	1228.39	7.74087	0.920127
Luk. t-norm	148.08	16.9293	0.989052
Idempotent	26.6825	24.372	0.998137
Representable	26.6826	24.378	0.998139

Table 2 MSE, SNR and SSIM for filtered images shown in Fig. 6 associated to the two experiments displayed in Fig. 4

Noise parameter	MSE	SNR	SSIM
0.02	26.6825	24.372	0.998137
0.04	41.1434	22.4912	0.9971357
0.06	50.7033	21.5839	0.996468
0.08	70.2527	20.1676	0.995104
0.1	102.487	18.5275	0.992877

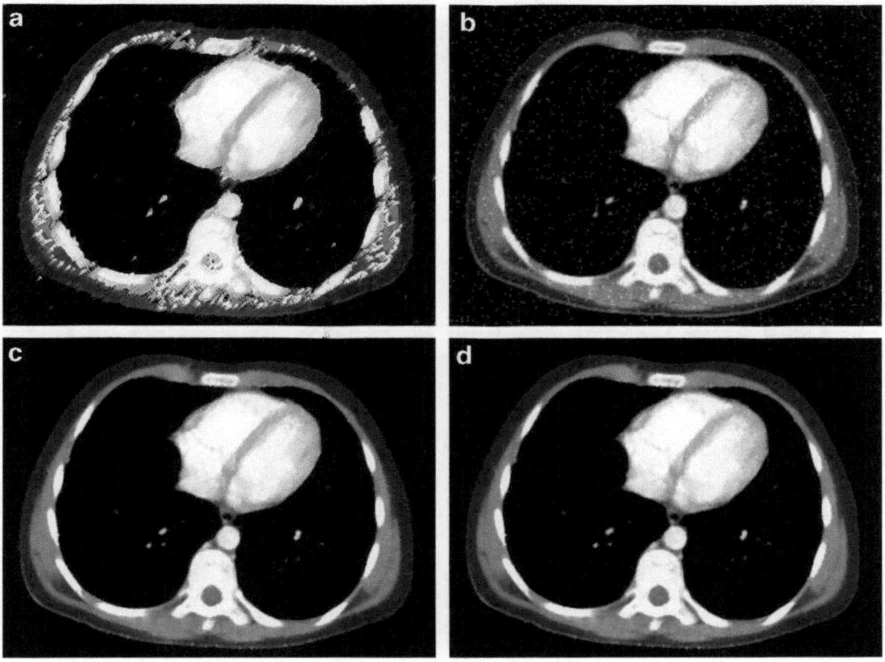

Fig. 5 Filtered image $C_{U,\mathcal{I}_U}(F, B)$ where $F = O_{U,\mathcal{I}_U}(C_{U,\mathcal{I}_U}(A, B), B)$, associated to the edge images displayed in Fig. 3, and obtained by the proposed morphological algorithm. (**a, b**) Filtered images obtained using the umbra approach and the Łukasiewicz t-norm respectively. (**c, d**) Filtered images obtained using an idempotent and representable uninorm respectively. The objective measures associated to these images are depicted in Table 1

In Fig. 7 we can see another CT scan image altered by salt and pepper of parameter 0.04 (Fig. 7a–b). The results obtained by the proposed algorithm are shown in Fig. 7c–d. Also, detailed features are detected in the CT image and many thin features are detected with a strong intensity.

Finally, Fig. 8 shows an experiment in which the original image is corrupted with Gaussian noise of parameter 0.005. A Wiener filter is applied, because it works better than the median filter in presence of Gaussian noise, previously to the classical edge detection method. In this case the structural element used by the morphological operators is a 5×5 matrix given by

$$\begin{pmatrix} 0 & 0 & 1 & 0 & 0 \\ 0 & 1 & 1 & 1 & 0 \\ 1 & 1 & 1 & 1 & 1 \\ 0 & 1 & 1 & 1 & 0 \\ 0 & 0 & 1 & 0 & 0 \end{pmatrix} \cdot e \tag{10}$$

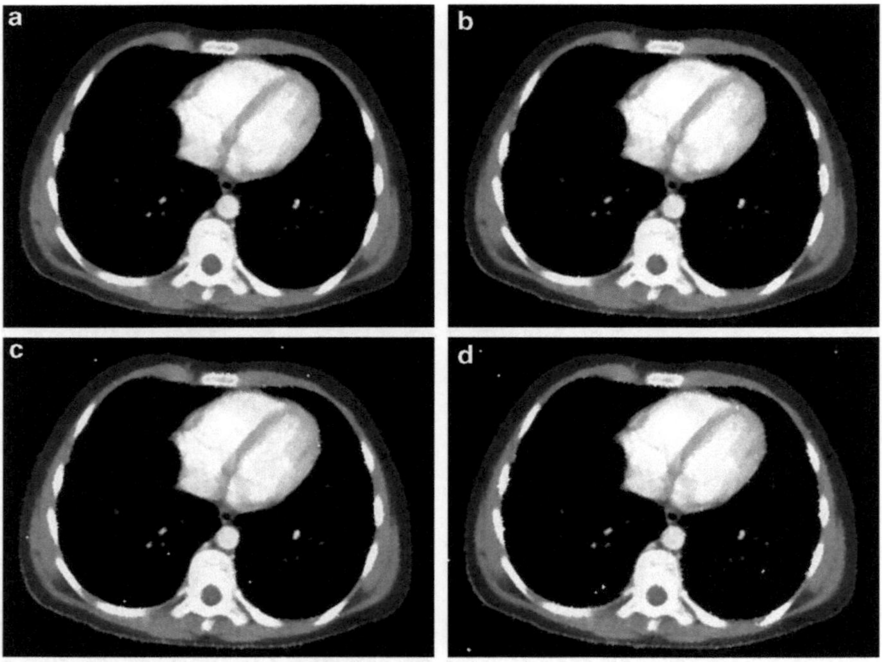

Fig. 6 From *left* to *right* and from *top* to *bottom*, filtered image $C_{U,\mathcal{I}_U}(F, B)$ where $F = O_{U,\mathcal{I}_U}(C_{U,\mathcal{I}_U}(A, B), B)$, obtained by the proposed algorithm using the same idempotent uninorm and structural element than in Fig. 3h, when we corrupted the original image with 0.04 (**a**), 0.06 (**b**), 0.08 (**c**) and 0.1 (**d**) salt and pepper noise, respectively. The objective measures associated to these images are depicted in Table 2

where e is the neutral element of the uninorm. It can be seen how the edge images obtained using the fuzzy proposed approach produce a good edge detection performance. Observe that the classical approaches fail to detect some main edge features of the image.

5 Conclusions and Future Work

In this work, an edge detection algorithm based on the fuzzy morphology using uninorms, derived as a residual operator from the basic morphological operations, has been proposed. Such algorithm is able to detect the features in low contrast regions, and preserve them as well as other apparent edges. To evaluate the performance of the algorithm, comparison experiments with other well known approaches were carried out. The results indicate that the proposed algorithm is robust against noisy images. Experimental results show that it outperforms other edge detection methods in detecting detailed edges features and thin edge features, in the displayed medical images. Moreover, these edges can be preserved even though the image is

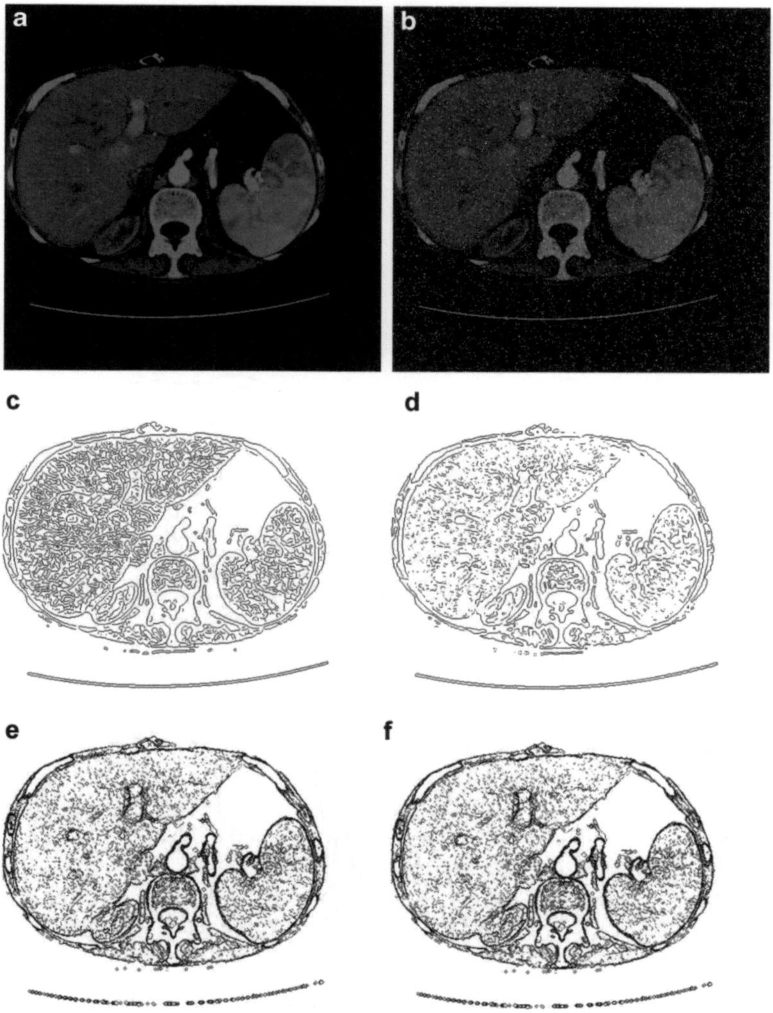

Fig. 7 (**a**) Original CT scan image. (**b**) Corrupted with salt and pepper noise of parameter 0.04. (**c**, **d**) Results obtained by Canny and zero-cross edge detectors, respectively. (**e**, **f**) Edge detection results obtained by the proposed algorithm using the representable and idempotent uninorm, respectively

corrupted by noise. Future work consists on one hand, in the study of the behaviour of the algorithm when we increase the Gaussian noise and, on the other hand in the selection of the size, shape, direction of the structuring element adapted to the edge features of the image and how we can improve performance.

Acknowledgements This work has been supported by the Government Spanish Grant MTM2009-10320 and TIN2007-67993, with FEDER support.

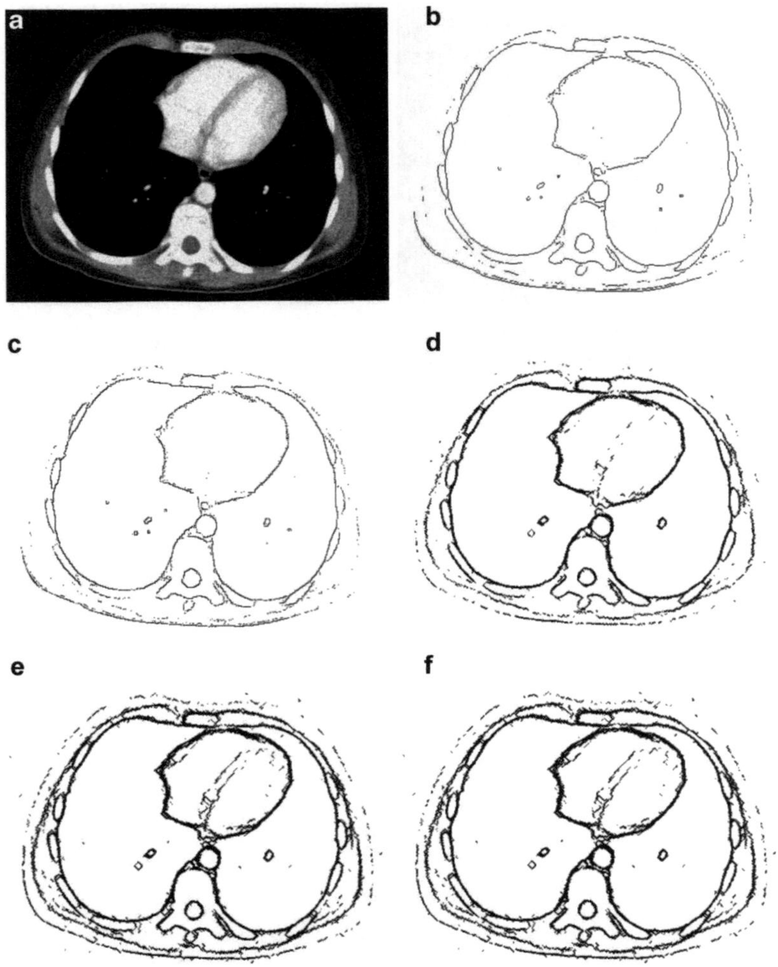

Fig. 8 (**a**) Image corrupted with 0.005 Gaussian noise. (**b, c**) Edge images obtained using Prewitt and Roberts edge detectors, respectively. (**d–f**) Results obtained by the proposed algorithm using the Łukasiewicz t-norm, a representable and an idempotent uninorm, respectively

References

1. Bloch, I., Maître, H.: Fuzzy mathematical morphologies: a comparative study. Pattern Recogn. **28**, 1341–1387 (1995)
2. Bustince, H., Barrenechea, E., Pagola, M., Fernandez, J.: Interval-valued fuzzy sets constructed from matrices: Application to edge detection. Fuzzy Set. Syst. **160**(13), 1819–1840 (2009)
3. Canny, J.: A computational approach to edge detection. IEEE Trans. Pattern Anal. Mach. Intell. **8**(6), 679–698 (1986)
4. Chen, T., Wu, Q.H., Rahmani-Torkaman, R., Hughes, J.: A pseudo top-hat mathematical morphological approach to edge detection in dark regions. Pattern Recogn. **35**(1), 199–210 (2002)

5. De Baets, B.: Fuzzy morphology: A logical approach. In: Ayyub, B.M., Gupta, M.M. (eds.) Uncertainty Analysis in Engineering and Science: Fuzzy Logic, Statistics, and Neural Network Approach, pp. 53–68. Kluwer Academic Publishers, Norwell (1997)
6. De Baets, B., Fodor, J.: Residual operators of uninorms. Soft Comput. **3**, 89–100 (1999)
7. De Baets, B., Kerre, E., Gupta, M.: The fundamentals of fuzzy mathematical morfologies part i: basics concepts. Int. J. Gen. Syst. **23**, 155–171 (1995)
8. De Baets, B., Kwasnikowska, N., Kerre, E.: Fuzzy morphology based on uninorms. In: Proceedings of the 7th IFSA World Congress, pp. 215–220. Prague (1997)
9. Fodor, J., Yager, R., Rybalov, A.: Structure of uninorms. Int. J. Uncertainty, Fuzziness, Knowledge-Based Systems **5**, 411–427 (1997)
10. González, M., Ruiz-Aguilera, D., Torrens, J.: Algebraic properties of fuzzy morphological operators based on uninorms. In: Artificial Intelligence Research and Development, Frontiers in Artificial Intelligence and Applications, vol. 100, pp. 27–38. IOS Press, Amsterdam (2003)
11. González-Hidalgo, M., Mir-Torres, A., Ruiz-Aguilera, D.: A robust edge detection algorithm based on a fuzzy mathematical morphology using uninorms (ϕMM-U morphology). In: Tavares, J.M.R., Jorge, R.M.N. (eds.) Computational Vision and Medical Image Processing: VipIMAGE 2009 09, pp. 630–635. CRC Press, Taylor & Francis, Inc., Bristol, PA, USA (2009)
12. González-Hidalgo, M., Mir-Torres, A., Ruiz-Aguilera, D., Torrens, J.: Edge-images using a uninorm-based fuzzy mathematical morphology: Opening and closing. In: Tavares, J., Jorge, N. (eds.) Advances in Computational Vision and Medical Image Processing. Computational Methods in Applied Sciences, vol. 13, pp. 137–157. Springer, Netherlands (2009)
13. González-Hidalgo, M., Mir-Torres, A., Ruiz-Aguilera, D., Torrens, J.: Image analysis applications of morphological operators based on uninorms. In: Carvalho, P., Dubois, D., Kaymak, U., Sousa, J.M.C. (eds.) Proceedings of the Joint 2009 International Fuzzy Systems Association World Congress and 2009 European Society of Fuzzy Logic and Technology Conference (IFSA-EUSFLAT 2009), pp. 630–635. EUSFLAT Society, Lisbon, Portugal (2009) http://www.eusflat.org/publications/proceedings/IFSA-EUSFLAT%_2009/
14. González-Hidalgo, M., Mir-Torres, A., Sastre, J.T.: Noise reduction using alternate filters generated by fuzzy mathematical operators using uninorms (ϕMM-U morphology). In: Burillo, P., Bustince, H., Baets, B.D., Fodor, J. (eds.) EUROFUSE WORKSHOP 09, Preference Modelling and Decision Analysis, pp. 233–238. Public University of Navarra, Pamplona, Spain (2009)
15. Guimarães, S.J.F., Leite, N.J., Couprie, M., de Albuquerque Araújo, A.: A directional and parametrized transition detection algorithm based on morphological residues. In: Proceedings of the 15th Brazilian Symposium on Computer Graphics and Image Processing, SIBGRAPI'02, pp. 261–268. IEEE Computer Society, Washington, DC, USA (2002)
16. Jiang, J.A., Chuang, C.L., Lu, Y.L., Fahn, C.S: Mathematical-morphology-based edge detectors for detection of thin edges in low-contrast regions. IET Image Process. **1**(3), 269–277 (2007)
17. Nachtegael, M., Kerre, E.: Classical and fuzzy approaches towards mathematical morphology. In: Kerre, E.E., Nachtegael, M. (eds.) Fuzzy Techniques in Image Processing. Studies in Fuzziness and Soft Computing, vol. 52, pp. 3–57. Physica-Verlag, New York (2000)
18. Pastore, J.I., Moler, E., Ballarin, V.: Multiscale morphological operators and geodesic distance applied to computer axial tomography segmentation. Lat. Am. Trans. IEEE **5**(1), 28–31 (2007)
19. Pratt, W.K.: Digital Image Processing, 4th edn. Wiley (2007)
20. Ruiz-Aguilera, D., Torrens, J.: Residual implications and co-implications from idempotent uninorms. Kybernetika **40**, 21–38 (2004)
21. Serra, J.: Image Analysis and Mathematical Morphology, vols. 1, 2. Academic, London (1982, 1988)
22. Wang, Z., Bovik, A.C., Sheikh, H.R., Simoncelli, E.P.: Image quality assessment: From error visibility to structural similarity. IEEE Trans. Image Process. **13**(4), 600–612 (2004)
23. Yu-qian, Z., Wei-hua, G., Zhen-cheng, C., Jing-tian, T., Ling-yun, L.: Medical images edge detection based on mathematical morphology. In: Proceedings of the 2005 IEEE Engineering in Medicine and Biology 27th Annual Conference, pp. 6492–6495. Shanghai, China (2005)

Leveraging Graphics Hardware for an Automatic Classification of Bone Tissue

Manuel Jesús Martín-Requena and Manuel Ujaldón

Abstract Zernike moments are fundamental digital image descriptors used in many application areas due to their good properties of orthogonality and rotation invariance, but their computation is too expensive and limits its application in practice, overall when real-time constraints are imposed. The contribution of this work is twofold: Accelerate the computation of Zernike moments using graphics processors (GPUs) and assess its expressiveness as descriptors of image tiles for its subsequent classification into bone and cartilage regions to quantify the degree of bone tissue regeneration from stem cells. The characterization of those image tiles is performed through a vector of features, whose optimal composition is extensively analyzed after testing 19 subsets of Zernike moments selected as the best potential candidates. Those candidates are later evaluated depending on its ability for a successful classification of image tiles via LDA, K-means and KNN classifiers, and a final rank of moments is provided according to its discriminative power to distinguish between bone and cartilage. Prior to that study, we introduce a novel approach to the high-performance computation of Zernike moments on GPUs. The proposed method is compared against three of the fastest implementations performed on CPUs over the last decade using recursive methods and the fastest direct method computed on a Pentium 4, with factor gains up to 125× on a 256 × 256 image when computing a single moment on a GPU, and up to 700× on a 1024 × 1024 image when computing all repetitions for a given order using direct methods.

Keywords Bone tissue classification · Digital image descriptors · Zernike moments · Graphics processors

M.J. Martín-Requena and M. Ujaldón (✉)
Computer Architecture Department, University of Málaga, Spain
e-mail: martinrequena@uma.es; ujaldon@uma.es

J.M.R.S. Tavares and R.M.N. Jorge (eds.), *Computational Vision and Medical Image Processing: Recent Trends*, Computational Methods in Applied Sciences 19,
DOI 10.1007/978-94-007-0011-6_12,

1 Introduction

Image segmentation is one of the most fundamental yet difficult problems in computer vision [20] and image analysis [17]. A driving application for segmentation is medical imaging, where the goal is to identify a 3D region within a volume obtained as a set of consecutive images or slides. Different approaches have been proposed to deal with this challenge [16]: Histogram thresholding, edge detection, region-based, artificial neural networks, fuzzy logic-based methods, and feature clustering. Within this last set of methods, a number of techniques [24] have been used for obtaining the vector of features required as input to the clustering process: Statistical (based on co-occurrence matrices and autocorrelation functions), geometrical (Voronoi tessellation), structural (tree grammars), model based (random fields and fractals) and signal processing (spatial and frequency domain filters, Legendre and Zernike moments, Gabor and wavelet models). Among them, spatial domain filters are the most direct way to characterize edges, granularity and shape as global features in many application areas, including aircraft identification [4], scene matching [18] and character recognition [23].

An important subset of spatial domain filters are based on moment functions of pixel intensity values [22]. Moment functions are expressed as discrete sums, which can be interpreted as a convolution of the image with a mask. However, moments are more attractive than convolutions because some are invariant to image translation, scale change and rotation [3, 10]. Derived from the general concept, moments with orthogonal basis functions such as Legendre and Zernike polynomials can be used to represent the image by a set of mutually independent descriptors, with a minimal amount of information redundancy [21]. The orthogonality property enables the separation of the individual contribution of each order moment, allowing the image reconstruction from a linear addition of such contributions. The greater the number of moments considered, the better the reconstructed image, and we have to go beyond order 50 to obtain a reasonable output [8], which results in a significant computational cost.

In general, the calculation of Zernike moments with order up to M for an $N \times N$ image by a straightforward method requires $O(M^2N^2)$ sums and products. These sophisticated formulas, combined with a frequent use in high resolution images, lead to a severe computational cost which impedes a feasible application in many areas demanding a quick or even real-time response. To deal with this issue, we may distinguish two solutions depending on applications:

1. Industrial control systems with real-time constraints focus on low-order moments [9], which also allow them to stay away from noise sensitivity of high order moments.
2. Image processing and pattern recognition applications rely on several methods recently proposed to speed-up the computation. Those methods are summarized in Sect. 2.1.

Our work provides an implementation of Zernike moments on high-performance emerging architectures like graphics processors (GPUs) which is closer to real-time response regardless of the source application. The motivation of our work entails a step forward in performance duet to the current capabilities of GPUs with respect to GFLOPS (arithmetic intensity for the fast computation of a heavy workload) and GB/s (memory bandwidth for the fast data retrieval on a vast memory use).

The rest of this paper is organized as follows. We start with a description of Zernike moments in Sect. 2. Then, Sect. 3 briefly introduces the GPU hardware platform and its underlying CUDA software execution model. Section 4 describes our GPU implementation and the performance attained versus existing methods. Section 5 illustrates the usefulness of certain Zernike moments for the segmentation of image samples taken from our biomedical survey, and assess their skill to differentiate between bone and cartilage tissue regenerated from stem cells. Finally, Sect. 6 summarizes our contribution and concludes.

2 Zernike Moments

In order to define Zernike moments, we first introduce Zernike functions, a set of complex orthogonal functions with a simple rotational property which forms a complete orthogonal basis over the class of square integrable functions introduced by F. Zernike in 1934. The (p, q) order Zernike function, $V_{pq}(x, y)$, is defined as:

$$V_{pq}(x, y) = R_{pq}(\rho) \cdot e^{jq\theta}, \quad x^2 + y^2 \leq 1 \tag{1}$$

where $\rho = \sqrt{x^2 + y^2}$ is the length of the vector from the origin to the pixel (x,y), $\theta = arctan(y/x)$ is the angle between the vector and the x axis, and $R_{pq}(\rho)$ is a polynomial in ρ of degree $p \geq 0$, containing no power of ρ lower than $|q|$ (see [22] for an explicit formula). The integer q represents the repetition index for a given order p, and is required to satisfy $|q| \leq p$, where $p - |q|$ is an even number.

Any polynomial of degree p will be invariant with respect to rotations of axes about the origin if and only if the polynomial is of the form given by (1).

The completeness and orthogonality of $V_{pq}(x, y)$ allow us to represent any square integrable image function $f(x, y)$ defined on the unit disk in the following series:

$$f(x, y) = \sum_{p=0}^{\infty} \sum_{q=-p}^{p} \rho_p A_{pq} V_{pq}(x, y), \quad p - |q| = even \tag{2}$$

where $\rho_p = \frac{p+1}{\pi}$ is the normalizing constant and A_{pq} is the Zernike moment of order p with repetition q, i.e.,

$$A_{pq} = \int\int_D f(x, y) V_{pq}(x, y) dx dy \tag{3}$$

The fundamental feature of the Zernike moments is their rotational invariance. If f(x,y) is rotated by an angle α, then we can obtain that the Zernike moment A'_{pq} of the rotated image is given by

$$A'_{pq} = A_{pq} e^{-jq\alpha} \tag{4}$$

Zernike moments are also invariant to linear transformations, which makes them more suitable for image analysis than other existing approaches like Legendre moments [22, 23], but always at the expense of a higher computational cost [14].

2.1 Optimizations

The computation of Zernike moments has been extensively improved over the years. The three following methods summarize all major optimizations:

1. Mukundan et al. [14] use a recursive algorithm for the calculation of Zernike polynomial coefficients through a square-to-circular image transformation scheme which minimizes the computation involved in Zernike moment functions.
2. Hwang et al. [9] have developed a fast recursive computation that depends on the symmetry properties of a point in the first octant, where the reduction in operations is accomplished by making use of similar terms derived for the symmetrical points in the remaining seven octants.
3. Al-Rawi [1] recently implemented on a CPU a wide range of Zernike moment orders via geometric moments which clearly outperforms the best methods based on Zernike polynomials.

2.2 Input Images

During our experimental analysis the source for our input data set consisted of real biomedical images used for cartilage and bone regeneration. We tried images with different stainings to study the influence of image contents over the execution time (see Fig. 1). The workload of our image processing algorithms was strongly

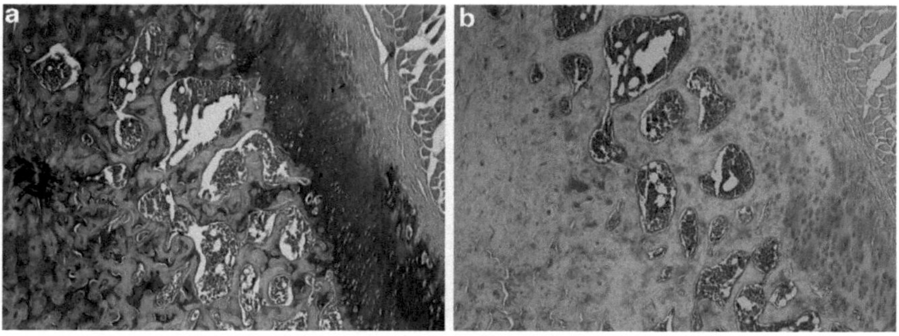

Fig. 1 The input images to our experimental survey were taken from biomedical studies on stem cells to quantify the degree of cartilage and bone regeneration. (**a**) Astral-safranin blue, with a good balance of red, green and blue channels. (**b**) Alcian blue, where cyan tones predominate and the analysis may be reduced to a single color channel, like the role played by luminance in grayscale images

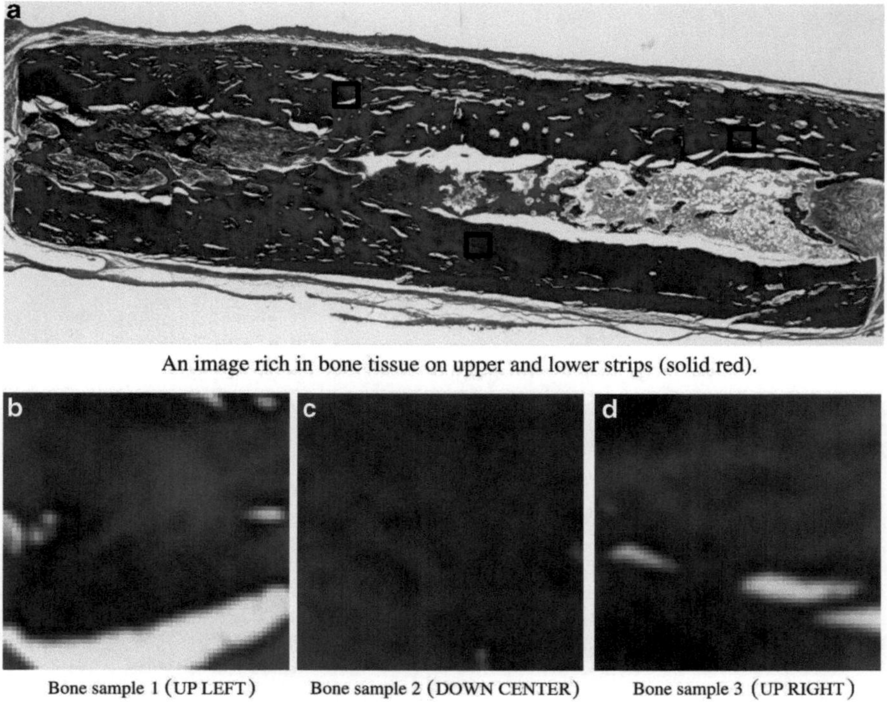

Fig. 2 Biomedical tissue image stained with picrosirius, where a strong and solid red reveals the successful transformation of stem cells into bone tissue. From the 2560×1920 original image, three samples of 64×64 pixels were selected to characterize bone tissue for the computation of Zernike moments

affected by image resolution and loosely affected by image contents, after which we selected image tiles of 64×64 pixels stained with picrosirius for the characterization of bone and cartilage regeneration (see Figs. 2 and 3). Since X-ray images or images captured by an electronic microscope work with grayscale images, we convert to grayscale images in a preprocessing stage prior to the actual computation of Zernike moments over the luminance channel.

3 Using GPUs to Compute Zernike Moments

Modern GPUs are powerful computing platforms recently devoted to general-purpose computing [7] using CUDA (Compute Unified Device Architecture) [15].

As a hardware interface, CUDA started by transforming the G80 microarchitecture related to the GeForce 8 series from Nvidia into a parallel SIMD architecture endowed with up to 128 cores, where a collection or threads run in parallel. Figure 4

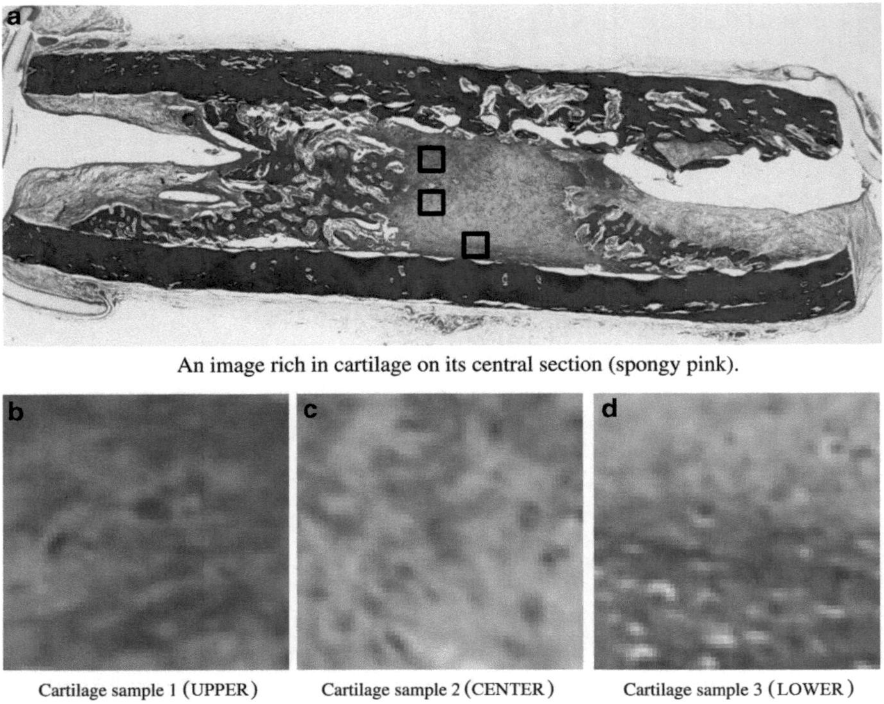

Fig. 3 Biomedical tissue image stained with picrosirius, where the central region reveals the presence of cartilage tissue as spongy pink. Within this area, three samples of 64×64 pixels were selected for the further computation of Zernike moments

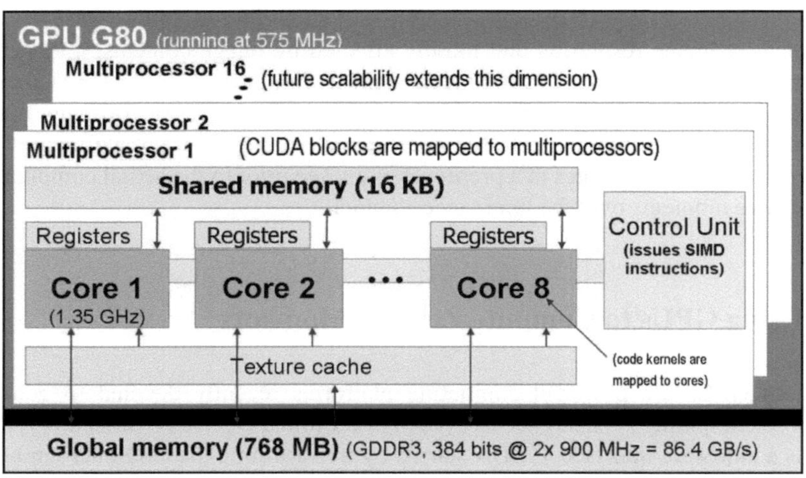

Fig. 4 The CUDA hardware interface for the G80

Table 1 Summary of hardware features for the set of hardware processors used during our experiments

Processor	Core 2 Q9450	GeForce 9800 GX2	Tesla C1060
Type and manufacturer	CPU by Intel	GPU by Nvidia	GPU by Nvidia
# Cores and speed	Four @ 2.66 GHz	One @ 600 MHz	One @ 575 MHz
Streaming processors	Does not apply	128 @ 1.35 GHz	240 @ 1.296 GHz
Memory speed	2 × 900 MHz	2 × 1 GHz	2 × 800 MHz
Memory bus width	384 bits	256 bits	512 bits
Memory bandwidth	86.4 GB/s	64 GB/s	102 GB/s
Memory size and type	768 MB GDDR3	512 MB GDDR3	4 GB GDDR3
Bus to video memory	Does not apply	PCI-e x16 2.0	PCI-e x16 1.0

outlines the block diagram of this architecture. Later, the GeForce 9800 GX2 would be released from the 9 series, and the Tesla C1060 from the 10 series, the platforms used during our experiments (see Table 1). From the CUDA perspective, cores are organized into a set of multiprocessors, each having a set of 32-bit registers and 16 KB of on-chip shared memory as fast as local registers (one cycle latency). At any given cycle, each core executes the same instruction on different data (SIMD), and communication between multiprocessors is performed through global memory (the video memory tied to the graphics card, whose latency is around 400–600 cycles).

As a programming interface, CUDA consists of a set of C language library functions, and the CUDA-specific compiler generates the executable for the GPU from a source code where we find elements like computational blocks, threads, kernels and grids [15]. All of the threads can access all of the GPU memory, but, as expected, there is a performance boost when threads access data resident in shared memory, which is explicitly managed by the programmer.

4 Performance Analysis

4.1 Hardware Resources

To demonstrate the effectiveness of our techniques, we have conducted a number of experiments on different CPU and GPU platforms (see Table 1 for hardware details). Stream processors (cores) outlined in Fig. 4 are built on a hardwired design for a much faster clock frequency than the rest of the silicon area (1.296–1.35 GHz versus 575–600 MHz). We decided to use two different video cards to quantify the benefits of a newer GPU generation and additional video memory.

4.2 GPU Implementation

This section describes our implementation on a GPU and evaluates the performance of our image analysis algorithms on emerging architectures as compared to existing methods running on regular PCs.

The computation of Zernike moments was implemented up to order $p = 50$. In general, low order moments keep most of the image features for image analysis and classification, whereas moments of high order are used for image reconstruction, being more sensitive to noise and computationally demanding. We compute the full set of Zernike moments (that is, all repetitions) under different orders set to $p = 4, 8, 12, ..., 48$. For example, three moments are computed for the fourth order: $A_{4,0}$, $A_{4,2}$ and $A_{4,4}$.

4.3 Performance Against Existing Methods

In order to compare execution times for the computation of Zernike moments, it is important to distinguish between recursive methods and direct methods:

Recursive Methods They are more convenient when a set of chained moments have to be computed, because new coefficients are calculated as functions of the previous ones and the weight of evaluating complex mathematical formulas is partially amortized on each additional order it is computed on top of the existing ones. An illustrative example here is image reconstruction, where all moments (repetitions) are required up to a given order.

Direct Methods They are faster when moments are computed partially or individually to become features characterizing an image after a selection of the most discriminant coefficients. This situation arises more often on image classifiers, and being the one we are interested for our biomedical analysis, it brings our attention and priority from now on.

The computation of a single order moment and an isolated repetition within an order cannot be computed by recursive methods without sweeping over all previous repetitions and orders. Hwang et al. [9] developed individual formulas to skip this significant overhead, but despite this effort, our results on the GPU are much faster than the CPU when processing the same non-recursive algorithm on both sides (see Table 2). The first column on that table shows execution times obtained by Hwang et al. on a Pentium 4 1.7 GHz CPU (2006) to obtain three different coefficients by direct methods. We then show our execution times extended to ten different cases on a newer CPU (2009), and two counterpart GPUs. Speed-up factors up to 125x are attained in the best case scenario, which corresponds to the higher moment order, $p = 48$, and the lower repetition, $q = 0$.

Additional optimizations based on task-level parallelism and symmetry can be performed on both sides:

Table 2 Execution times (in ms) for computing Zernike moments on a 256 × 256 image. A single repetition for a given order is calculated as shown on each row, with all the computation performed through direct methods. The final column reflects the performance factor gained by the best GPU platform versus the fastest CPU counterpart hardware

A single moment of an order	On CPUs Hwang (2006)	Core 2 Q9450	On GPUs GeForce 9800	Tesla C1060	GPU/ CPU gain
$A_{0,0}$	n.a.	41.22	5.28	5.45	7.56×
$A_{6,2}$	225	109.53	5.54	5.55	19.73×
$A_{12,0}$	282	179.42	5.75	5.49	32.68×
$A_{25,13}$	408	231.79	5.75	5.65	41.02×
$A_{36,0}$	n.a.	584.02	6.40	6.04	96.63×
$A_{36,18}$	n.a.	353.55	5.81	5.76	61.38×
$A_{36,36}$	n.a.	85.34	5.58	5.36	15.92×
$A_{48,0}$	n.a.	856.17	6.85	6.31	124.98×
$A_{48,24}$	n.a.	514.87	6.49	5.77	89.23×
$A_{48,48}$	n.a.	89.78	5.50	5.34	16.81×

Parallelism Traditionally, the CPU exploits instruction-level parallelism using pipelining and superscalar executions, so does the GPU with data parallelism through a SIMD execution over 128/240 stream processors. Parallelism may be enhanced on both sides using a more novel approach based on task-level parallelism: On CPUs, using multiple cores (up to four in our platform); on GPUs, using multiple graphics cards (also limited to four in our case). In both cases, the code must be parallelized declaring four threads and partitioning input data into four symmetric chunks. With a similar programming effort, preliminary results for our code reveal a good scalability in both cases, CPU and GPU, to conclude that the gap in performance still maintains after this optimization step.

Symmetry An expensive computing stage in Zernike formulas is a term involving the distance from each pixel to the image center. An optimization performed in [9] and also ported to the GPU by our implementation consists of calculating eight coefficients at a time, all those that keep a symmetry within the image origin and thus share this distance. [9] reported almost an 8x factor gain by using this strategy, which is similar to the speed-up factor we achieved on the GPU using CUDA.

We now move to the computation of a whole set of orders and repetitions, the scenario where recursive methods show its usefulness. Table 3 shows the execution times for a set of implementations performed on different CPUs using mostly Microsoft Visual C++ 2005 and Windows XP, together with our results on GPUs using CUDA. Note that these executions are performed on a 1024 × 1024 image, whereas the previous results were using 256 × 256 images to be able to compare with existing implementations on each particular case.

On the CPU side, this time we show the best three recursive methods introduced in Sect. 2.1. Due to the way the GPU processes data through rendering passes, the direct method is faster than any other recursive method on the GPU. This also

Table 3 Execution times (in ms) for computing Zernike moments on a 1024 × 1024 image. All repetitions of a given order are calculated, with the required number of moments shown between parenthesis on each row. The final column reflects the performance factor gained by the best GPU platform computing direct methods versus the fastest CPU using recursive methods

All moments, m, for a given order, N	Recursive methods on CPU platforms			Direct methods			Direct vs. recursive speed-up
	Mukundan (1995)	Hwang (2006)	Al-Rawi (2008)	on a CPU Core 2 Q9450	on a GPU GeForce 9800 GX2	on a GPU Tesla C1060	
$A_{4,*}$ (3)	1391.00	258.00	62.50	2725.02	97.86	91.14	0.68×
$A_{8,*}$ (5)	3820.50	859.00	54.50	6725.49	110.63	97.83	0.55×
$A_{12,*}$ (7)	7703.00	1969.00	62.50	12563.06	130.50	104.90	0.59×
$A_{16,*}$ (9)	13187.50	3836.00	78.00	20410.76	147.59	113.70	0.68×
$A_{20,*}$ (11)	20109.50	6586.00	93.50	30612.76	169.58	125.64	0.74×
$A_{24,*}$ (13)	28719.00	10617.00	117.50	43354.13	195.34	140.60	0.83×
$A_{28,*}$ (15)	39078.00	15359.00	133.00	59023.90	224.69	155.85	0.85×
$A_{32,*}$ (17)	51039.00	22773.00	156.00	77622.09	258.76	173.55	0.89×
$A_{36,*}$ (19)	64945.50	30617.50	179.50	99562.33	294.06	193.94	0.92×
$A_{40,*}$ (21)	80625.00	40390.50	203.50	125124.62	333.62	217.58	0.93×
$A_{44,*}$ (23)	98570.50	52765.50	219.00	153914.94	376.97	240.18	0.91×
$A_{48,*}$ (25)	120899.00	67125.00	250.00	187060.00	425.84	266.99	0.93×

introduces the advantage of a much higher degree of parallelism when running on multiprocessors, together with a promising scalability in future GPU generations. Unfortunately, this decision assumes a much higher workload, which can be quantified on the CPU side when moving from existing recursive implementations on older platforms to our results collected by a direct method on a newer Intel Core 2 Quad (see the fourth and fifth columns in Table 3). Despite this much higher computational workload, GPU execution times are similar to those obtained on CPUs, and we expect GPUs to evolve in a more favorable way in the near future due to its higher scalability, leading to a winner strategy for all studied cases.

5 Classification of Bone Tissue Using Zernike Moments

5.1 The Biomedical Problem

A wide variety of histologically stained images in cell biology require deep analysis to characterize certain features for the tissue being analyzed. A good example is cartilage and bone regeneration, where a specific microenvironment has been reported to induce the expression of skeletal matrix proteins, playing a regulatory role in the initiation of cartilage differentiation and the induction of bone-forming cells from pluripotent mesenchymal stem cells [2].

We have developed algorithms for tracking such biomedical evolution at image level as a preliminary step for converting the complete analysis process to a semi-automatic task: the medical expert interacts with the computer to attain a number of image descriptors and attributes that help to understand the biomedical features and lead to an automatic classification of image tiles into bone or cartilage, to later quantify the degree of bone regeneration depending on culture conditions.

The skeletal cartilage and bone regeneration image data set is obtained from implants on seven month old male rats. After 17 days of culture, in-vivo stem cells are implanted on animals into demineralized bone matrix or diffusion chambers. Four weeks later, rats are sacrificed, six chambers excised and tissues analyzed biochemically or processed for light microscopy after the appropriate fixation and sectioned at 7μm thickness. From each chamber, approximately 500 slices of tissue sample are obtained, each being a microscopic image composed of 2560×1920 pixels which is then decomposed into 40×30 tiles of 64×64 pixels for its subsequent classification into bone and cartilage classes.

The ultimate goal for computing Zernike moments within our biomedical application is to use them as features for characterizing every image tile so that we can perform an accurate image segmentation into bone and cartilage regions at tile level.

5.2 A Preliminary Selection of Zernike Moments

The orthogonality property of Zernike moments enables the separation of the individual contribution of each order moment, so after a preliminary inspection, the candidate moments were limited as follows:

1. We handle information for low order moments only, more precisely up to order $N = 16$, since higher moments were found to be increasingly costly and irrelevant (those moments are traditionally useful within the scope of image reconstruction).
2. We ignore the imaginary part of all moments, using the real side only.

When these two restrictions meet, the set of Zernike moments considered for each image tile shown in Figs. 2 and 3 are listed in Tables 4 and 5, respectively, for all even orders and repetitions (odd orders are omitted due to space constraints). These selected values are promising as long as we detect several properties characterizing bone and cartilage by simple visual inspection. Just to mention a local and a global indicator, we may point out the following ones:

1. The $A_{0,0}$ moment (the upper coefficient in all tables) stays below the 100 value in all bone samples, whereas it goes well above this mark in all cartilage samples.
2. The sum of moments with negative value is higher in cartilage samples (32, 32 and 33 negative values, for each of the three tiles) than in bone samples (28, 31 and 26 negative values, respectively). This indicator is also more stable when applied to cartilage samples, with higher variance on bone counterparts. Finally, note that cartilage tiles tend to look more homogeneous in color, and there is only one bone tile with such property, which is precisely the one with a higher number of negative moments (31).

Table 4 Zernike moments (real components only, imaginary not shown) for even orders between 0 and 16 for our three samples of bone tissue. Different orders (p) listed on consecutive rows; repetitions (q) spread over columns

Bone 1	$q = 0$	$q = 2$	$q = 4$	$q = 6$	$q = 8$	$q = 10$	$q = 12$	$q = 14$	$q = 16$
$p = 0$	75.19	–	–	–	–	–	–	–	–
$p = 2$	35.55	−21.16	–	–	–	–	–	–	–
$p = 4$	4.78	−1.62	9.02	–	–	–	–	–	–
$p = 6$	−20.23	9.17	−9.73	10.50	–	–	–	–	–
$p = 8$	−8.74	1.25	−5.12	−4.69	4.72	–	–	–	–
$p = 10$	−1.40	−5.96	1.68	0.94	−10.36	14.06	–	–	–
$p = 12$	−12.15	−1.02	−6.61	−0.97	−2.38	−6.30	0.59	–	–
$p = 14$	−17.02	4.49	−6.32	−3.58	−1.53	−0.05	−7.39	2.93	–
$p = 16$	−8.07	1.96	−0.15	−0.07	−4.48	0.47	−11.71	3.80	−4.74
Bone 2	$q = 0$	$q = 2$	$q = 4$	$q = 6$	$q = 8$	$q = 10$	$q = 12$	$q = 14$	$q = 16$
$p = 0$	44.80	–	–	–	–	–	–	–	–
$p = 2$	0.11	0.64	–	–	–	–	–	–	–
$p = 4$	−0.54	0.00	−0.01	–	–	–	–	–	–
$p = 6$	−1.54	−0.86	−0.13	−0.05	–	–	–	–	–
$p = 8$	−3.04	0.21	−0.44	0.43	−1.41	–	–	–	–
$p = 10$	−3.44	0.32	−2.35	0.09	−0.62	1.67	–	–	–
$p = 12$	−4.42	0.17	−1.10	−0.38	−1.33	−0.05	−4.64	–	–
$p = 14$	−3.61	−0.22	−1.01	−0.45	−1.23	−0.64	−3.24	0.00	–
$p = 16$	−5.03	−0.54	−0.78	0.56	−0.25	−0.82	−2.42	0.13	−2.21
Bone 3	$q = 0$	$q = 2$	$q = 4$	$q = 6$	$q = 8$	$q = 10$	$q = 12$	$q = 14$	$q = 16$
$p = 0$	56.52	–	–	–	–	–	–	–	–
$p = 2$	−4.86	6.57	–	–	–	–	–	–	–
$p = 4$	−9.17	1.01	−5.98	–	–	–	–	–	–
$p = 6$	6.09	−8.85	5.39	−4.22	–	–	–	–	–
$p = 8$	−7.18	5.91	−9.02	3.15	1.68	–	–	–	–
$p = 10$	−4.29	−0.18	3.55	−1.11	−0.94	2.43	–	–	–
$p = 12$	−0.38	−4.14	1.19	−2.65	0.78	−1.18	−5.97	–	–
$p = 14$	−7.61	3.96	−4.69	5.80	−4.08	1.35	−2.36	−3.94	–
$p = 16$	0.01	−2.99	1.55	−5.22	−0.50	0.43	−4.58	0.66	−2.03

5.3 Searching for the Optimal Vector of Features

Once the number of candidate moments was restricted, the final selection of features for the vector used as input to the classifier was driven by maximization accuracy when testing several combinations of Zernike moments under different classifiers. Our goal here is to determine those Zernike moments which are more discriminant during the classification process.

Table 5 Zernike moments (real components only, imaginary not shown) for even orders between 0 and 16 for our three samples of cartilage tissue. Different orders (p) listed on consecutive rows; repetitions (q) spread over columns

Cartilage 1	$q=0$	$q=2$	$q=4$	$q=6$	$q=8$	$q=10$	$q=12$	$q=14$	$q=16$
$p=0$	140.97	–	–	–	–	–	–		–
$p=2$	−4.42	3.35	–	–	–	–	–		–
$p=4$	−1.96	−2.76	−4.18	–	–	–	–		–
$p=6$	−1.94	−1.67	1.87	−1.02	–	–	–		–
$p=8$	−13.20	1.00	−4.41	1.61	−5.13	–	–		–
$p=10$	−8.24	0.80	−4.70	−0.38	0.80	−1.51	–		–
$p=12$	−12.35	−0.04	−1.28	0.30	−3.76	0.05	−11.32	–	–
$p=14$	−13.94	2.08	−4.46	0.41	−6.25	3.00	−9.38	−1.17	–
$p=16$	−9.71	−3.43	−1.83	−0.27	−3.85	−3.32	−10.91	2.30	−5.91

Cartilage 2	$q=0$	$q=2$	$q=4$	$q=6$	$q=8$	$q=10$	$q=12$	$q=14$	$q=16$
$p=0$	186.90	–	–	–	–	–	–	–	–
$p=2$	−1.27	0.63	–	–	–	–	–	–	–
$p=4$	−15.64	0.38	−3.43	–	–	–	–	–	–
$p=6$	−3.81	2.22	−0.61	0.33	–	–	–	–	–
$p=8$	−12.18	−3.87	−4.89	2.85	3.25	–	–	–	–
$p=10$	−6.79	1.71	−6.81	−2.85	−2.35	2.29	–	–	–
$p=12$	−21.91	−0.94	−2.00	−0.41	−10.18	−1.25	−10.81	–	–
$p=14$	−10.65	0.94	−5.03	1.34	−0.38	0.34	−18.35	0.95	–
$p=16$	−18.50	−2.19	−1.15	−3.09	−2.99	−1.54	−13.35	−4.32	−6.40

Cartilage 3	$q=0$	$q=2$	$q=4$	$q=6$	$q=8$	$q=10$	$q=12$	$q=14$	$q=16$
$p=0$	168.50	–	–	–	–	–	–	–	–
$p=2$	3.79	−5.94	–	–	–	–	–	–	–
$p=4$	−15.14	8.63	−6.22	–	–	–	–	–	–
$p=6$	−6.41	0.08	−2.63	−1.15	–	–	–	–	–
$p=8$	−7.79	−2.71	−2.11	1.47	−3.80	–	–	–	–
$p=10$	−9.36	−2.80	−2.20	0.05	−4.40	−0.53	–	–	–
$p=12$	−8.85	−0.78	−1.07	−1.85	−1.38	0.81	−14.14	–	–
$p=14$	−18.36	2.56	−5.27	0.88	−3.85	0.13	−12.01	−0.77	–
$p=16$	−16.30	3.35	−3.40	−0.44	−3.67	−0.57	−12.97	0.80	−8.90

5.3.1 Candidate Vectors

After an extensive analysis on a broad set of images and tile samples, we realize that the first and last repetition of each order were capturing most of the relevant information (note that those are the moments placed on the first column and main diagonal for the matrices shown in Tables 4 and 5). This observation was then validated using mathematical methods coming from the theory of eigenvalues and Principal Component Analysis (PCA) [12].

The result of this analysis phase was the selection of the 19 potential vectors shown in Table 7 (the particular set of A_{pq} moments selected for each test run is indicated using the • symbol, showing candidate moments on rows and potential vectors on columns). Note that the moments for the last repetition of each order are listed first, followed by the first repetitions, and ending with those three moments which we found to be more relevant from all remaining ones.

5.3.2 Classifiers Used

For the classification process of our candidate vectors, we have used the following three classifiers:

1. **Linear discriminant analysis** [5]. This is a feature extraction method which can automatically extract a low-dimensional feature representation where data can be easily separated according to their class labels [13]. The algorithm assumes that sample vectors of each of the C classes are generated from underlying multivariate Normal distributions of common covariance matrix but different means. In our work, we use the extension proposed by Rao [19] to find the (C-1)-dimensional subspace which minimizes the Bayes error. Since we have two classes (bone and cartilage), our subspace is one-dimensional.
2. **K-means** [11]. This is an unsupervised clustering method where an iterative process aims at minimizing a cost function which measures the distance from the vector of features representing the tile to be classified to the center of each of the C candidate classes. After an estimation for the initial center of each class, tiles are assigned to classes having the closest center and new centers are recomputed. This process is repeated until the cost function converges to a local minimum. As it is a heuristic algorithm, there is no guarantee that it will converge to the global optimum, and the result may depend on the initial guess for the centers.
3. **K nearest neighbors (KNN)** [6]. This is a supervised clustering method which estimates the probability for the tile to belong to a class using the information provided by the training sets. For each tile, the distance between the vector for the tile to classify and each stored sample is calculated, and the K closest samples are selected. The tile is then assigned to the class which contains more elements in those selected samples. Throughout our analysis, we have used three values for K: 5, 10 and 20. A higher K increases the computational cost, but also the probability for a correct classification when all features have the same relevance in the classification process.

5.3.3 Training Samples and Input Tiles

Our benchmark for testing the classification accuracy consisted of four biomedical tissue images consecutively extracted from a 3D volume and stained with picrosirius (see Fig. 5). Overall, we selected 130 tiles for each type of tissue (either bone or cartilage), 30 or them for training our classifiers and the remaining 100 for subsequently running the classification tests.

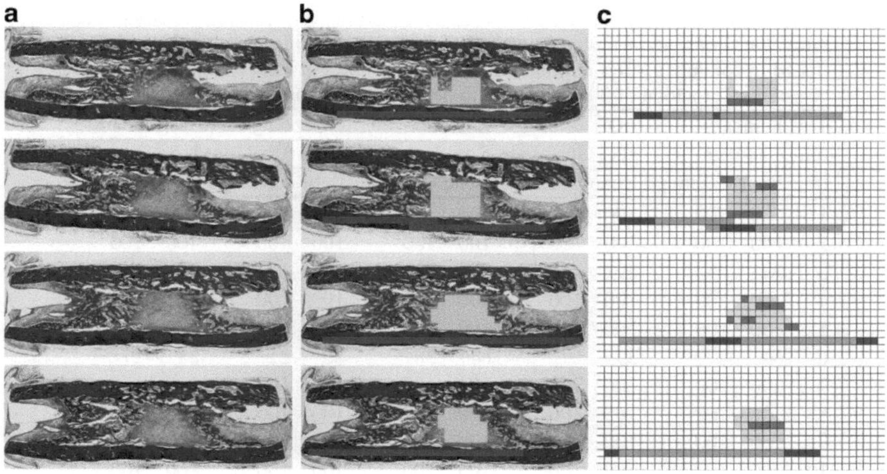

Fig. 5 Four biomedical tissue images consecutively extracted from a 3D volume and stained with picrosirius were involved in our training and classification phases. We illustrate here (**a**) the original images, (**b**) the bone and cartilage regions (lower strip and central area, respectively), and (**c**) the training samples (darker tiles) and the tiles used during the classification process. Overall, there are 130 samples for each type of tissue, 30 of them used for training our classifiers and the remaining 100 used for running the classification tests. The image size is 2560 × 1920 pixels, whereas the tile size is 64 × 64 pixels (most of the tiles containing only white background are not shown)

5.3.4 Classification Results

Once the classifiers were trained, we feed them with 200 tiles, 100 of each tissue class, to determine the accuracy of the classification process for each candidate vector of features composed solely of Zernike moments. The selection of moments characterizing each potential vector (or test run) is shown as columns in Table 7, whereas Table 6 lists those vectors on rows to assess the accuracy achieved by each classifier as a percentage of correct class assignment for each of the input tiles.

From these results, we can extract the following conclusions as far as the behavior of Zernike moments is concerned:

1. The $A_{0,0}$ moment is a crucial feature for the success of the classification, since all of the thirteen tests which use it do not miss any single correct assignment. On the other hand, any of the remaining six tests which do not use it are able to reach 100%.
2. The size for the vector of features becomes almost irrelevant for succeeding, as few moments may retain core information, while many other moments may be more correlated.
3. Zernike moments for the last repetition of each order retain a similar amount of information than the set of moments corresponding to the first repetition (in both

Table 6 Accuracy for the classification process of our set of potential vectors of features (listed in rows as test runs) when being used under different clustering methods (listed in columns). After a training phase, 100 samples of each class were fed to the classifiers, for a total of 200 input tiles to be tagged either as bone or cartilage

Test run	K-means classifier		LDA classifier		KNN classifier (depending on K neighbours)					
					K = 5		K = 10		K = 20	
(#)	Bone	Cartilage	Bone	Cartilage	Bone	Cartilage	Bone	Cartilage	Bone	Cartilage
1	100	100	100	100	100	100	100	100	100	100
2	100	100	100	100	100	100	100	100	100	100
3	93	99	49	48	70	29	81	17	90	3
4	100	100	100	100	100	100	100	100	100	100
5	100	100	100	100	100	100	100	100	100	100
6	64	47	39	57	64	38	80	21	88	27
7	100	100	100	100	100	100	100	100	100	100
8	100	100	100	100	100	100	100	100	100	100
9	100	100	100	100	100	100	100	100	100	100
10	100	100	100	100	100	100	100	100	100	100
11	100	100	100	100	100	100	100	100	100	100
12	100	100	100	100	100	100	100	100	100	100
13	95	96	95	96	95	97	95	97	96	97
14	100	100	100	100	100	100	100	100	100	100
15	100	100	100	100	100	100	100	100	100	100
16	87	51	24	92	73	71	83	57	65	79
17	100	100	100	100	100	100	100	100	100	100
18	100	100	100	100	100	100	100	100	100	100
19	100	100	100	100	100	100	100	100	100	100

cases, five out of the fifteen test runs which only use those set of moments scored 100% for all classifiers).

4. Under that restricted number of low order moments, the lowest Zernike moments do not retain more information than highest ones. Apart from the $A_{0,0}$ element, all remaining moments appear to contribute similarly to the classification success.

A couple of final observations refer to the behavior of the classifiers: K-means exhibits better results than LDA and KNN, and KNN becomes quite unstable when increasing K from 5 to 10 and 20 (as it favors accuracy on bone samples but worsen results on cartilage ones).

5.3.5 The Rank of Favorite Zernike Moments

At this point of our experimental study, there is a clear winner as the best Zernike moment for classifying tiles in our biomedical application: $A_{0,0}$. However, its primacy has somehow shadowed all remaining moments. In order to shed some light on them, we have conducted an additional experiment to apply the K-means classifier to a vector of features composed of a single Zernike moment. The classification

Table 7 Our selection of A_{pq} Zernike moments (listed as rows) for each test run or potential vector of features used for classification purposes (listed as columns). The penultimate column indicates as "Avg." the mean percentage of classification success achieved when using the set of classifiers summarized in Table 6, and as "Appear.", the number of tests in which each particular moment was involved. Finally, the last column shows as "Alone" the percentage of classification success obtained when a particular moment is used as a single feature on a K-means classifier, and as "Rank", the position occupied by that moment on a ranking built when sorting all candidate moments from highest to lowest successful percentage

p	q	1	2	3	4	5	6	7	8	9	10	11	12	13	14	15	16	17	18	19	Avg. (Appear.)	Alone – Rank
0	0	•	•	-	•	•	-	•	•	•	•	•	•	-	•	•	-	•	•	•	100% (15)	100% – #01
1	1	•	-	•	•	-	•	•	•	-	-	-	•	-	•	-	•	-	-	-	86.51% (9)	51.5% – #30
2	2	-	-	-	•	•	-	•	-	•	-	-	•	-	•	-	•	-	-	-	95.46% (7)	52.5% – #28
3	3	-	-	-	•	-	•	•	-	-	-	-	•	-	•	-	•	-	-	-	86.78% (6)	58.5% – #18
4	4	-	-	-	•	•	-	-	•	-	•	•	-	-	-	-	-	-	-	-	100% (5)	68.5% – #12
5	5	-	-	-	•	-	•	-	•	-	-	-	-	-	-	-	-	-	-	-	84.17% (3)	51.0% – #32
6	6	-	-	-	•	•	-	•	-	•	-	-	•	-	-	-	-	-	-	-	100% (5)	53.5% – #24
7	7	-	-	-	•	-	•	•	-	-	-	-	•	-	-	-	-	-	-	-	88.12% (4)	59.5% – #16
8	8	-	-	-	•	•	-	-	•	-	•	-	-	-	-	-	-	-	-	-	100% (4)	65.0% – #13
9	9	-	-	-	•	-	•	-	•	-	-	-	-	-	-	-	-	-	-	-	84.17% (3)	59.5% – #16
10	10	-	-	-	•	•	-	•	-	•	-	-	-	•	-	-	-	-	-	-	99.18% (5)	60.5% – #14
11	11	-	-	-	•	-	•	•	-	-	-	•	-	•	-	-	-	-	-	-	89.68% (5)	52.5% – #28
12	12	-	-	-	•	•	-	-	•	-	•	-	-	-	-	-	-	-	-	-	100% (4)	93.5% – #04
13	13	-	-	-	•	-	•	-	•	-	-	-	-	-	-	-	-	-	-	-	84.17% (3)	55.0% – #23
14	14	-	-	-	•	•	-	•	-	•	-	-	-	•	-	-	-	-	-	-	91.58% (5)	51.5% – #30
15	15	-	-	-	•	-	•	•	-	-	-	-	-	•	-	-	-	-	-	-	87.10% (4)	56.0% – #22
16	16	-	-	-	•	•	-	-	•	-	•	-	-	-	-	-	-	-	-	-	100% (4)	86.5% – #07
2	0	•	•	-	-	-	-	-	•	-	•	-	-	-	-	-	-	-	-	-	100% (4)	57.0% – #20
3	1	•	-	•	-	-	-	-	•	-	-	-	-	-	-	-	-	-	-	-	85.97% (3)	53.5% – #24
4	0	•	•	-	-	-	-	•	-	•	-	-	•	-	•	-	•	-	-	-	95.46% (7)	73.0% – #11
5	1	•	-	•	-	-	-	•	-	-	-	-	•	-	-	-	-	-	-	-	89.47% (4)	50.0% – #33
6	0	•	•	-	-	-	-	-	•	-	•	-	-	-	-	-	-	-	-	-	100% (4)	78.0% – #09
7	1	•	-	•	-	-	-	-	•	-	-	-	-	-	-	-	-	-	-	-	85.97% (3)	53.5% – #24
8	0	•	•	-	-	-	-	•	-	•	-	-	•	-	-	-	-	-	-	-	100% (5)	86.0% – #08
9	1	•	-	•	-	-	-	•	-	-	-	-	•	-	-	-	-	-	-	-	89.47% (4)	53.0% – #27
10	0	•	•	-	-	-	-	-	•	-	•	-	-	-	-	-	-	-	-	-	100% (4)	87.5% – #06
11	1	•	-	•	-	-	-	-	•	-	-	-	-	-	-	-	-	-	-	-	85.97% (3)	56.5% – #21
12	0	•	•	-	-	-	-	•	-	•	-	•	-	•	-	-	-	-	-	-	97.75% (6)	88.0% – #05
13	1	•	-	•	-	-	-	•	-	-	-	-	-	•	-	-	-	-	-	-	88.45% (4)	50.0% – #33
14	0	•	•	-	-	-	-	-	•	-	•	-	-	-	-	-	-	-	-	-	100% (4)	94.5% – #02
15	1	•	-	•	-	-	-	-	•	-	-	-	-	-	-	-	-	-	-	-	85.97% (3)	58.0% – #19
16	0	•	•	-	-	-	-	•	-	•	-	•	-	•	-	-	-	-	-	-	97.75% (6)	94.5% – #02
7	3	-	-	-	-	-	-	-	-	-	-	-	-	-	-	-	-	-	•	•	100% (2)	50.0% – #33
10	2	-	-	-	-	-	-	-	-	-	-	•	-	-	-	-	-	•	•	•	100% (4)	60.0% – #15
12	4	-	-	-	-	-	-	-	-	-	-	-	-	-	-	-	-	•	•	-	100% (2)	76.0% – #10

accuracy obtained on each case completes its corresponding row in Table 7 (see last column), where we have also ranked them from highest to lowest accuracy.

These results confirm the first two conclusions drawn within the last section, and allows us to nuance the last two as well:

1. Six of the top ten moments in the rank belong to the first repetition for each moment order, which becomes more meaningful than the last repetition, where only two moments are located within the top ten.
2. Zernike moments of higher orders are more discriminant than lower ones, since all nine of the top ten moments that follow $A_{0,0}$ in the rank are or sixth order or higher. Also, all those moments belong to even orders and repetitions, and subsequently, moments of an odd order may be discarded without affecting the classification accuracy. That was the ultimate reason for limiting that way the set of values shown in Tables 4 and 5.

6 Summary and Conclusions

In this work, we analyze the expressiveness of Zernike moments as image descriptors within a biomedical imaging application for quantifying the degree of bone tissue regeneration from stem cells, and introduce a novel approach to the high-performance computation of Zernike moments on graphics processors (GPUs). The proposed method is compared against three of the fastest implementations performed on CPUs over the last decade using recursive methods and the fastest direct method computed on a Pentium 4, with factor gains up to 125× on a 256×256 image when computing a single moment on a GPU, and up to 700× on a 1024×1024 image when computing all repetitions for a given order using direct methods. This is extraordinarily valuable in computational domains like real-time imaging or microscopic and biomedical imaging where large-scale images predominate. We also find that recursive methods become more effective on CPUs when a large amount of repetitions within an order or a wide list of consecutive orders need to be computed.

Despite of the workload burden, direct methods on the GPU are rewarded with a higher scalability to become a solid alternative for computing Zernike moments in the years to come. They are also more attractive in real-time or high-resolution imaging versus recursive methods due to its inherent capability to limit the computation to a small number of selected moments which may retain the bulk of the information required for the successful classification of small tiles into image regions.

In this respect, we have identified those Zernike moments which are more relevant for image segmentation into bone and cartilage regions within the context of our biomedical application. Our findings can be summarized as follows:

1. The real component is more meaningful than the imaginary side, which can be discarded.
2. Moments of even orders retain most of the information, so all odd orders may be discarded as well.

3. The first and the last repetitions are the most important features within a given order, with the former being slightly more relevant.
4. The moment of order 0 encapsulates most of the information. Therefore, when dealing with high resolution images and/or real-time constraints, our vector of features may be reduced to this single feature without suffering a significant reduction in the segmentation accuracy.

GPUs are evolving towards general-purpose architectures [7], where we envision image processing as one of the most exciting fields able to benefit from its impressive computational power. This work demonstrates that Zernike moments are a valid alternative for integrating the vector of features required to classify image tiles into regions characterizing bone and cartilage tissue, and distinguishes those relevant orders and repetitions for a reliable segmentation in computer-aided biomedical analysis.

Acknowledgements This work was supported by the Junta de Andalucía of Spain, under Project of Excellence P06-TIC-02109. We want to thank Silvia Claros, José Antonio Andrades and José Becerra from the Cell Biology Department at the University of Malaga for providing us the biomedical images used as input to our experimental analysis.

References

1. Al-Rawi, M.: Fast zernike moments. J. Real-Time Image Process. **3**(1-2), 89–96 (2008)
2. Andrades, J.A., Santamaría, J., Nimni, M., Becerra, J.: Selection, amplification and induction of a bone marrow cell population to the chondroosteogenic lineage by rhOP-1: An *in vitro* and *in vivo* study. Int. J. Dev. Biol. **45**, 683–693 (2001)
3. Bin, Y., Jia-Ziong, P.: Invariance analysis of improved Zernike moments. J. Opt. A: Pure Appl. Opt. **4**(6), 606–614 (2002)
4. Dudani, S., Breeding, K., McGhee, R.: Aircraft identification by moment invariants. IEEE Trans. Comput. **26**(1), 39–46 (1977)
5. Fisher, R.: The statistical utilization of multiple measurements. Ann. Eugenics **8**, 376–386 (1938)
6. Fix, E., Hodges, J.: Discriminatory Analysis – Nonparametric Discrimination: Consistency Properties. Project Number 21-49-004, USAF School of Aviation Medicine 4, University of California, Berkeley, Randolph Field, Texas (USA) (1951)
7. GPGPU: General-Purpose Computation Using Graphics Hardware (2009) http://www.gpgpu.org
8. Gu, J., Shu, H., Toumoulin, C., Luo, L.: A novel algorithm for fast computation of Zernike moments. Pattern Recogn. **35**, 2905–2911 (2002)
9. Hwang, S., Kim, W.: A novel approach to the fast computation of Zernike moments. Pattern Recogn. **39**(11), 2065–2076 (2006)
10. Khotanzad, A., Hong, Y.: Invariant image recognition by Zernike moments. IEEE Trans. Pattern Anal. Mach. Intell. **12**(5), 489–497 (1990)
11. MacQueen, J.: Some methods for classification and analysis of multivariate observations. In: Proceedings of 5th Berkeley Symposium on Mathematical Statistics and Probability, vol. 1, pp. 281–297. University of California Press (1967)
12. Martínez, A., Avinash, C.: PCA versus LDA. IEEE Trans. Pattern Anal. Mach. Intell. **23**(2), 228–233 (2001)

13. McLachlan, G.: Discriminant Analysis and Statistical Pattern Recognition. Wiley, New York (1992)
14. Mukundan, R., Ramakrishnan, K.: Fast computation of Legendre and Zernike moments. Pattern Recogn. **28**(9), 1433–1442 (1995)
15. Nvidia: CUDA Home Page (2009) http://developer.nvidia.com/object/cuda.html
16. Pal, N., Pal, S.: A review on image segmentation techniques. Pattern Recogn. **26**, 1277–1294 (1993)
17. Pratt, W.: Digital Image Processing. Fourth Edition. Ed. Wiley-Interscience (2007)
18. Prokop, R., Reeves, A.: A survey of moment based techniques for unoccluded object representation. Graph. Model Image Process. **54**(5), 438–460 (1992)
19. Rao, C.: Linear Statistical Inference and its Applications, second edn. Wiley, New York (2002)
20. Sofou, A., Evangelopoulos, G., Maragos, P.: Soil image segmentation and texture analysis: A computer vision approach. Geosci. Rem. Sens. Lett. IEEE **2**(4), 394–398 (2005)
21. Teague, M.: Image analysis via the general theory of moments. J. Opt. Soc. Am. **70**(8), 920–930 (1980)
22. Teh, C., Chin, R.: On image analysis by the methods of moments. IEEE Trans. Pattern Anal. Mach. Intell. **10**, 496–512 (1988)
23. Trier, O., Jain, A., Taxt, T.: Feature extraction methods for character recognition – A survey. Pattern Recogn. **29**, 641–701 (1996)
24. Tuceryan, M., Jain, A.K.: Texture Analysis. World Scientific Publishing Co (1998)

A Novel Template-Based Approach to the Segmentation of the Hippocampal Region

M. Aiello, P. Calvini, A. Chincarini, M. Esposito, G. Gemme, F. Isgrò, R. Prevete, M. Santoro, and S. Squarcia

Abstract The work described in this document is part of a major work aiming at a complete pipeline for the extraction of clinical parameters from MR images of the brain, for the diagnosis of neuro-degenerative diseases. A key step in this pipeline is the identification of a box containing the hippocampus and surrounding medial temporal lobe regions from T1-weighted magnetic resonance images, with no interactive input from the user. To this end we introduced in the existing pipeline a module for the segmentation of brain tissues based on a constrained Gaussians mixture model (CGMM), and a novel method for generating templates of the hippocampus. The templates are then combined in order to obtain only one template mask. This template mask is used, with a mask of the grey matter of the brain, for determining the hippocampus. The results have been visually evaluated by a small set of experts, and have been judged as satisfactory. A complete and exhaustive evaluation of the whole system is being planned.

Keywords Magnetic resonance · Image analysis · Hippocampus segmentation

---

M. Aiello (✉), M. Esposito, F. Isgrò, and R. Prevete
Dipartimento di Scienze Fisiche, Università di Napoli Federico II, and Istituto Nazionale di Fisica Nucleare, Sezione di Napoli, Italy
e-mail: aiello@na.infn.it

P. Calvini and S. Squarcia
Dipartimento di Fisica, Università di Genova, and Istituto Nazionale di Fisica Nucleare, Sezione di Genova, Italy

A. Chincarini and G. Gemme
Istituto Nazionale di Fisica Nucleare, Sezione di Genova, Italy

M. Santoro
Dipartimento di Informatica e Scienze dell'Informazione, Università di Genova, Italy

J.M.R.S. Tavares and R.M.N. Jorge (eds.), *Computational Vision and Medical Image Processing: Recent Trends*, Computational Methods in Applied Sciences 19,
DOI 10.1007/978-94-007-0011-6_13,

1 Introduction

The hippocampus is a structure of the Medial Temporal Lobe (MTL) that plays an essential role in the learning and memory capabilities of the brain. It is involved in Alzheimer's disease (AD) and other neurodegenerative diseases (see [7, 12, 17, 22]). For this reason the hippocampus is targeted in the analysis of neuro-images. In particular, the analysis of the shape of the hippocampus is a well accepted indicator in the diagnosis of the Alzheimer's disease, and the analysis of its changes over time can be useful for controlling the evolution of the disease. The problem to find relations between the hippocampus and clinical variables has been studied for some time already: [1, 2, 5, 11, 20].

A step preliminary to the analysis of the shape of the hippocampus is the segmentation of the hippocampus in MRIs, that in the last years has been tackled by many researchers following different approaches. Among the various works more interesting to the realisation of an automated system are two classes of methods: semi-automated and fully automated methods.

An interesting example of semi-automated method is described in [15]: a pipeline that combines the use of low-level image processing techniques such as thresholding and hole-filling with the technique of the geometric deformable models [13, 16]. This process is regarded as semi-automated since the starting step is the labelling of some points on the hippocampal contour by the user; this is necessary to constrain the segmentation process to avoid the inclusion of some other grey matter structures, as the amigdala, in the hippocampal region. This kind of intervention by an expert is also present in [18].

A fully automated approach to the hippocampus segmentation based on the a priori anatomical knowledge of the hippocampus is described in [6]. The a priori knowledge is modelled by statistical information on the shape [14, 18] and by the deformation on a single atlas [8].

The approaches just mentioned are too sensible to the initialisation step, in the first case (i.e. the semi-automated methods), the labelling of the deformation constraints (landmarks) by the user is not exhaustive to describe the morphological variability of the hippocampal shape and is sensible to the specific MRI modality.

In the case of the fully automated method, the use of a single atlas to obtain the a priori knowledge not take in account the anatomical variability between various degrees of the atrophy of the hippocampus.

The work presented in this document is part of a pipeline, see [3, 4], the goal of which is the extraction of clinical variables from the hippocampus automatically segmented in MR images. What is presented in this document is a method for the segmentation of the brain tissues based on a constrained Gaussians mixture model, and a method for the generation of templates of the hippocampus that is novel respect to what was done in the pipeline presented in previous papers [3, 4].

In the remainder of this document first we will review the system implemented (Sect. 2); Sect. 3 is dedicated to the brain tissues segmentation module based on a constrained Gaussian mixture model; then we will give details of the novel procedure for generating the hippocampus templates (Sect. 4), and finally we will show some results; the last section is left to some final remarks.

2 The Pipeline

In this section we briefly review how the pipeline implemented works. Further details can be found in [3,4].

The pipeline consists of three main modules. The first one extracts from the MR two boxes containing the left and the right hippocampus plus a portion of the adjacent tissues and cavities. The second module, still under development, performs the automatic segmentation of the hippocampus, using a set of template masks manually segmented by expert radiologists. The last one, that is being studied, is dedicated to the computation of clinical variables that are related to the atrophic state of the hippocampus.

The pipeline accepts MR images and extracts two hippocampal boxes (HB) containing respectively the left and the right hippocampus, plus a portion of the adjacent tissues and cavities. This is achieved by a rigid registration between the input MR and a set of template boxes previously determined. These template boxes result from a rather long and computational intensive extraction procedure, described hereafter.

The templates extraction basically relies on the fact that the grey level contrast displayed by the complex hippocampal formation plus contiguous ventricles and adjacent structures is so characteristic as to be unique all over the brain. No other structure exists in the brain mimicking the same grey level distribution. Therefore, a procedure can be prepared which, on the basis of some suitably chosen examples, is able to identify the hippocampal region unambiguously.

2.1 Images Dataset

The data-set of structural scans consists of $\approx$100 T1–TFE volumetric MR images, made available by the National Institute of Cancer (IST), Genoa, Italy, (1.5 T Gyroscan system, Philips Medical System) from a population of elderly people whose age, sex, neuropsychological evaluation and clinical evaluation (Normal, Mild Cognitive Impairment or MCI and AD) is known (ages between 56 and 86 years, 35% males, 65% females, clinical conditions ranging from good health state to dementia of AD type. The diagnosis of MCI or AD was made according to the Petersen's and the NINCDS–ADRDA criteria respectively and the images were acquired with isotropic voxels of 1 mm side. Neuroanatomical considerations, verified by the inspection of some images of the data-set, permit to decide the size of a Hippocampal Box (HB) as a $30 \times 70 \times 30\,\text{mm}^3$ parallelepiped-shaped box (sizes of right-to-left, posterior-to-anterior and inferior-to-superior directions respectively). The hippocampal formation and a fraction of the adjacent structures can be easily contained in a HB of that size, provided the original MR image is given the correct orientation by rotating it mainly on the sagittal plane. The extraction of the 200 HBs (100 right and 100 left HBs) from the set of the 100 available MR images was performed by applying a procedure which requires minimal interactive intervention. As an example, let us briefly illustrate the process for the extraction of the

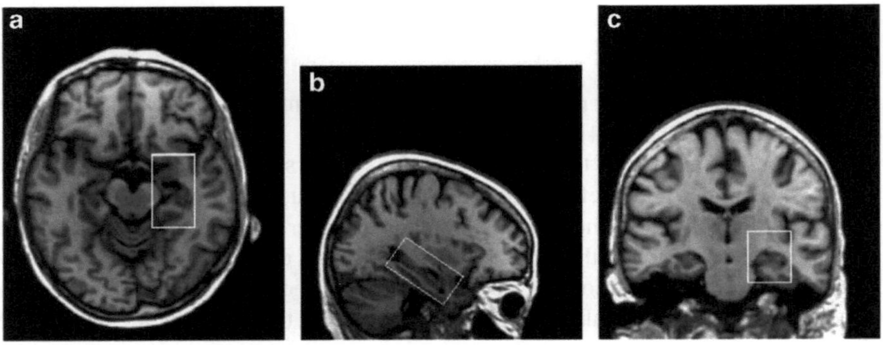

Fig. 1 (**a**) Axial, (**b**) sagittal, and (**c**) coronal views of an image after alignment with the ICBM152 template. On the three slices an outline of the right hippocampal box is also shown

right HBs, the procedure for the extraction of the left ones being the same. Firstly, the images are spatially normalised to stereotactic space (ICBM152, see Fig. 1) via a 12-parameters affine transformation [9] which normalises the images so that the hippocampi all share a similar position and orientation.

2.2 Extraction of the Hippocampal Boxes

The extraction procedure is based on the registration of the first, manually defined HB (denoted in the following as the *fixed* image) on the 100 images (the *moving* images) via a 6-parameters rigid transform. The registration procedure is based on the definition of a distance between two HBs. The distance provides a measure of how well the fixed image is matched by the transformed moving image. This measure forms the quantitative criterion to be optimised over the search space defined by the parameters of the transform. In our procedure we adopted a definition of distance given in terms of the normalised correlation coefficient $\mathcal{C}$. Assigned the HBs A and B, each one consisting of N voxels ($N = 63{,}000$ in our case), the corresponding $\mathcal{C}$ is given by

$$\mathcal{C}_{A,B} = \frac{\sum_{\alpha=1}^{N} \left(A_\alpha - \overline{A}\right)\left(B_\alpha - \overline{B}\right)}{\sqrt{\sum_{\alpha=1}^{N} \left(A_\alpha - \overline{A}\right)^2} \sqrt{\sum_{\alpha=1}^{N} \left(B_\alpha - \overline{B}\right)^2}} \tag{1}$$

where A_α and B_α, of HBs A and B are voxel intensities and the average intensity $\overline{I}$ is given by

$$\overline{I} = \frac{1}{N} \sum_{\alpha=1}^{N} I_\alpha \tag{2}$$

where $I = A, B$.

From this quantification of similarity, one derives the following definition of distance between A and B

$$d_{A,B} = 1 - \mathcal{C}_{A,B} \tag{3}$$

which will be used in the following. This distance is insensitive to multiplicative factors between the two images and produces a cost function with sharp peaks and well defined minima. On the other hand, it has a relatively small capture radius. This last feature, however, is not a severe limitation in our case because all the images are aligned in the same stereotactic space and the hippocampal formations span a relatively small parameter space.

The success of the registration of each moving image to the fixed image is quantified by the minimum reached in distance values. With a moderate computational effort, one could extract all the 100 remaining right HBs by using the first manually defined HB alone, but the quality of the results is not homogeneously good. In fact the fixed image is successful in extracting the HBs which are not too dissimilar from it. However, due to the ample morphological variability contained in the population of MR images, some HBs exist which are unsatisfactorily extracted or not found at all. Therefore, a more exhaustive approach is required.

The population of the remaining 99 MR images is registered to the fixed image. Thus, for each given image j $(2 \leq j \leq 99)$ this operation produces the value of the score $d_{1,j}$, stored in the first row of an upper triangular matrices. We remark that no actual HB extraction is performed at this stage. On the basis of the presently available score list (the first row of matrix **d**), the second box is extracted from $\mathrm{MR}_{(j^*)}$ where j^* is the index of the minimum (non zero) value of $\delta_{1,j}$. Once the second HB is available, the remaining 98 moving images are registered on this new fixed image, and a new set of scores are obtained and stored in the second row of the matrix. The second extracted HB is selected from $\mathrm{MR}_{(k^*)}$ where now k^* is given by the index of the minimum (non zero) value of $d_{1,j}$ and $d_{2,j}$, not taking into account the scores of the already extracted HBs. The procedure for the progressive extraction of all HBs follows this scheme and the extension to an increasing number of HB examples is obvious.

The illustrated procedure is able to detect hippocampi at any atrophy stage and to extract the corresponding HBs. Except for the extraction of the first HB, the whole process runs automatically, without requiring any manual intervention, and no appreciable drift affecting hippocampus orientation or positioning in the HB is noticeable during the extraction process. Visual assessment by an expert reader of the whole set of 100 exhaustive extracted HBs shows that the level of spatial registration of similar anatomical structures is very high. Such stability is not surprising if one considers the way the whole procedure works. At the beginning, the early extractions exhaust the set of the HBs which are very similar to the manually defined HB. Then, the procedure starts extracting HBs which are progressively different from the first ones, but diversity creeps into the growing HB database very slowly thanks to the relevant size of the population of the available MR images. Thus the orientation and position of the essential geometrical features of the hippocampal formation are preserved during the whole process of HB extraction.

2.3 Selection of Templates

As far as computational costs are concerned, this procedure is rather demanding and it is unreasonable to run it over again for extracting the two HBs of any new MR image. Instead of proposing scenarios of n HBs hunting for the $n+1$th HB, we show that the same hunt can be successfully performed by a decidedly smaller number of properly chosen HBs, in the following named HB Templates (HBTs). The HBTs are selected among all HBs as representative cases of the wide morphological variability of the MTL in a large population of elderly people. This idea is consistent with the fact that in the research field on atrophy progression affecting the medial temporal lobe usually only five scores are considered on the basis of visual MRI inspection: absent, minimal, mild, moderate and severe.

The basic idea of the HBTs selection process is to create groups of HBs, or clusters. To classify the n HBs in homogeneous clusters we used hierarchical clustering. The centroid for each cluster is then used as representative (template). To determine the optimal number of templates we increased the number of clusters k, starting from $k = 3$ to $k = 20$. We then evaluated the performance of the different sets of HBTs in extracting all the $n = 100$ right HBs. The test consisted in extracting all n HBs from all MR images given the set of k HBTs. Each MR image was registered to all the k HBTs and actual HB extraction was performed on the basis of the best score obtained (among the k available scores). The test was repeated for $k = 3/20$. The procedure generated eighteen sets of n HBs (for each $k = 3/10$) to be compared to the original set extracted with the exhaustive procedure. To quantify the capability of the HBT sets in extracting the n HBs, we calculated the average distance between the newly extracted elements and the original ones. As the average distance decreases as the number of templates gets larger and larger, we chose the minimum number of templates whose extraction performance (average distance) is less than a given threshold.

With these templates we find the right and left hippocampal formations in any new MR image, using statistical indicators to assess the precision on this volume extraction. MR images ranging from normality to extreme atrophy can be successfully processed. We plan to obtain a set of clinical parameters useful for monitoring the progress of the disease from the analysis of the hippocampal formations.

A different analysis performed directly on the hippocampal boxes can allow the diagnosis of the disease. The boxes are analysed both with linear and non linear methods such as Voxel Based Morphometry and neural networks classifiers. The computed features are chosen to maximise the area under the ROC curve between Normal and AD cohorts. The same features are then used to classify MCI patients into likely AD converters and non-converters. The procedure predictions are subsequently verified by clinical follow-ups data, and the sensitivity/specificity against early detection of AD is computed.

3 Constrained Gaussian Mixture Model Segmentation of the Brain

The constrained Gaussian mixture model (CGMM henceforth) is a procedure for the segmentation of the tissues of the brain based on a constrained Gaussian mixture modelling of the voxel's intensity distribution constrained by the spatial distribution of the tissues. In particular, the voxels distribution can be modelled as

$$f\left(v_t|\Theta\right) = \sum_{i=1}^{n} \alpha_i f_i\left(v_t|\mu_i, \Sigma_i\right) \qquad (4)$$

where v_t is the space-intensity feature vector associated to the t-th voxel, n is the number of Gaussians components of the mixture, μ_i, Σ_i e α_i are, respectively, mean, covariance matrix and mixture coefficient of the i-th Gaussian f_i. Further technical details can be found in [10].

To adapt the CGMM framework to our case where we need to segment grey matter in the hippocampal box the following parameters must be set:

- Number of tissues in which we want to segment the MRI box, in our case we are interested to cerebrospinalfluid (CSF), grey matter (GM) and white matter (WM).
- Number of Gaussians used for modelling the distribution of the intensity feature.
- Number of clusters associated to each Gaussian.
- Number of Gaussians which model each tissue.

In order to find the best values for this parameters it has been adopted a strategy based on the analysis of boxes histogram. Let us observe the four histograms shown in Fig. 2: they do show a similar grey levels distribution for the four HBs. This suggests that it can be suitable to use a number of Gaussians equal to the number of clusters. A discussion on the *experimental* choice of the best values is postponed to Sect. 5.

4 Hippocampal Mask Template Generation

Since there is no statistical atlas of the hippocampus, a set of template masks, i.e. HBs where the hippocampus has been manually segmented, can be used for the segmentation. What we present here is a method for combining the set of template masks in order to obtain only one template mask. The template mask thus found is then used together with a mask of the grey-matter for determining the hippocampus in the input hippocampal box. The grey-matter mask is obtained by a three class classifier (white matter, grey matter). Our pipeline includes different classifiers for performing this task.

More precisely our problem is to create only one hippocampal mask template from a set $M = \{M_1, M_2, \ldots, M_n\}$ of n manually segmented raw hippocampal

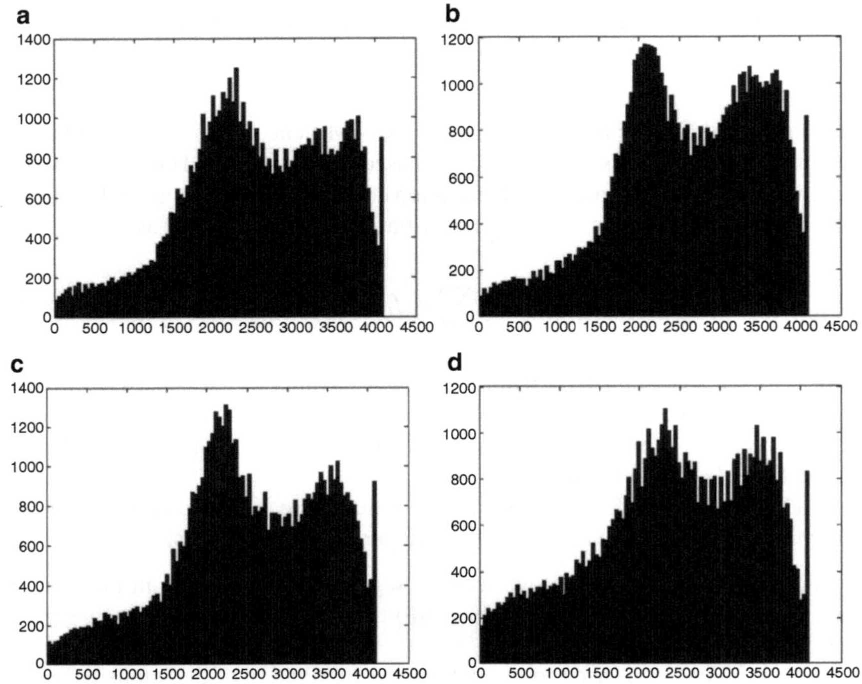

Fig. 2 (**a–d**): Grey level histograms of four different Hippocampal Boxes

boxes (RHB) [3], and use this derived mask for the hippocampus segmentation from the current hippocampal box H_0.

The first step is to warp all the M_is onto H_0 (using the Thirion's Demons registration algorithm [19]). This produces a set of n morphed RHB $M'\{M'_1, M'_2, \ldots, M'_n\}$ and a set of n vectorial fields which can measure the magnitude of the deformation. At this point we want to generate the template representative of the set M'. To achieve this we adopted the STAPLE algorithm.

4.1 STAPLE

STAPLE (Simultaneous Truth and Performance Level Estimation) [21] is an algorithm for the simultaneous ground truth and level performance of various classifiers. A probabilistic estimation of the ground truth is produced with an optimal combination of all classifiers weighting any classifier with his performance level. The algorithm is formulated as an instance of Expectation Maximisation (***EM***) where:

- The segmentation of any classifier for all voxels is an observable.
- The "true" segmentation is an hidden binary variable for all voxels.

- The performance level is represented by the **sensitivity** and **specificity** parameters:
  - **sensitivity** $\boldsymbol{p}$: true positives rate.
  - **specificity** $\boldsymbol{q}$: true negatives rate.

4.1.1 The Algorithm

Let us consider a volume of N voxel and a set of R binary segmentations of this volume, let us assume that:

- $p = (p_1, p_2, \ldots, p_R)^T$ is a column vector R elements, where each element is the sensitivity of the corresponding classifier.
- $q = (q_1, q_2, \ldots, q_R)^T$ is a column vector R elements, where each element is the specificity of the corresponding classifier.
- D is a matrix $N \times R$ of the classifiers decisions for any of N voxel of the R segmentations.
- T is a vector of N elements which represent the hidden true segmentation.

Now, we can consider:

- (D, T): the complete data.
- $f(D, T \mid p, q)$: the probability function of the complete data.

We want to determine the pairs (p, q) maximising the logarithm of the likelihood of the complete data:

$$(\hat{p}, \hat{q}) = \arg\max_{p,q} \ln f(D, T \mid p, q) \tag{5}$$

Now let be:

- $\theta_j = (p_j, q_j)^T \;\; \forall j \in 1 \ldots R$: the performance parameters of the classifier j.
- $\theta = [\theta_1 \theta_2 \ldots \theta_R]$: the complete set of performance parameters.
- $f(D, T \mid \theta)$: the probability function of the vector of the complete data.

Then,

$$\ln L_c\{\theta\} = \ln f(D, T \mid \theta) \tag{6}$$

the EM algorithm can solve this problem:

$$\ln L\{\theta\} = \ln f(D \mid \theta) \tag{7}$$

This is solved iterating the following EM steps:

E-step: estimation of $Q(\theta \mid \theta^{(k)}) = \sum_T \ln f(D, T \mid \theta) f(T \mid D, \theta^k)$.
A compact expression for this step is:

$$W_i^{(k)} \equiv f\left(T_i = 1 \mid D_i, p^{(k-1)}, q^{(k-1)}\right) = \frac{a_i^{(k-1)}}{a_i^{(k-1)} + b_i^{(k-1)}} \tag{8}$$

where $W_i^{(k)}$ indicate the probability of the voxel i, on the true segmentation, be labelled as 1. $a_i^{(k-1)}$ and $b_i^{(k-1)}$ are defined as follow:

$$\begin{aligned} a_i^{(k-1)} &\equiv f(T_i = 1) \prod_j f\left(D_{ij} \mid T_i = 1, p_j^{(k-1)}, q_j^{(k-1)}\right) \\ &= f(T_i = 1) \prod_{j:D_{ij}=1} p_j^{(k-1)} \prod_{j:D_{ij}=0} \left(1 - p_j^{(k-1)}\right) \end{aligned}$$

and

$$\begin{aligned} b_i^{(k-1)} &\equiv f(T_i = 0) \prod_j f\left(D_{ij} \mid T_i = 0, p_j^{(k-1)}, q_j^{(k-1)}\right) \\ &= f(T_i = 0) \prod_{j:D_{ij}=0} q_j^{(k-1)} \prod_{j:D_{ij}=1} \left(1 - q_j^{(k-1)}\right) \end{aligned}$$

where $j : D_{ij} = 1$ is the set of indexes for which the decision of classifier j for the voxel i is 1; $f(T_i = 1)$ and $f(T_i = 0)$ are the a priori probabilities of $T_i = 1$ and $T_i = 0$ respectively; $f(D_{ij} \mid T_i = 1, p_j^{(k-1)}, q_j^{(k-1)})$ represents the conditional probability of the jth labeling for the voxel i given the parameters and the true segmentation label equal to 1.

M-step: maximisation of $Q(\theta \mid \theta^{(k)})$ on the space of the parameters θ, i.e., $\theta^{(k+1)}$ such that:

$$Q(\theta^{(k+1)} \mid \theta^{(k)}) \geq Q(\theta \mid \theta^{(k)}) \quad \forall \theta$$

Using $W_i^{(k-1)}$ estimated in the E-step, is possible to find the optimal parameters by this formulae:

$$\begin{aligned} p_j^{(k)} &= \frac{\sum_{i:D_{ij}=1} W_i^{(k-1)}}{\sum_i W_i^{(k-1)}} \\ q_j^{(k)} &= \frac{\sum_{i:D_{ij}=0} \left(1 - W_i^{(k-1)}\right)}{\sum_i \left(1 - W_i^{(k-1)}\right)} \end{aligned} \tag{9}$$

4.2 *Our Strategy*

4.2.1 Initialisation Strategy

A blind use of the above procedure for determining a single template mask can lead to errors. This is because each one of the original template masks M_i is representative of a class of hippocampus, therefore using all of them on each input H_0 is not

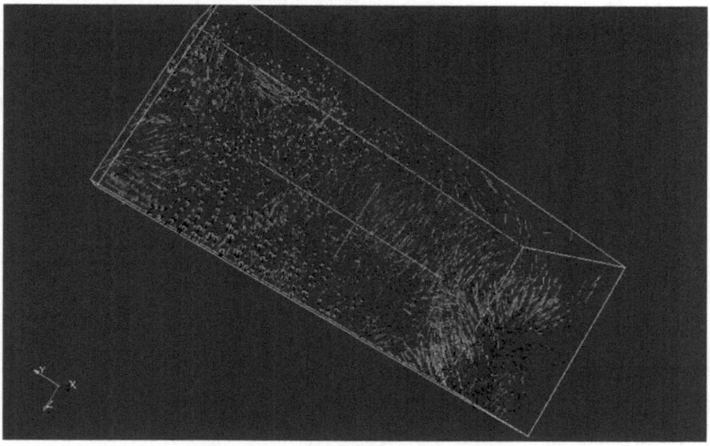

Fig. 3 Deformation matrix. The vector magnitude increases from dark to light

correct. We solve this problem taking into account the different degree of deformation of each M_i on H_0 to weight the contribution of each template mask M_i.

The registration step produces a deformation matrix which can be viewed as composed by deformation vectors (see Fig. 3).

According to the deformation matrix of an HB template we can measure its similarity to the hippocampal box H_0. For this purpose, we use the average modulus of the vector field and these values, are translated in specificity and sensitivity values (p_i^0,q_i) using the following rules:

- To the HB template with lower average modulus (*minHB*) will be assigned the following values: $p_{best}^0 = q_{best}^0 = 0.99$.
- To the HB template with higher average modulus (*maxHB*) will be assigned the following values: $p_{worst}^0 = q_{worst}^0 = 0.01$.
- To the remaining HB template will be assigned the values according to the following formula : $\forall i \neq best, i \neq worst, i = 1, \ldots, classifiers$

$$p_i^0 = q_i^0 = 0.99 - \frac{HB_i - minHB}{maxHB - minHB}. \qquad (10)$$

In Table 1 we show the pairs (p, q) calculated for eight HB templates. In the our case, differently respect to the strategy described in [21] we don't need to initialise the initial reference W^0 with the average volume of the RHB, then we set W^0 to a zero matrix. In Table 2 we show a summary of the algorithm for the template generation procedure.

4.2.2 Convergence Check

The use of the EM algorithm guarantees the convergence to a local minimum: since STAPLE estimates both the ground truth and the level performance of the classifiers,

Table 1 p and q calculated according to our strategy

	Mean norm	p	q
HB Template 1	**1.70052**	0.99	0.99
HB Template 2	**1.83688**	0.72	0.72
HB Template 3	2.03555	0.33	0.33
HB Template 4	2.21146	0.01	0.01
HB Template 5	1.97187	0.45	0.45
HB Template 6	2.14845	0.11	0.11
HB Template 7	2.15173	0.10	0.10
HB Template 8	2.04179	0.32	0.32

Table 2 Summary of the algorithm

```
[TEMPLATE GENERATION PROCEDURE]
-----------------------------------------------------------------
[INPUT:] A set of n RHB.
[OUTPUT:] The hippocampal template W.
-----------------------------------------------------------------

[INITIALISATION]

Sort the HBs in ascending  wrt their average modulus

//Set p^0, w^0 and W^0 according to the indications of section 3.2.
 p_0^0 = q_0^0 = 0.99
 p_n^0 = q_n^0 = 0.01
for i=0 to n
   p_n^0 = q_n^0 = 0.99 - (HB_i - minHB)/(maxHB - minHB)
end

[EM algorithm]
for k= 1...until S_k does not change significantly
    [E-STEP] Compute W^k according to equation 8
    [M-STEP] Compute p^k and q^k according to the equation 9
    S_k = sum_{i=1}^{k} W^k
end

return W^k
```

then convergence can be controlled simply monitoring these three variables. A simple measure of convergence is the variation of the sum over the voxels of the probability of the true segmentation

$$S_k = \sum_{i=1}^{N} W_i$$

computed for each iteration k. The iterations can be stopped when the difference $S_k - S_{K-1}$ is small enough.

4.2.3 Model Parameters

The selection of different a priori probabilities $f(T_i = 1)$, that can vary spatially or globally, can move the local maxima to which the algorithm converges. A probability $f(T_i = 1)$ that changes spatially is a good choice for those structures for which a probabilistic atlas is available.

The interest in our case is oriented towards those structure for which non probabilistic atlas is available: in this case we can use a single global a priori probability $\gamma = f(T_i = 1) \forall i$. Such probability encodes all the available information before knowing the results of the segmentations relative to the probability of the structure we want to segment. In practise such information are not easily available, and therefore it is more convenient to estimate γ form the segmentations, as

$$\gamma = \frac{1}{RN} \sum_{j=1}^{R} \sum_{i=1}^{N} D_{ij}$$

5 Experimental Assessment

In this section we first discuss how the number of Gaussians for the CGMM segmentation module has been experimentally determined, and the we show a result of the hippocampal mask template generation module.

The hippocamp is composed by GM which has mean value of the intensity between the mean value of CSF and the mean value of the WM. To find a good number of Gaussians for modelling the histograms we note that the right number is larger than three. In Fig. 4 the histograms obtained as a Gaussian mixture of the histogram in Fig. 4a using an increasing number of Gaussians for the model. Here we focus our attention only on the histogram of a particular HB, but we found that the same arguments hold for any other HB.

First of all we can note that the use of three (Fig. 4b) or four (Fig. 4c) Gaussians leads to a bad matching. A much better result is obtained when using five Gaussians (Fig. 4d). In particular, moving from left to right on the x axis, we can assign the first Gaussian to the CSF, the second and the third to the GM. More difficult is to decide if the fourth Gaussian should be assigned to the GM or to the WM. In fact, if it is assigned to the GM we risk to over-sample the GM; on the other hand if it is assigned to the WM, then the GM might be under estimated, leading to errors in the hippocampus segmentation, as the hippocampus is part of the grey matter. The extraction process makes use of the GM segmentation for refining the results from the STAPLE module, that often expands on areas that have not been classified as grey matter. Therefore, it is much better to assign more Gaussians to the grey matter.

In Fig. 4f the outcome of modelling the histogram using seven Gaussians. The results is better than when using only five Gaussians, however there is the problem

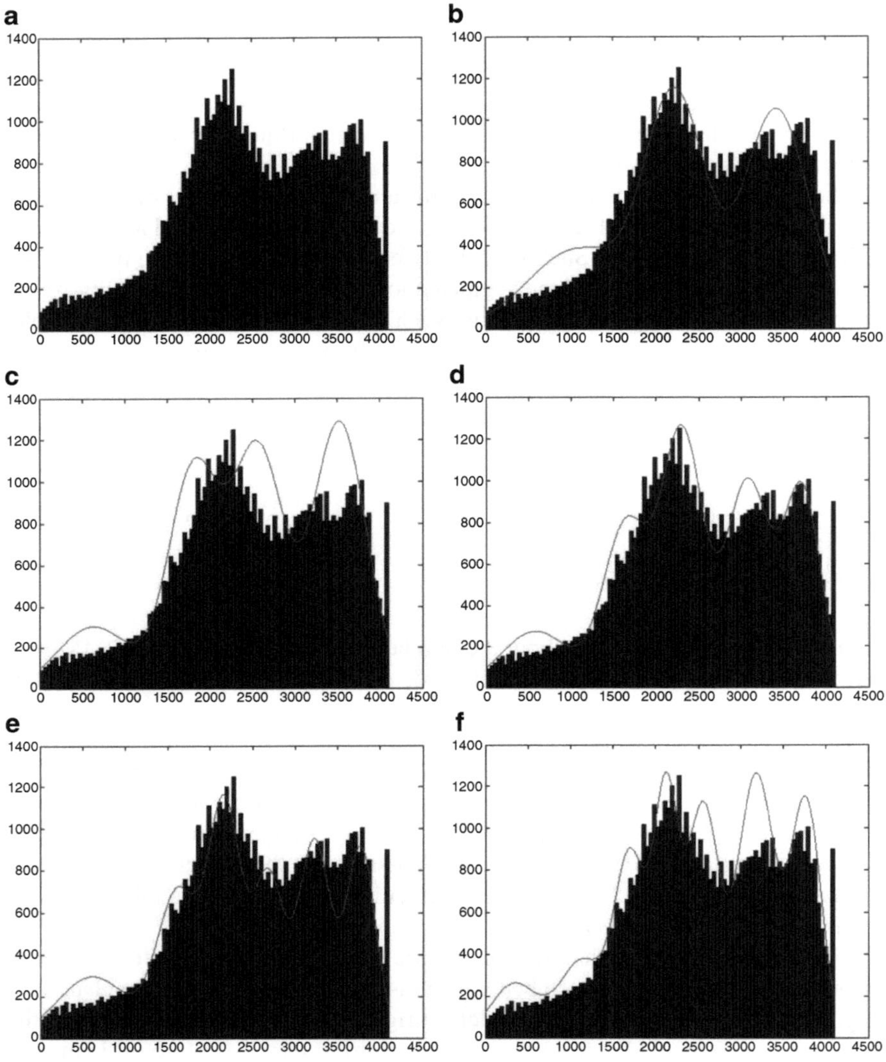

Fig. 4 Histogram modelling with the Gaussian mixture model. (**a**) Original histogram; (**b**) Result using three Gaussians; (**c**) Result using four Gaussians; (**d**) Result using five Gaussians; (**e**) Result using six Gaussians; (**f**) Result using seven Gaussians

if the second Gaussian from the left is assigned to the CSF or to the GM should be assigned to the CSF or to the GM: either ways we end up with a down-sampling or a over-sampling of the GM respect to the CSF.

The result when using six Gaussians is shown in Fig. 4e: in this case there is no uncertainty for assigning the Gaussians on the left of the histogram, as for the case of Fig. 4f. Therefore the best choice is to model the histogram of the hippocampal box using six histogram. The result of CGMM segmentation of a HB using the parameter reported in Table 3 is shown in Fig. 5.

We used the hippocampus template determined with the method described above to actually refine a segmentation of the grey matter obtained with the constrained mixture of Gaussians method described earlier in this chapter.

Since there is no ground truth, the results have been visually evaluated by a small set of experts, and have been judged as satisfactory. However we are planning a complete and exhaustive evaluation of the whole pipeline. Results are shown in Figs. 6–8.

Table 3 Parameters of the CGMM segmentation used for our experiments

Tissue	Number of clusters	Number of Gaussians
GM	3	3
WM	2	2
CSF	1	1

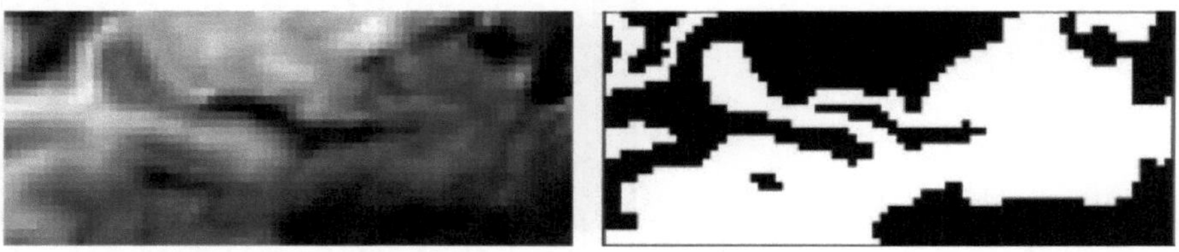

Fig. 5 *Left*: Sagittal view of a HB. *Right*: Segmentation obtained by the CGMM framework with the parameters in Table 3

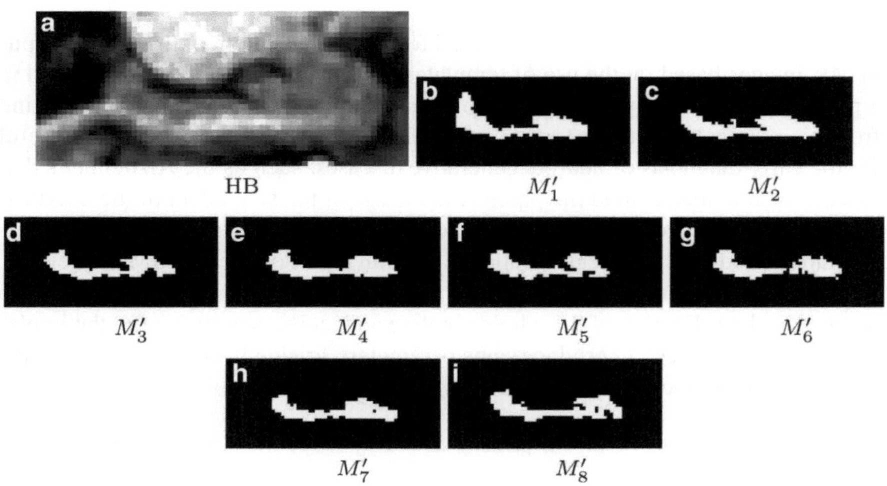

Fig. 6 (**a**) Box HB; (**b–i**) Template boxes M_is warped onto the box HB

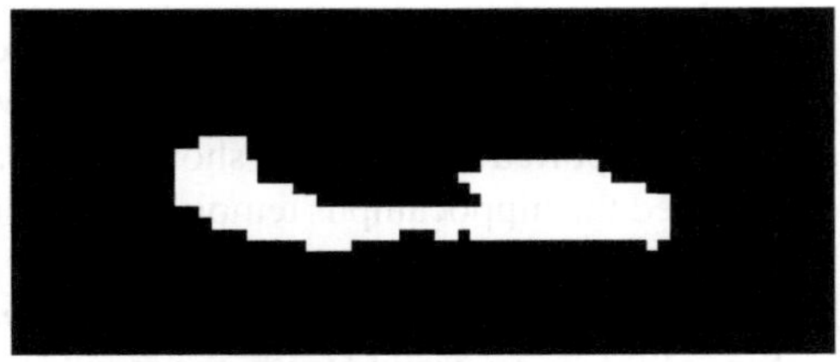

Fig. 7 Hippocampal Mask Template obtained combining the eight template M_i' in Fig. 6

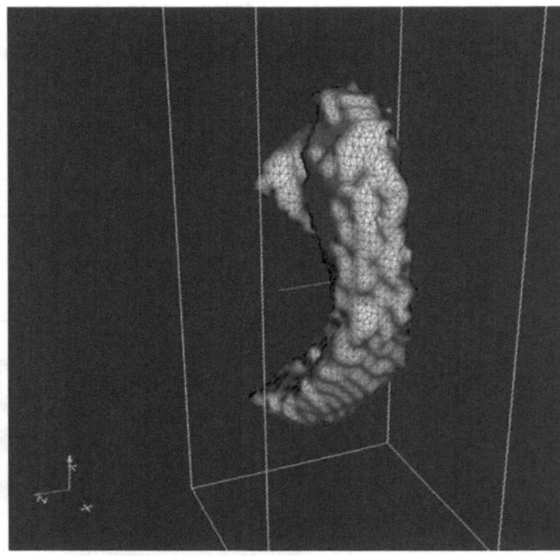

Fig. 8 3D rendering of the Hyppocampal box template in Fig. 7. *The mesh* indicates the STAPLE result which cover the grey matter segmentation of the hyppocampal box

6 Conclusions

In this work it is presented a novel method for the segmentation of the hippocampus in MR images based on the use of template masks. Our method is implemented in a pipeline that aims to perform an automated analysis of the hippocampus starting from his segmentation to perform a morphological analysis that can be very useful for the early diagnosis of neurodegenerative diseases, such as the Alzheimer's disease. The main idea behind the pipeline is the use of the side effect of the STAPLE algorithm to produce a single, meaningful template which can refine a rough segmentation produced by a segmentation algorithm based on the CGMM framework. The next steps of our work aim to get a ground truth of segmented hippocampi to proceed to the validation of the whole pipeline and, consequently, aim to the implementation of a strategy to produce some parameters, arising from the morphological analysis of the hippocampus, such as clinical scores.

Acknowledgements This work was partially funded by INFN within the MAGIC-5 research project.

References

1. Atiya, M., Hyman, B., Albert, M., Killiany, R.: Structural magnetic resonance imaging in established and prodroaml Alzheimer disease: a review. Alz. Dis. Assoc. Dis. **17**(3), 177–195 (2003)
2. Braak, H., Braak, E.: Neuropathological staging of Alzheimer-related changes. Acta. Neuropathol. **82**, 239–259 (1991)
3. Calvini, P., Chincarini, A., Donadio, S., Gemme, G., Squarcia, S., Nobili, F.N., Rodriguez, G., Bellotti, R., Catanzariti, E., Cerello, P., Mitri, I.D., Fantacci, M.: Automatic localization of the hippocampal region in mr images to asses early diagnosis of Alzheimer's disease in MCI patients. In: Nuclear Science Symposium Conference Record, pp. 4348–4354 (2008)
4. Calvini, P., Chincarini, A., Gemme, G., Penco, M., Squarcia, S., Nobili, F., Rodriguez, G., Bellotti, R., Catanzariti, E., Cerello, P., Mitri, I.D., Fantacci, M.: Automatic analysis of medial temporal lobe atrophy from structural MRIs for the early assessment of Alzheimer disease. Med. Phys. **36**(8), 3737–3747 (2009)
5. Chetelat, G., Baron, J.: Early diagnosis of Alzheimer disease: contribution of structural neuroimaging. Neuoroimage **18**(2), 525–541 (2003)
6. Chupin, M., Chételat, G., Lemieux, L., Dubois, B., Garnero, L., Benali, H., Eustache, F., Lehéricy, S., Desgranges, B., Colliot, O.: Fully automatic hippocampus segmentation discriminates between early Alzheimer's disease and normal aging. In: Proceedings of the 5th IEEE International Symposium on Biomedical Imaging: From Nano to Macro, pp. 97–100 (2008)
7. Dubois, B., Albert, M.: Amnestic MCI or prodromal Alzheimer disease? Lancet Neurol. **3**(4), 246–248 (2004)
8. Duchesne, S., Pruessner, J.C., Collins, D.L.: Appearance-based segmentation of medial temporal lobe structures. Neuroimage **17**(2), 515–531 (2002)
9. Evans, A., Kambler, M., Collins, D., MacDonald, D.: An MRI-based probabilistic atlas of neuroanatomy. In: Shorvon, S., Fish, D., Andermann, F., Bydder, G., Stefan, H. (eds.) Magnetic Resonance Scanning and Epilepsy. NATO ASI Series A, Life Sciences, vol. 264, pp. 263–274. Plenum Press, New York (1994)
10. Greenspan, H., Ruf, A., Goldberger, J.: Constrained Gaussian mixture model framework for automatic segmentation of MR brain images. IEEE Trans. Med. Imag. **25**(9), 1233–1245 (2006)
11. Joshi, S., Pizer, S., Fletcher, P., Yushkevich, P., Thall, A., Marron, J.: Multiscale deformable model segmentation and statistical shape analysis using medial description. IEEE Trans. Med. Imag. **21**(5), 538–550 (2002)
12. Kantarci, K., Jack, C.: Neuroimaging in Alzheimer disease: an evidence based review. Neuroimag. Clin. N. Am. **13**(2), 197–209 (2003)
13. Kass, W., Witkin, A., Terzopoulos, D.: Snakes: active contour models. Int. J. Comput. Vis. **1**(4), 321–331 (1988)
14. Kelemen, A., Székely, G., Gerig, G.: Elastic model-based segmentation of 3D neurological data sets. IEEE Trans. Med. Imag. **18**(10), 828–839 (1999)
15. Lee, W., Gow, K., Zhao, Y., Staff, R.: Hybrid segmentation of the hippocampus in mr images. In: Proceedings of the 13th European Signal Processing Conference, Antalya, Turkey (2005)
16. Miller, J., Lorensen, W., O'Bara, R., Wozny, M.: Geometrically deformed models: A method for extracting closed geometric models from volume data. SIGGRAPH Comput. Graph. **25**, 217–226 (1991)
17. Petersen, R., Smith, G., Waring, S., Tangalos, E., Kokmen, E.: Mild cognitive impairment: clinical characterization and outcome. Arch. Neurol. **56**(3), 303–308 (1999)
18. Shen, D., Moffat, S., Resnick, S.M., Davatzikos, C.: Measuring size and shape of the hippocampus in MR images using a deformable shape model. NeuroImage **15**, 422–434 (2002)
19. Thirion, J.: Image matching as a diffusion process: an analogy with maxwell's demons. Med. Image Anal. **2**(3), 243–260 (1998)
20. Thompson, P., Hayashi, K., de Zubicaray, G., Janke, A., Rose, S., Semple, J., Hong, M., Herman, D., Gravano, D., Doddrell, D., Toga, A.: Mapping hippocampal and ventricular change in Alzheimers's disease. Neuroimage **22**(4), 1754–1766 (2004)

21. Warfield, S., Zou, K., Wells, W.: Simultaneous truth and performance level estimation (STAPLE): an algorithm for the validation of image segmentation. IEEE Trans. Med. Imag. **23**, 903–921 (2004)
22. Winblad, B., Palmer, K., Kivipelto, M., Jelic, V., Fratiglioni, L., Wahlund, L., Nordberg, A., Backman, L., Albert, M., Almkvist, O., Arai, H., Basun, H., Blennow, K., de Leon, M., DeCarli, C., Erkinjuntti, T., Giacobini, E., Graff, C., Hardy, J., Jack, C., Jorm, A., Ritchie, K., van Duijn, C., Visser, P., Petersen, R.: Mild cognitive impairment–beyond controversies, towards a consensus: report of the international working group on mild cognitive impairment. J. Intern. Med. **256**(3), 240–246 (2004)

Model-Based Segmentation and Fusion of 3D Computed Tomography and 3D Ultrasound of the Eye for Radiotherapy Planning

M. Bach Cuadra, S. Gorthi, F.I. Karahanoglu, B. Paquier, A. Pica, H.P. Do, A. Balmer, F. Munier, and J.-Ph. Thiran

Abstract Computed Tomography (CT) represents the standard imaging modality for tumor volume delineation for radiotherapy treatment planning of retinoblastoma despite some inherent limitations. CT scan is very useful in providing information on physical density for dose calculation and morphological volumetric information but presents a low sensitivity in assessing the tumor viability. On the other hand, 3D ultrasound (US) allows a highly accurate definition of the tumor volume thanks to its high spatial resolution but it is not currently integrated in the treatment planning but used only for diagnosis and follow-up. Our ultimate goal is an automatic segmentation of gross tumor volume (GTV) in the 3D US, the segmentation of the organs at risk (OAR) in the CT and the registration of both modalities. In this paper, we present some preliminary results in this direction. We present 3D active contour-based segmentation of the eye ball and the lens in CT images; the presented approach incorporates the prior knowledge of the anatomy by using a 3D geometrical eye model. The automated segmentation results are validated by comparing with manual segmentations. Then, we present two approaches for the fusion of 3D CT and US images: (i) landmark-based transformation, and (ii) object-based transformation that makes use of eye ball contour information on CT and US images.

M. Bach Cuadra (✉), S. Gorthi, F.I. Karahanoglu, B. Paquier, and J.-Ph. Thiran
Signal Processing Laboratory (LTS5), Ecole Polytechnique Fédérale de Lausanne, Switzerland
e-mail: meritxell.bach@epfl.ch; subramanyan.gorthi@epfl.ch; isik.karahanoglu@epfl.ch; benoit.paquier@epfl.ch; jp.thiran@epfl.ch

A. Pica
Radiation Oncology Department, Lausanne University Hospital (CHUV), Switzerland
e-mail: alessia.pica@chuv.ch

H.P. Do
Institute of Applied Radiophysics, Lausanne, Switzerland
e-mail: dohuuphuoc@hotmail.fr

A. Balmer and F. Munier
Ophthalmic Hospital Jules Gonin, Lausanne, Switzerland
e-mail: aubain.balmer@fa2.ch; Francis.Munier@fa2.ch

J.M.R.S. Tavares and R.M.N. Jorge (eds.), *Computational Vision and Medical Image Processing: Recent Trends*, Computational Methods in Applied Sciences 19,
DOI 10.1007/978-94-007-0011-6_14,

Keywords Parametric Active Contours · Model-based segmentation · Multi-model image fusion · Ultrasound imaging · Computer tomography · Eye imaging · radiotherapy

1 Introduction

Retinoblastomas are one of the common primary ocular malignancies in childhood. They are very aggressive tumors appearing before the age of four years old, hereditary in 40% of the cases, and they account for 5% of childhood blindness [8]. Linear accelerator (LINAC) based conformal stereotactic radiotherapy (SRT) is one of the most precise radiotherapy treatments for retinoblastomas[1] to control advanced, often chemotherapy resistant, intra-ocular tumors in progression after chemotherapy and focal ophthalmologic therapies in children. Thus, primary endpoint of such radiation therapy is the eye and visual function preservation following intra-ocular progression. Therefore, delineating the tumor in order to optimize radiation doses, allowing minimization of dose to adjacent developing tissues is a crucial goal. To this end, patients usually undergo a multi-modal imaging: First, Computed Tomography (CT) scan, which is very useful in providing information on physical density for dose calculation and morphological volumetric information, and second, ophthalmologic examination with 2D and 3D ultrasound (US) and fundus pictures, which allow a very accurate definition of the tumor volume thanks to its high spatial resolution. Actually, thanks to its improving quality, the use of US imaging is increasing in ophthalmology [9, 19]. Note that such multi-modal CT-US imaging framework has been already suggested for the therapy of other organs like the liver and kidney [15, 18] but, as far as we know, this is the first attempt of combining these two modalities in the radiotherapy planning of the eye.

In the current therapy planning, 2D and 3D ultrasound imaging and fundus photographs are qualitatively used for diagnosis, gross tumor volume definition and follow-up but they are not integrated in the treatment planning. Notice that tumor is not always visible un CT images and thus the use of ultrasound or fundus photographs is crucial. Our ultimate goal is the fusion of 3D US imaging, optimal for tumor volume delineation, and CT imaging, optimal for dose calculation and treatment planning. Through an automated segmentation of gross tumor volume (GTV) in the 3D US along with the registration to the CT, the rather inaccurate and time-consuming manual volume definition[2] could be shortened and the volume definition would become highly reproducible and comparable, overcoming the intrinsic problems of inter- and intra-user variability, thus making radiation treatment techniques amenable to standardization.

[1] This treatment has been developed at the Lausanne University Hospital (CHUV) in collaboration with the Jules Gonin University Eye Hospital. It reduces the risk of long term complications in external beam radiation therapy [12].

[2] By manual volume definition we mean the manual segmentation of organs at risk and tumor, when possible, in the CT that defines the treatment planning. However, in some cases, the gross tumor volume cannot be manually segmented since it is not visible.

The overall framework is represented in Fig. 1: Input images are represented on the left side, the methodology is described inside the dashed box and the resulting treatment planning, including the tumor, is shown as output on the right hand side. The methodology goes from top to bottom and from left to right: first, eye segmentation is done in the CT, second, through image registration we can find the eyeball area and lens in the US and then, we will proceed to the tumor segmentation in the US. Finally tumor-segmentation in US is transferred to the radiotherapy planning on the CT through the image fusion.

In this paper we present the first steps towards this multi-modal imaging framework for the radiotherapy planning of the eye. We present an automated segmentation of the eye exploiting the prior knowledge that we have on eye's anatomy; the prior knowledge about the eye is incorporated by parameterizing the active contour with a 3D geometrical model. Then, we will present the fusion of these two modalities using landmark-based and object-based transformations. This work is an extended version of our previous work in [1]. The paper is organized as follows. In Sect. 2, a brief state-of-the-art on eye segmentation techniques will be presented, focusing on the ones that exploit a geometrical eye model. In Sect. 3, the parametric Active Contour segmentation of the eye ball and lens in the CT image will be shown. Results from the automated segmentation will be compared with manual segmentations done by an expert. In Sect. 4, we will use landmark-based and object-based rigid registration to initially fusion the CT and 3D US images along with qualitatively results. Finally, discussion and future works will be summarized in Sect. 5.

2 Related Works on Eye Segmentation

Related works on segmentation of organs of sight are very sparse in time as well as in methodology (see Table 1). Souza et al. [17] segmented the extraocular muscles in CT images with mathematical morphology; D'Haese et al. [6] segmented the eyeball, lens and optic nerve by atlas-based registration in MR images; Cates et al. [5] segmented the eyeball and optic nerve on Visible Human Female data using

Table 1 Summary of related works on segmentation of organs of sight

Works	Image modality	Segmentation target	Segmentation method	Eye model
Bondiau (1997), [3]	CT, Fundus	Hough transform	Sclera, lens, optic nerve, clips	Yes
Souza (2000), [17]	CT	Mathematical morphology	Extra ocular muscles	No
Dobler (2002), [7]	CT, MR, Fundus	–	Tumor and complete eye anatomy	Yes
D'Haese (2003), [6]	MR	Atlas-based registration	Sclera, lens, optic nerve, chiasm	Yes
Cates (2005), [5]	VHF	Watershed	Eyeball, optic nerve	No
Bekes (2008), [2]	CT	Soft classification	Sclera, lens, optic nerve, chiasm	Yes

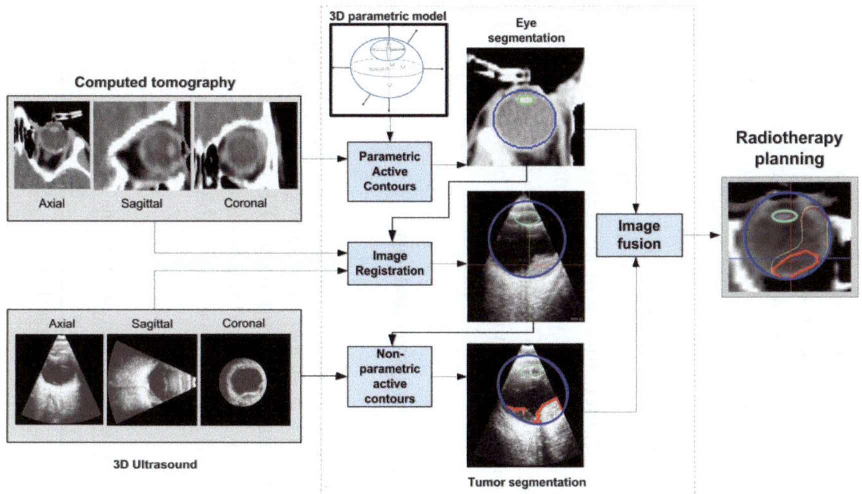

Fig. 1 Global framework for model-based segmentation and image fusion of 3D CT and 3D ultrasound of the eye for radiotherapy planning. Input images are represented on the left side, with axial, coronal and sagittal views of each. Methodology is described inside the dashed box. From *top-bottom* and *left-right*: First, eye segmentation is done in the CT, using the parameterized active contours; second, through image registration we can find the eyeball area and lens in the US; third, we will proceed to the tumor segmentation. By fusion, tumor will be superposed to the treatment planning in the CT

watershed method. Other works have explicitly taken into account the particular geometrical shape of the eye. The use of a geometrical eye model was suggested very early by Bondiau et al. [3] in 1997. Their goal was the eye reconstruction to improve protontherapy treatment of ocular tumors. Their approach consisted in building an eye model (sclera, lens, optic nerve and tantalum clips) and adapting each structure of the model to the CT image through a Hough transform. They also presented preliminary results of the fusion of CT with retinographies. Later, Dobler and Bendl [7] presented a very precise 3D geometric and hierarchical model of the eye composed in total of nine structures (sclera, vitreous body, cornea, anterior chamber, lens, iris, macula, optical nerve, and optical disc) with each structure described either by an ellipsoid or an elliptic cylinder. Their goal was to combine the 3D geometrical eye model along with the 3D CT, the 3D MR and the 2D fundus diagram for a new proton therapy system planning called *OCTOPUS* [13]. The setting of the model parameters was done by manual measurements on ultrasound images. Then, the model was adapted to the CT and MR images by registration[3] and 3D to 2D projections were used to adapt the model to the fundus photographs. Recently, in Bekes et al. [2] introduced a simplified eye model consisting in sclera (modeled as a sphere), the lens (modeled as an ellipsoid), the optic nerve and chiasm (cylinder). In their approach the selection of parameters was almost completely automated to minimize user interaction. Their model-based segmentation was performed on CT images based on thresholding and soft classification methods.

As in [2, 3, 7], our method makes use of a 3D geometrical eye model. Our main contribution regarding the existing approaches is the use of parameterized active contours (AC) to represent the eye. This will allow us to take advantage of this mathematically well-formulated framework and exploit the edge and region characteristics from the CT scan to adapt the model for every patient. Unlike [2, 3], we will represent the eye structures by ellipsoids. We are currently interested in the segmentation of eye ball and lens only, but other structures can be easily included in such framework either by parametric or non-parametric active contours. The idea of a multi modal framework for improving therapy planning [3, 7] is not new neither. However, as far as we know, our work is the first one that attempts in combining 3D ultrasound and CT scans.

3 Eye Segmentation in the Active Contour Framework

The CT image properties and the very well known geometry of the eye lead to an adaptation of the active contours theory [4] which aims at finding a curve C that minimizes the energy functional E, designed to be minimal when C has found the desired contour. The general expression of E is given by

$$E(C) = E_{image}(C) + E_{smooth}(C), \tag{1}$$

[3] The type of registration process used in [7] for adapting the model to the 3D images was not explicitly mentioned in that paper.

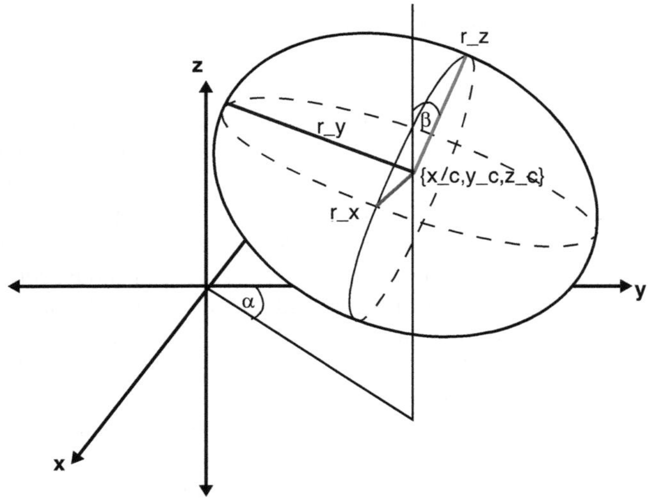

Fig. 2 The proposed 3D parametric model of the eye consisting of ellipsoids for the eye ball and the lens. The model parameters for the eye lens are $\theta_{lens} = \{x_c, y_c, z_c, r_x, r_y, r_z, \alpha, \beta\}$ corresponding to the center coordinates, the length of the axes and the rotation angles. Model parameters for the eye ball are $\theta_{ball} = \{x_c, y_c, z_c, r_x, r_y, r_z\}$ thus α and β angles are neglected since these values are going to be varying around 0

Here, we take advantage of using a parameterized model, which means that the analytical expression of C is known everywhere on the domain of the image and is defined by a set of parameters θ. Thus, C is a parameterized model based on the ellipsoid parameters $\theta = \{x_c, y_c, z_c, r_x, r_y, r_z, \alpha, \beta\}$ corresponding to the center coordinates, the length of the axes and the rotation angles (see Fig. 2).

Obviously, we will not impose any E_{smooth} term since our parameterized curve is already smooth. Then, the E_{image} term can be expressed in two sub-terms:

$$E_{image}(C(\theta)) = E_{boundary}(C) + E_{region}(C), \tag{2}$$

which are computed from the image features.

$E_{boundary}$ attracts the curve towards the object boundaries using an edge detecting function f, and in this work is given by:

$$E_{boundary} = \int_C f(C, s)ds. \tag{3}$$

Such edge detection function works fine in CT images but other gradient-based functions should be used for other images. Once applied to the image I, $f(C, s)$ has to return an optimum value (minimum in our case) when its variables, which are the curve spatial coordinates $(x(\theta, s), y(\theta, s), z(\theta, s))$ mapped by the model on the image, are matching the edges of the object to be delineated. Therefore, f can be of the form:

$$f(C,s) = \begin{cases} -(I_{eq}(C,s) * G_\sigma) & \text{if } I_{eq}(C,s) > T_h, \\ 0 \text{ otherwise.} \end{cases} \quad (4)$$

where T_h is a threshold applied on the equalized image intensity and empirically set to 0.8, G is the Gaussian function with standard deviation σ and $I_{eq} * G_\sigma$ represents the smoothed version of the equalized image histogram I.

E_{region} captures the regional statistics to drive C towards homogeneous regions. The idea here is to maximize the difference between two statistical descriptors (the mean value of intensities) related to two regions of the image, Ω_{in} and Ω_{out}, in our case, respectively the inside and the outside of an ellipsoid within a selected region of interest around the lens. Formally

$$E_{region} = -|\text{mean}(\Omega_{in}) - \text{mean}(\Omega_{out})|. \quad (5)$$

The segmentation problem is now reduced to an energy optimization problem. Thus, the parameter-set θ that results in minimum energy provides the segmentation of the objects of interest.

$$\theta_{\text{object}} = \arg\min_\theta E(C(\theta)). \quad (6)$$

From our experiments, we found that boundary-based term ($E_{boundary}$) alone is sufficient for the accurate segmentation of the eye ball. Similarly for the lens, we found that region-based term (E_{region}) alone is sufficient. Hence, for the results that we present in the Sect. 3.2, we use only $E_{boundary}$ term for the eye ball, and only E_{region} term for the lens segmentation.

3.1 Practical Implementation and Optimization Strategy

3.1.1 Eyeball Segmentation

We observed from our experiments that rotation angles for the eye ball are always varying around 0 (this particularly linked to the CT image acquisition protocol used here). Hence, we simplified the eye ball segmentation by neglecting these angles: $\{\alpha, \beta\}$. As a result, the number of parameters to be optimized for the eye ball are 6. We do not apply the optimization directly to the CT scan but to an *edge detected image* (see Fig. 3a). This image is obtained as defined previously in (4): First, histogram is equalized to expand intensity values and enhance sharp edges; second, a threshold of 0.8 is applied to extract the eyeball contours; third, we smooth by a Gaussian filter.

3.1.2 Lens Segmentation

As mentioned previously, we will use region information to segment the lens. Using the edge information similar to the eyeball is not preferred since lens boundary

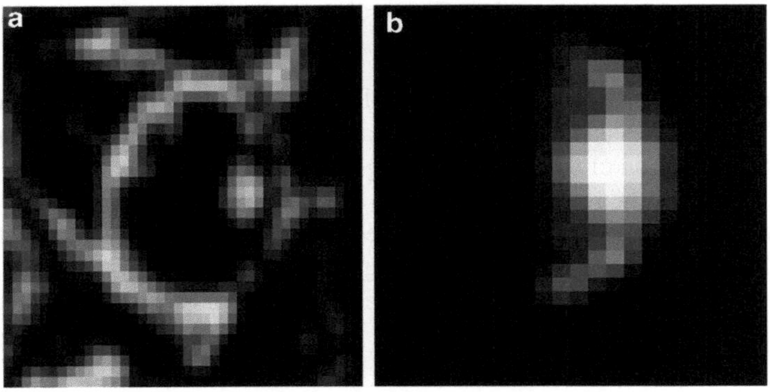

Fig. 3 Input images for the eyeball (**a**) and lens (**b**) segmentation for one of the patients

is located near the eyeball edge. Here, eight parameters defining the ellipsoid will be used. We will proceed in a small region of interest corresponding to the upper part of the eyeball where the lens is located (see Fig. 3b). This is done to obtain a comparable volume inside and outside the lens and ensure the good behavior of the regional energy term.

3.1.3 Optimization

The optimization is implemented with a Nelder-Mead simplex search included in the Matlab *fminsearch* function. Note that a set of parameters such as θ includes elements of different nature and therefore their range is very different. For example a semi-axis of the eye ball ranges from 5 to 20 mm while an angle ranges from 1 to 360 degrees. To overcome this problem we proceed to the optimization iteratively using three subsets of parameters, $[x_c, y_c, z_c]$, $[r_x, r_y, r_z]$, and $[\alpha, \beta]$ (actually only the first two subsets for the eye ball). Moreover the algorithm is applied twice per object (first expanding the ellipsoid and later shrinking it). Histogram equalization of the image is performed as a pre-processing step. Eye ball optimization is initialized by user clicks, (center coordinates x_c, y_c, z_c and the radius in z direction, r_z). Lens optimization is restricted to one half of the eyeball only. The overall optimization algorithm is summarized as follows:

1. **Input data**
   Image with smoothed edges (lens) or threshold image (eyeball) (see Fig. 3)
2. **Ellipsoid initialization**
   Smaller (eyeball)/Bigger (lens)

3. **Iterative loop**
   Three iterations loop optimizing two subsets of parameters for the eyeball, three subsets for the lens
4. **Security check**
   To avoid too much deviation from solution (axes length can be neither longer nor shorter than usual eye size)
5. **Stopping conditions**
   After $N = 15$ iterations or if the ellipsoid is outside normal anatomy size
6. **Go back** to 2
   Bigger than eyeball/lens, now ellipsoid shrinks instead of growing

3.2 Segmentation Results and Validation

Segmentation results for three patients are presented in this section. Fore each patient, only the eye under radiotherapy planning is considered. CT images are acquired in the Lausanne University Hospital, on a LightSpeed VCT General Electric Medical Imaging scanner. Images have a resolution of $0.7 \times 0.7 \times 2\,\text{mm}^3$ and volume of interest around the eye area is of $90 \times 90 \times 30$ voxels. Results are shown in Fig. 4. By visual inspection on axial and sagittal views we can conclude that the segmentation is good for both lens and eyeball. 3D view reconstruction is also shown, note that the segmentation of the skull has been done simply by threshold for visualization purposes. Fitted ellipsoid parameters (the radii for both eyeball and lens and the rotational angles of the lens) are shown Table 2. Quantitative evaluation is done by comparison with manual segmentations done by an expert. We used the Dice Similarity Measure (DSM) as relative index of similarity between manual (m) and automated (a) segmentations. DSM is defined as

$$DSM^{o}_{a,m} = \frac{2 \cdot N_{a \cap m}}{N_a + N_m}, \tag{7}$$

where N_a and N_m are the voxels belonging to the object (ball and lens) o according to the automated and manual segmentation methods a and m, respectively, and $N_{a \cap m}$ is the number of voxels belonging to the object according to both methods. Although $DSM > 0.7$ is considered as an excellent agreement between the two segmentations, DSM is hardly interpreted as an absolute value but as a value to compare the similarities between pairs of methods. Resulting DSM values are shown in Table 3 presenting a very high agreement between the manual and the automated segmentation for the eyeball and the lens.

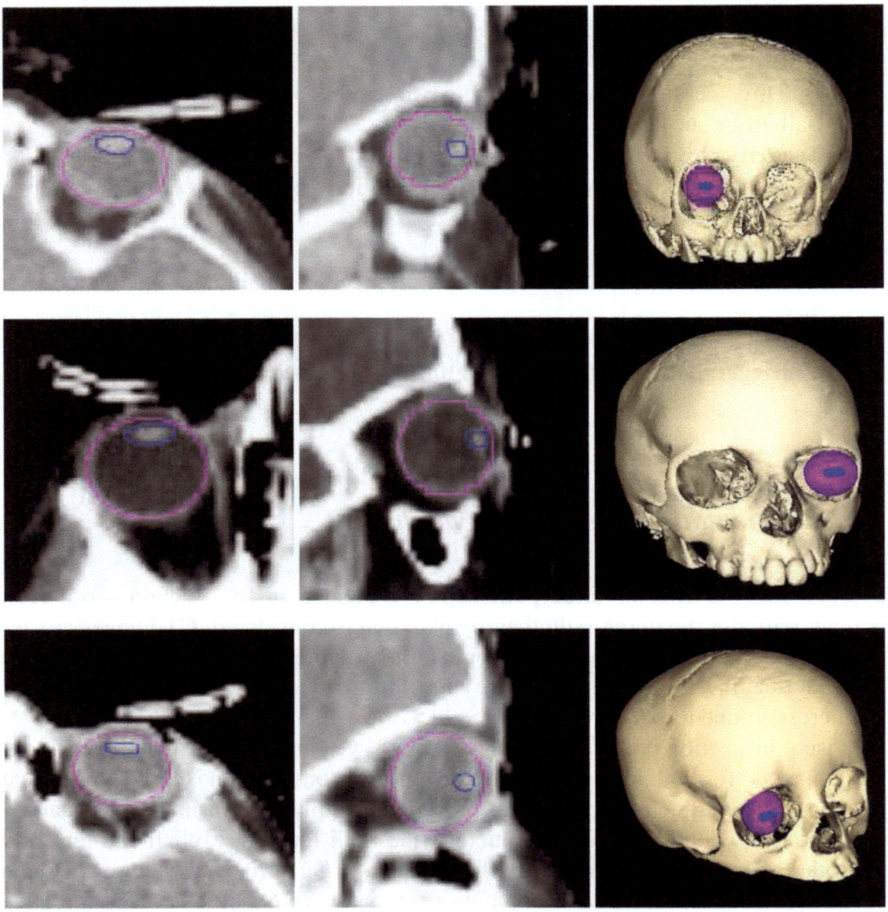

Fig. 4 Axial, sagittal and 3D views of the automated segmentation results of the eye ball and the lens, for three patients

Table 2 Computed radii and rotational angles for the eye ball and the lens, obtained from the automated CT image segmentation

	Eye ball	Lens	
	(r_x, r_y, r_z) in mm	(r_x, r_y, r_z) in mm	(α, β) in degrees
Patient 1	(10.0, 9.1, 10.0)	(3.6, 1.8, 2.0)	(186.6, 165.4)
Patient 2	(12.3, 10.6, 12.6)	(3.1, 1.5, 1.5)	(181.7, 181.1)
Patient 3	(10.5, 9.8, 11.0)	(4.9, 2.2, 2.4)	(185.3, 177.0)

Table 3 Quantitative evaluation for the eyeball and the lens

	Volume (mm^3)			
	Manual	Automated	Error	DSM
Eyeball				
Patient 1	4764	4827	1.33%	89.9%
Patient 2	7758	7798	0.52%	92.6%
Patient 3	6114	5543	9.33%	90.2%
Lens				
Patient 1	141	102	−27.7%	78.4%
Patient 2	205	215	4.9%	76.9%
Patient 3	217	219	0.9%	76.8%

4 Image Fusion

As introduced earlier, one of our goals is the fusion of CT and 3D ultrasound images. Other approaches in the literature have already suggested the fusion of multi-modal images such as CT and fundus photographs [3, 7] to improve the treatment planning precision, specifically to better define the gross tumor volume in the CT space. To proceed to this fusion, they computed the flattening geometrical distortion from 3D (the CT scan) to 2D (the fundus photograph) spaces. However, the nature of our problem is slightly different. In our case, we do have two 3D volumes to match, thus we have a volume-to-volume registration problem.

The ophthalmic 3D ultrasound images used here are acquired with OTI Ophthalmic Technologies Inc. [14]. The OTI-Scan 3D is one of the most advanced ophthalmic ultrasound system available today. The internal rotator assembly generates a 3D image in less than 2 s with a 0.1 mm resolution in each X, Y, and Z direction. An example of such acquisition is shown in Fig. 1.

Multi-modal volume registration is a widely studied problem in medical imaging [10]. There exists however few studies related to the 3D ultrasound registration with any other modality [15, 16, 18] and none of them is dedicated to the eye. Multi-modal registration is often applied on image volumes coming from the same subject. Its registration aims at compensating for difference in positions of the patient during the image acquisition process of both modalities. Thus, a rigid registration (three translations and three rotations) is often enough to this end. Often, prior to voxel-based registration, a global supervised initialization is computed to ensure a better convergence of any further registration. This is particularly needed in our case since CT and US images are acquired with very different fields of view. Note that while the CT contains the whole head, the US image only presents partially one eye.

In this section we present two *supervised* registration approaches for an initial fusion of CT and US. By *supervised* we mean that both methods needs user interaction.

4.1 Landmark-Based Registration

We choose a landmark based transformation with six parameters (three rotations and three translations) that will give the best fit mapping between corresponding point sets of the moving (US) and the target (CT) images, in a least squares sense. Landmarks selection, particularly in US image, is not an easy task and must be done by an expert. Landmark selection and registration has been done with the MITK application [11].

Three landmarks per patient and image have been selected. It is not always possible to select the same landmarks between patients. If the tumor is visible in the CT (this is not the case for Patient 2) it becomes a good landmark since its localization is easy in both modalities. The head of the optic nerve is a good landmark as well but it can be sometimes behind a tumor and thus not clearly visible in the US where a shadow behind the tumor mass appear (as it occurs for Patient 1). The summary of selected landmarks for each patient is shown in Table 4.

At this point we can proceed to the fitting of the rigid parameters that best approximate these three locations. Resulting transformation parameters (rotational angles in degrees and translations in mm) are shown in Table 5. Visualization of resulting registration is done by superposing transformed US image and moving landmarks (M1, M2 and M3) onto the CT and are shown in Fig. 5. Eyeball contour and lens have been superposed as well. Visual inspection shows a good initialization but it is difficult to quantify the accuracy of this registration. The root mean square error

Table 4 Summary of selected landmarks for each patient and Root Mean Square Error (RMSE) before (*top row*) and after (*bottom row*) registration

	Landmark 1	Landmark 2	Landmark 3	RMSE
Patient 1	Lens	Tumor 1	Tumor 2	16.32
				0.95
Patient 2	Optic nerve	Lens	Eye center	23.30
				0.36
Patient 3	Optic nerve	Lens	Tumor	16.27
				1.36

Table 5 Rigid transformation parameters estimated by the landmark-based registration. X, Y, Z are the axis directions, rotation angles are in degrees and translations are in mm

		X	Y	Z
Patient 1	*Rotation*	46.94	−60	161.32
	Translation	11.51	−57.19	24.10
Patient 2	*Rotation*	5.41	89.56	−84.95
	Translation	40.82	−12.36	51.58
Patient 3	*Rotation*	−3.49	−32.31	3.46
	Translation	−80.00	−144.11	179.37

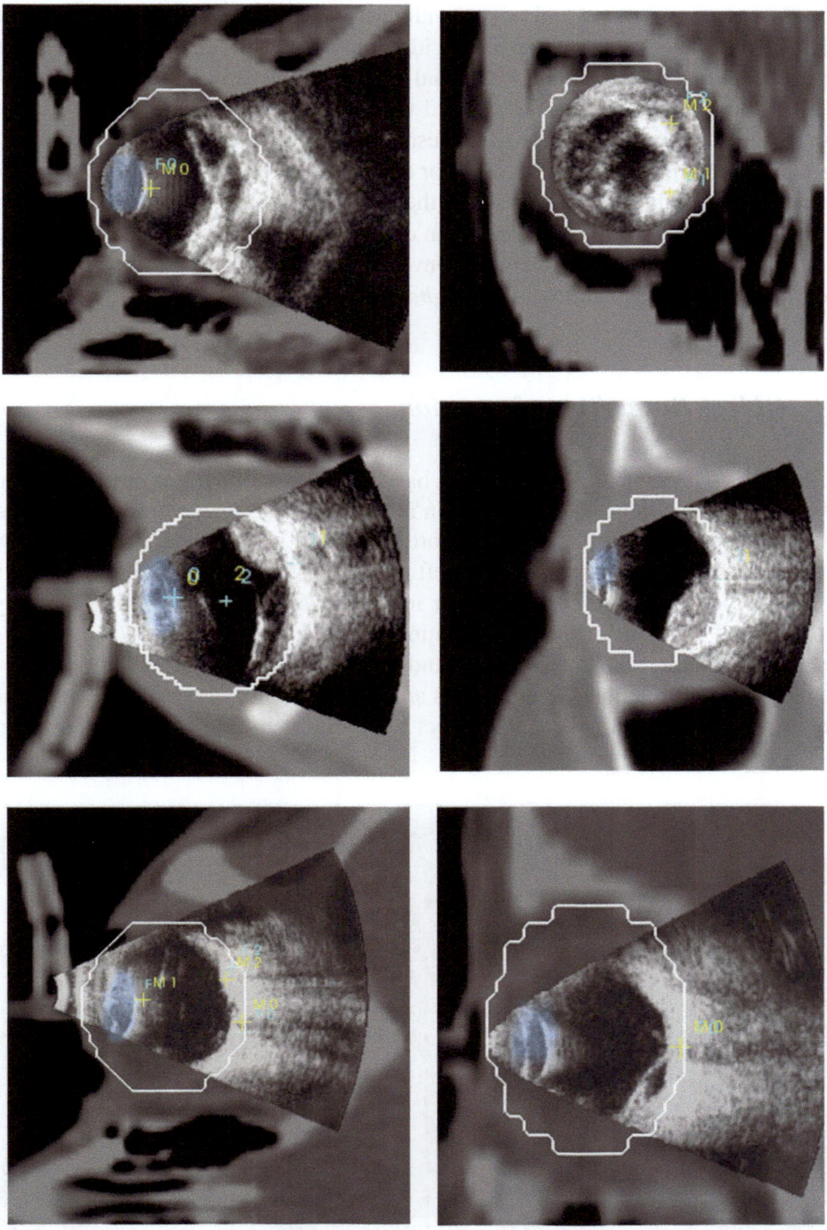

Fig. 5 Landmark-based registration results for three patients. Ultrasound is superposed to the CT image. Moving landmarks are in yellow, fixed landmarks are in cyan. The lens mask in blue and the eyeball contour in black. (**Top row**) Patient 1: Axial (*left*) and coronal (*right*) views of superposition. Landmarks are in the back of the lens (0), and in tumors (1 and 2). (**Middle row**) Patient 2: Axial (*left*) and sagittal (*right*) views of superposition. Landmarks are in the back of the lens (0), head of the optic nerve (1) and center of the eye ball (2). (**Bottom row**) Patient 3: Axial (*left*) and sagittal (*right*) views of superposition. Landmarks are in the head of the optic nerve (0), back of the lens (1) and small calcified tumor (2)

(RMSE) between moving and target landmarks before and after the transformation is shown in Table 4. This gives us an idea only about the accuracy in fitting the selected landmarks but about not the quality of the transformation.

The main problem that we have faced with the current landmark-based approach is that identification of anatomical corresponding landmarks on CT and US images is a tedious and time consuming task. For example, it took around 30 min per patient for an expert ophthalmologist to select the landmarks. Thus, landmark-based registration will always need the intervention of an expert for identifying corresponding point sets. In order to avoid these inconveniences, we propose in the next Section another type of initialization, an *object-based registration*.

4.2 Object-Based Transformation

As mentioned previously, initial images have different acquisition orientation. Thus, first step in the object-based registration is to change US orientation to CT. This is done by simply rotating the image accordingly. Still both images are not precisely in the same space as shown in Fig. 6 (left panel). We apply a second transformation by roughly selecting the eyeball center in both images and then fitting them by a translation. The result of this initialization is shown in Fig. 6 (right panel). Then, we create from the segmented eyeball and lens (CT) a mesh that will now represent the target object to match. These points are represented in Fig. 7 (left panel). Then, even a non expert user proceed to select few points (around 25) corresponding to

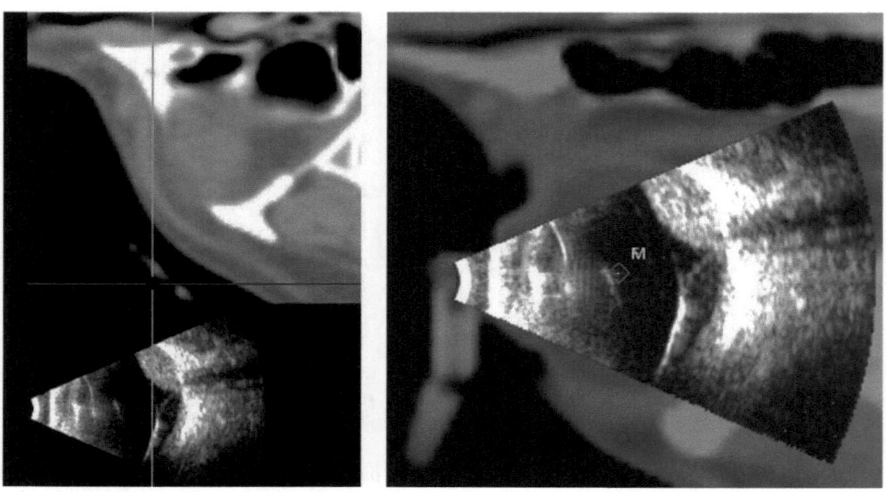

Fig. 6 Object-based initialization: *left* panel is the original position of both modalities after changing acquisition orientation of US image; *right* panel is the result of the rigid transform computed from eyeball center landmarks

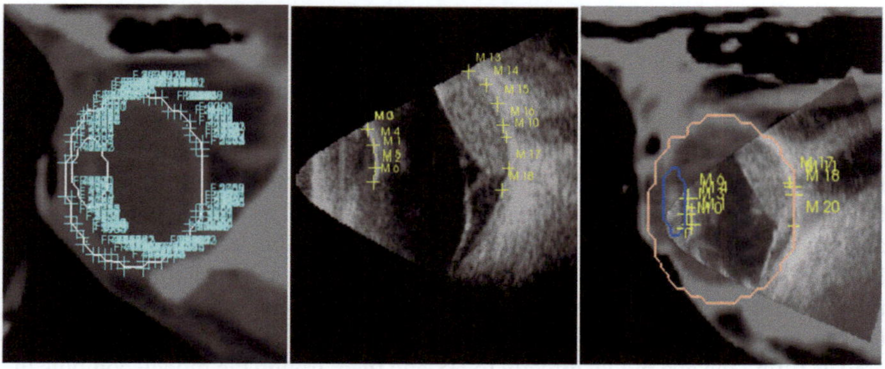

Fig. 7 Object-based registration: *left* panel are the mesh points of the eyeball and lens in the CT space; *middle* panel are the selected points on the US corresponding to the back of the lens and the back of the eye; *right* panel is the final positioning after ICP rigid registration

the back edges of the eyeball in the US, as well as some points in the back border of the lens. An example of such points are shown in Fig. 7 (middle panel)[4]. The whole procedure takes only few minutes. Finally, ICP algorithm is applied to compute the rigid transformation between these two sets of points. The resulting registration is shown in Fig. 7 (right panel).

At this point we cannot conclude whether landmark-based or object-based registration is better since we do not have a gold standard to compare with. Moreover, the object-based registration presented here is rather preliminary: mesh creation should be improved and more patients should be tested. Qualitatively, results of both transformations are very similar and we consider both initializations as good for a further voxel-based volume registration. However, object-based registration is performed in 2 or 3 min by even a non-expert user while landmark-based registration takes around 30 min and needs from an expert.

5 Discussion

In this paper, we have presented our preliminary work towards a multi-modal framework for the radiotherapy planning of retinoblastomas. To our knowledge, this is the first attempt to combine 3D CT and 3D US for the eye radiotherapy. In the present work we have presented a model-based segmentation of the eye ball and the lens on the CT images. The main difference compared to the existing model-based segmentation methods is that here we proceed by using the well formulated

[4] Every point is represented by a cross and tags enumerating it. However since for this mesh we have a lot of points the tags appear all superposed and make the visualization a little strange.

active contour framework. Evaluation in comparison with manual segmentation has shown a good accuracy of our segmentation model. Moreover, we have also computed a first required initialization of the rigid transformation that brings the CT, and thus the eye model, and the US into the same space. Two procedures have been suggested for the initial alignment: landmark-based and object-based registration. Landmark-based registration requires an expert user interaction for selecting the landmarks and this takes a considerable amount of time. The suggested object-based approach overcome this problem and resulting registration seems very close to the landmark-based one. Further research will be on creating a ground truth for registration assessment. For instance by creating simulated US data from CT or being able to scan an eye *phantom*. Also, as in [7], other registration strategies could be considered as fitting the eye model directly to US and then, trough the model, compute the transformation between both images. As well, we believe that the optic nerve should be included in the model. Finally, tumor segmentation on the US image should be investigated.

Acknowledgements This work is supported by the Centre d'Imagerie BioMédicale (CIBM) of the University of Lausanne (UNIL), the Swiss Federal Institute of Technology Lausanne (EPFL), the University of Geneva (UniGe), the Centre Hospitalier Universitaire Vaudois (CHUV), the Hôpitaux Universitaires de Genève (HUG) and the Leenaards and the Jeantet Foundations.

References

1. Bach Cuadra, M., Gorthi, S., Karahanoglu, F.I., Salvador, F., Pica, A., Do, H., Balmer, A., Munier, F., Thiran, J.P.: Model-based segmentation and image fusion of 3D computed tomography and 3D ultrasound of the eye for radiotherapy planning. In: Second ECCOMAS Thematic Conference on Computational Vision and Medical Image Processing, pp. 53–58 (2009)
2. Bekes, G., Máté, E., Nyúl, L.G., Kuba, A., Fidrich, M.: Geometrical model-based segmentation of the organs of sight on CT images. Med. Phys. **35**, 735–743 (2008)
3. Bondiau, P.Y., Malandain, G.: Eye reconstruction and CT-retinography fusion for proton treatment planning of ocular diseases. In: CVRMed-MRCAS'97, *LNCS*, vol. 1205, pp. 705–714. Springer (1997)
4. Caselles, V., Kimmel, R., Sapiro, G.: Geodesic active contours. Int. J. Comput. Vis. **22**(1), 61–79 (1997)
5. Cates, J.E., Whitaker, R.T., Jones, G.M.: Case study: an evaluation of user-assisted hierarchical watershed segmentation. Med. Image Anal. **9**(6), 566–578 (2005)
6. DHaese, P., Duay, V., Li, R., du Bois dAische, A., Merchant, T., Cmelak, A., Donnelly, E., Niermann, K., Macq, B., Dawant, B.: Automatic segmentation of brain structures for radiation therapy planning. In: Medical Imaging: Image Processing, ISCAS. SPIE (2003)
7. Dobler, B., Bendl, R.: Precise modelling of the eye for proton therapy of intra-ocular tumours. Phys. Med. Biol. **47**(4), 593–613 (2002)
8. Donaldson, S., Smith, L.: Retinoblastoma: biology, presentation, and current management. Oncology **3**(10), 45–51 (1989)
9. Fenster, A., Downey, D., Cardinal, H.: Three-dimensional ultrasound imaging. Phys. Med. Biol. **46**(5), 67–99 (2001)
10. Maintz, J., Viergever, M.A.: A survey of medical image registration. Med. Image Anal. **2**(1), 1–36 (1998)
11. Maleike, D., Nolden, M., Meinzer, H.P., Wolf, I.: Interactive segmentation framework of the medical imaging interaction toolkit. Comput. Meth. Programs Biomed. **96**(1), 72–83 (2009)

12. Munier, F., Verwey, J., Pica, A., Balmer, A., Zografos, L., Abouzeid, H., Timmerman, B., Goitein, G., Moeckli, R.: New developments in external beam radiotherapy for retinoblastoma: from lens to normal tissue-sparing techniques. Clin. Exp. Ophthalmol. **36**(1), 78–89 (2008)
13. OCular TumOur Planning UtilitieS (OCTOPUS). http://www.dkfz.de/en/medphys/therapy_planning_development/projects/octopus.html
14. Ophthalmic Technologies Inc. (OTI), Canada. http://www.opko.com/
15. Penney, G., Blackall, J., Hamady, M., Sabharwal, T., Adam, A., Hawkes, D.: Registration of freehand 3D ultrasound and magnetic resonance liver images. Med. Image Anal. **8**, 81–91 (2004)
16. Roche, A., Pennec, X.M.G.A.N.: Rigid registration of 3-D ultrasound with MR images: a new approach combining intensity and gradient information. IEEE Tran. Med. Imag. **20**(10), 1038–1049 (2001)
17. Souza, A., Ruiz, E.: Fast and accurate detection of extraocular muscle borders using mathematical morphology. In: Engineering in Medicine and Biology Society, 2000. Proceedings of the 22nd Annual International Conference of the IEEE, vol. 3, pp. 1779–1782 (2000)
18. Wein, W., Brunke, S., Khamene, A., Callstrom, M., Navab, N.: Automatic CT-ultrasound registration for diagnostic imaging and image-guided intervention. Med. Image Anal. **12**, 577–585 (2008)
19. Yannuzzi, L.A., Ober, M.D., Slakter, J.S., Spaide, R.F., Fisher, Y.L., Flower, R.W., Rosen, R.: Ophthalmic fundus imaging: today and beyond. Am. J. Ophthalmol. **137**(3), 511–524 (2004)

Flow of a Blood Analogue Solution Through Microfabricated Hyperbolic Contractions

P.C. Sousa, I.S. Pinho, F.T. Pinho, M.S.N. Oliveira, and M.A. Alves

Abstract The flow of a blood analogue solution past a microfabricated hyperbolic contraction followed by an abrupt expansion was investigated experimentally. The shape of the contraction was designed in order to impose a nearly constant strain rate to the fluid along the centerline of the microgeometry. The flow patterns of the blood analogue solution and of a Newtonian reference fluid (deionized water), captured using streak line imaging, are quite distinct and illustrate the complex behavior of the blood analogue solution flowing through the microgeometry. The flow of the blood analogue solution shows elastic-driven effects with vortical structures emerging upstream of the contraction, which are absent in Newtonian fluid flow. In both cases the flow also develops instabilities downstream of the expansion but these are inertia driven. Therefore, for the blood analogue solution at high flow rates the competing effects of inertia and elasticity lead to complex flow patterns and unstable flow develops.

Keywords Blood analogue fluid · Extensional flow · Microfluidics · Viscoelasticity · Flow visualization · Hyperbolic contraction

1 Introduction

The Human blood is a complex fluid consisting of a suspension of cellular elements, 98% of which are erythrocytes (red blood cells, RBCs) suspended in an aqueous matrix, the plasma, containing also proteins and other solutes. In healthy human

P.C. Sousa, I.S. Pinho, M.S.N. Oliveira (✉), and M.A. Alves
Faculdade de Engenharia da Universidade do Porto, Departamento de Engenharia Química, Centro de Estudos de Fenómenos de Transporte, Rua Dr. Roberto Frias, 4200–465 Porto, Portugal
e-mail: deq06010@fe.up.pt; bio06019@fe.up.pt; monica.oliveira@fe.up.pt; mmalves@fe.up.pt

F.T. Pinho
Faculdade de Engenharia da Universidade do Porto, Centro de Estudos de Fenómenos de Transporte, Departamento de Engenharia Mecânica, Rua Dr. Roberto Frias, 4200–465 Porto, Portugal
e-mail: fpinho@fe.up.pt

J.M.R.S. Tavares and R.M.N. Jorge (eds.), *Computational Vision and Medical Image Processing: Recent Trends*, Computational Methods in Applied Sciences 19,
DOI 10.1007/978-94-007-0011-6_15,

blood the white blood cells (leukocytes) and platelets represent about 2% of the suspended cellular elements. The ratio between the volume of the RBCs and the total volume of blood is the so-called hematocrit, an important physiological parameter to be considered in the characterization of human blood. Although we can consider plasma as a Newtonian fluid, the deformable RBCs and its structures confer non-Newtonian properties to this rheologically complex fluid. In effect, at low shear rates RBCs may form aggregated structures, named rouleaux, the dynamics of which impact severely on blood rheology [19]. The aggregation of blood cells depends on the protein concentration in plasma (a good example that minor amounts of an additive can have a large impact in fluid structure and rheology) and on the shear rate and is a reversible process that leads to a viscoelastic, shear-thinning and thixotropic behavior of blood [16, 17]. As such, blood shear viscosity depends on a number of variables, namely, hematocrit, the shear rate and even the vessel diameter, the latter known as the Fåhraeus–Lindqvist effect [10].

Despite the wealth of information on the complex rheology of blood [10, 17], the vast majority of research on hemodynamics assumes that blood behaves as a Newtonian fluid. This can be acceptable when blood is flowing through major arteries [5] however, non-Newtonian characteristics become important in small vessels or when the characteristic times of the flow and fluid become comparable, and in this respect it is also important to realize that the flow is time-dependent essentially everywhere. Furthermore, viscoelastic effects are enhanced when the vessel geometry exhibits fluid features such as contractions/expansions (e.g. due to fatty deposits), taper or bifurcations in addition to local time dependency. One such relevant feature is the *stenosis*, a local constriction of a blood vessel, usually defined as the percentage of vessel diameter reduction, due to the adherence and accumulation of cells, especially of fatty material. This accumulative process has a shear-rate dependent positive feedback mechanism, since more deposition takes place at higher shear rates and shear rates increase as the diameter of the vessel is reduced. Studies reported so far show that flow separation occurs in the expansion region of the *stenosis* at Reynolds numbers on the order of 10 for a 70% *stenosis* [5].

Since the use of blood in experimental studies is not always practical, primarily due to safety reasons, viscoelastic fluids with rheological characteristics similar to human blood are a good and safe alternative. Vlastos et al. [16] studied the combination of steady and oscillatory shear on the human blood flow behavior. For this purpose, they also used blood analogue solutions made from high molecular weight polymers dissolved in water, namely aqueous solutions of polyacrylamide and xanthan gum at different concentrations. The polyacrylamide and xanthan gum solutions have a rheological behavior similar to that of human blood at concentrations of 125 and 500 ppm (w/w), respectively, especially at low shear rates whereas at high shear rates they tend to exhibit higher viscosity and elasticity than blood. Still, these are adequate analogue fluids in a variety of flow conditions.

In this work, we compare the flows of a Newtonian fluid and a viscoelastic blood analogue through microfluidic contraction/expansion geometries to highlight the non-Newtonian effects at the microscale. The Newtonian fluid is water and the blood analogue is an aqueous xanthan gum solution (500 ppm w/w) as proposed in [14, 16].

2 Experimental

2.1 Microchannel Geometry

In this study three different microgeometries were studied. In all cases, the microchannels used are planar and have a contraction with a hyperbolic shape, followed by an abrupt expansion. The hyperbolic shape was chosen in order to provide a nearly constant strain rate of the fluid flow along the centerline of the microgeometry, as proposed by Oliveira et al. [8]. Using this configuration, it is possible to study the response of the fluid under strong accelerations, for controlled extensional flow conditions.

The geometry and length scale of the microchannels studied are comparable to small human vessels with a constriction. In the human circulatory system, capillaries are the smallest blood vessels, having diameters of 4–8 μm and arterioles typically have internal diameters in the range from 50 up to 100 μm [2]. In Fig. 1 we show a microscopy image of a typical contraction–expansion geometry used in this study.

The total width, $D_1 = 400\,\mu\text{m}$ of the microchannels was kept constant for all geometries. The minimum width of the contraction, D_2, and the hyperbolic contraction length, L_c were varied in order to obtain different values of the total Hencky strain (ε_H), here defined as $\varepsilon_H = \ln(D_1/D_2)$. The depth, h, of the microchannels used varied slightly relative to the nominal value of 50 μm due to inaccuracies inherent to the fabrication procedure. In Table 1 we present the dimensions for each geometry.

The channels were fabricated in polydimethylsiloxane, PDMS (Sylgard 184, Dow Corning), from an SU-8 photoresist mold using standard soft lithography

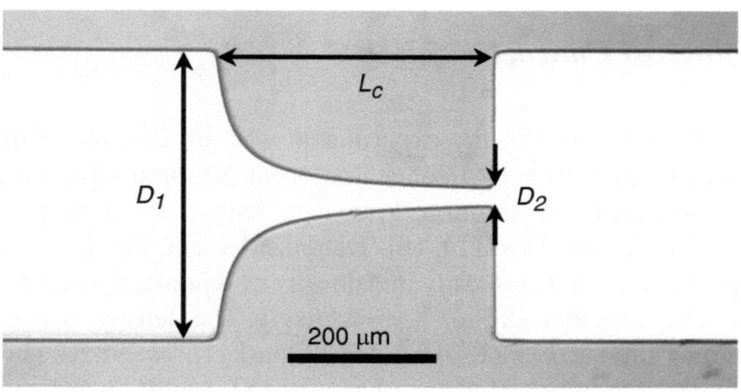

Fig. 1 Microchannel S_3 used in the experiments

Table 1 Geometry dimensions and corresponding Hencky strain

Channel	ε_H	D_2(μm)	L_c(μm)	h(μm)
S_1	0.76	187	34	47
S_2	1.86	62.4	128	45
S_3	2.75	25.5	380	44

techniques [6]. PDMS was utilized due to its transparency that permits optical access to the flow region, and also due to its simple and well-established fabrication techniques, which allow us to obtain geometries with well-defined features.

2.2 Flow Visualization

Visualizations of the flow patterns were carried out at room temperature, for a wide range of flow rates, using streak line photography. The optical setup consists of an inverted epi-fluorescence microscope (DMI 5000M, Leica Microsystems GmbH) equipped with a CCD camera (DFC350 FX, Leica Microsystems GmbH), a light source (100 W mercury lamp) and a filter cube (Leica Microsystems GmbH, excitation filter BP 530–545 nm, dichroic 565 nm and barrier filter 610–675 nm). A syringe pump (PHD2000, Harvard Apparatus) was used to inject the fluid and control the flow rate in the microchannel. Syringes with different volumes (50 μl–10 ml) were used according to the desired flow rate and connected to the microgeometries using Tygon tubing. The fluids were seeded with 1 μm fluorescent tracer particles (Nile Red, Molecular Probes, Invitrogen, Ex/Em: 520/580 nm) and sodium dodecyl sulfate (0.1 wt %, Sigma-Aldrich) was added in order to minimize adhesion of fluorescent tracer particles to the channels walls. The microgeometries containing the seeded fluid were continuously illuminated and the light emitted by the fluorescent tracer particles was imaged through the microscope objective (×10, NA = 0.25) onto the CCD array of the camera using "long" exposure times (∼1 s) in order to capture the particle pathlines. All streak line images presented here are centered at the mid-plane of the microchannel.

2.3 Rheological Characterization

The viscoelastic fluid used in the experiments was an aqueous solution of xanthan gum (Sigma-Aldrich) with a concentration of 500 ppm w/w, which is a well established blood analogue solution, known to have a shear rheology behavior similar to that of human blood [14, 16]. Deionized water was also used for comparison purposes. The shear viscosity and density of deionized water at 293.2 K are 1.003×10^{-3} Pa s and 998.3 kg m^{-3}, respectively. The density of the viscoelastic solution was measured at 293.2 K using density flasks ($\rho = 998.8$ kg m^{-3}).

The steady shear rheology of the xanthan gum (XG) solution was measured with a shear rheometer (Anton Paar, model Physica MCR301) using a cone-plate geometry (75 mm, 1° angle) under shear rate control. Figure 2 compares the measured shear viscosity of the XG solution at 293.2 K with reported values for human blood at 310.2 K [15].

In Fig. 2 we also show as dashed lines the lower and upper limits that should be considered for accurate measurements of the shear viscosity. The lower boundary

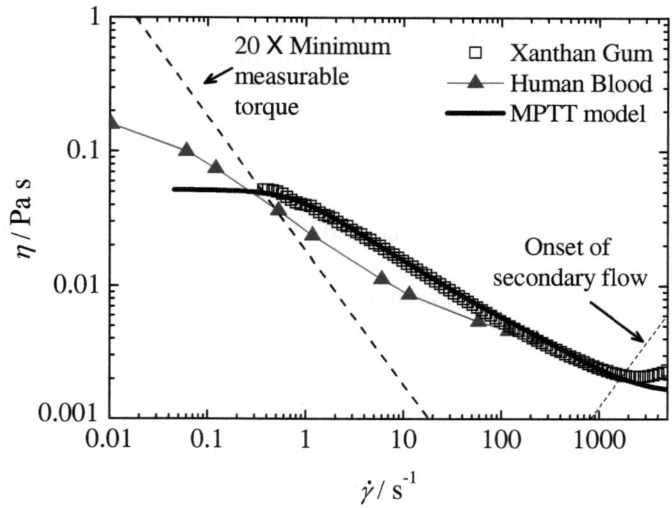

Fig. 2 Comparison of steady shear data of the xanthan gum solution at 293.2 K with reported values for human blood at 310.2 K [15]

of the shear viscosity was calculated considering 20 times the minimum resolvable torque specifications of the shear rheometer [1],

$$\eta(\dot{\gamma}) = \frac{3\,(20\Im_{\min})}{2\pi R^3}\frac{1}{\dot{\gamma}}, \tag{1}$$

where η is the shear viscosity, $\dot{\gamma}$ is the shear rate, $\Im_{\min}$ is the rheometer minimum resolvable torque (10^{-7}N m) and R is the radius of the cone geometry used in the measurements.

The laminar flow of a Newtonian fluid between a rotating cone and a fixed plate is a purely rotational steady shear flow when the following relation is valid [13]:

$$\frac{\omega\alpha^2\rho R^2}{12\eta} < 0.5, \tag{2}$$

where ω is the angular velocity and α is the angle between the cone and the plate. Therefore, the upper limit of the measurable shear viscosity, based on the onset of inertial instabilities (Taylor vortices) is given by

$$\eta = \frac{\omega\alpha^2\rho R^2}{6}. \tag{3}$$

Additionally, the shear viscosity curve was fitted using a modified Phan–Thien–Tanner model (MPTT) [18] with a Newtonian solvent contribution. The fit is also represented in Fig. 2. In this particular model, the total stress is $\boldsymbol{\sigma} = \boldsymbol{\tau} + \boldsymbol{\tau}_s - p\mathbf{I}$, where p is the pressure and $\boldsymbol{\tau}_s$ is the contribution of the Newtonian solvent given by $\boldsymbol{\tau}_s = \eta_{solvent}\,(\nabla\mathbf{u} + \nabla\mathbf{u}^T)$.

For an MPTT fluid, the constitutive equation for the polymer contribution ($\boldsymbol{\tau}$) to the extra stress tensor is given by,

$$f(\mathrm{Tr}\,\boldsymbol{\tau})\,\boldsymbol{\tau} + \lambda\left[\frac{\partial\boldsymbol{\tau}}{\partial t} + \nabla\cdot\mathbf{u}\boldsymbol{\tau}\right] = \eta_{polymer}(\nabla\mathbf{u} + \nabla\mathbf{u}^T) + \lambda(\boldsymbol{\tau}\cdot\nabla\mathbf{u} + \nabla\mathbf{u}^T\cdot\boldsymbol{\tau}) \quad (4)$$

Since we are using the linear form of the PTT model [11], f (Tr $\boldsymbol{\tau}$) becomes:

$$f(\mathrm{Tr}\,\boldsymbol{\tau}) = 1 + \frac{\lambda\varepsilon}{\eta_{polymer}}\mathrm{Tr}(\boldsymbol{\tau}), \quad (5)$$

where ε is the extensibility parameter and $\eta_{polymer}$ is the viscosity coefficient of the model, which is here given by a Carreau-type equation [18]:

$$\eta_{polymer} = \frac{\eta_p}{[1 + (\Gamma\dot{\gamma})^2]^{\frac{1-n}{2}}}. \quad (6)$$

In Eq. 6, Γ is a time parameter, n is the power-law index, η_p is the zero-shear-rate polymer viscosity and the shear-rate, $\dot{\gamma}$, is an invariant of the rate of deformation tensor ($\dot{\gamma} = \sqrt{(\dot{\boldsymbol{\gamma}} : \dot{\boldsymbol{\gamma}})/2}$ with $\dot{\boldsymbol{\gamma}} = \nabla\mathbf{u} + \nabla\mathbf{u}^T$).

The fitted viscosity is thus given by $\eta = (\tau + \tau_{solvent})/\dot{\gamma}$, where the parameters are: $\varepsilon = 0.05$, $\eta_p = 0.05$ Pa s, $\Gamma = 1.3$ s, $n = 0.5$ and the solvent viscosity is $\eta_{solvent} = 0.0015$ Pa s. The relaxation time considered in the fitting is the value determined using the CaBER measurements ($\lambda = 3.77$ ms) described below. The fit to the experimental shear data was done in order to allow for the calculations of the shear viscosity and possibly other rheological material functions that are a function of the shear rate, as well as to provide relevant information to be used in future numerical simulations of the flow of the blood analogue solution used in this study.

The relaxation time of the fluid was determined at 293.2 K under extensional flow conditions using a capillary-breakup extensional rheometer (Haake CaBER 1, Thermo Scientific). During CaBER measurements, the liquid is placed between two circular plates, which are separated by a distance h_i, and then an axial step strain is imposed until a final height (h_f) is reached. Subsequently, the liquid thread is left to relax and breakup under the combined action of capillary and extensional viscoelastic forces. The diameter of the filament $D(t)$ is monitored as a function of time, t, as shown in Fig. 3 for the xanthan gum solution. The circular plates used were $D_p = 6$ mm in diameter and the initial and final aspect ratios, defined as $\Lambda_i = h_i/D_p$ and $\Lambda_f = h_f/D_p$, were set as 0.33 and 1.39, respectively. The relaxation time, λ, can be determined by fitting the experimental data in the linear region of $\log[D(\mathrm{t})]$ as a function of t, since an elasto-capillary balance [4] leads to the relation $D(t)/D_0 \propto \exp[-t/(3\lambda)]$, where D_0 is the diameter of the filament at time $t = 0$. The average relaxation time obtained by CaBER measurements was 3.77 ms.

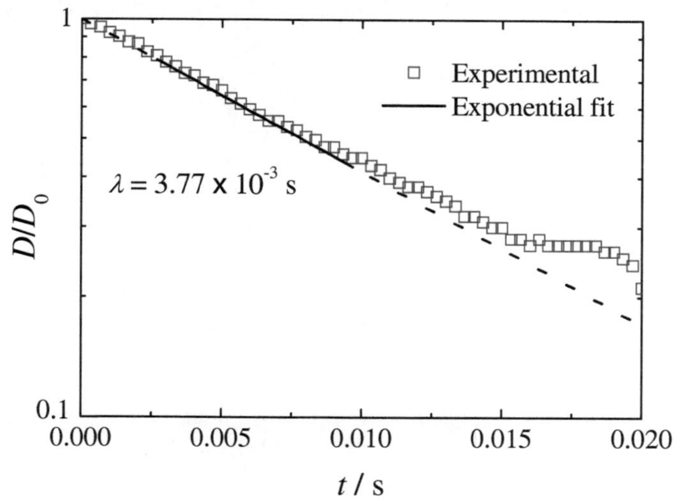

Fig. 3 Exponential decay of the xanthan gum filament diameter during a CaBER measurement at 293.2 K

The rheological model used exhibits shear-thinning behavior but does not contemplate the existence of a yield stress, which is usually associated with blood. At very low shear rates, the RBCs form a three-dimensional solid-like structure suggesting that blood may have a yield stress. Increasing the shear stress, blood begins to flow and the solid-like structure ruptures. Nevertheless, the reported yield stress for blood is very small, ranging from ~0.005 to ~0.01 N/m^2 [10] depending on the hematocrit and therefore, using a model without a yield stress is an acceptable approximation considering the high flow rate/shear rate conditions used in this work.

3 Results

3.1 Newtonian Fluid Flow Patterns

In this section, we present the results obtained with a Newtonian fluid (deionized water), flowing through the geometries described in Sect. 2.1. The investigation of the Newtonian fluid flow was carried out for comparison purposes.

Figures 4 and 5 show the flow patterns for two of the geometries studied (S_2 and S_3, respectively) as a function of the Reynolds number, here defined as:

$$Re = \frac{\rho V_2 D_2}{\eta(\dot{\gamma})}, \tag{7}$$

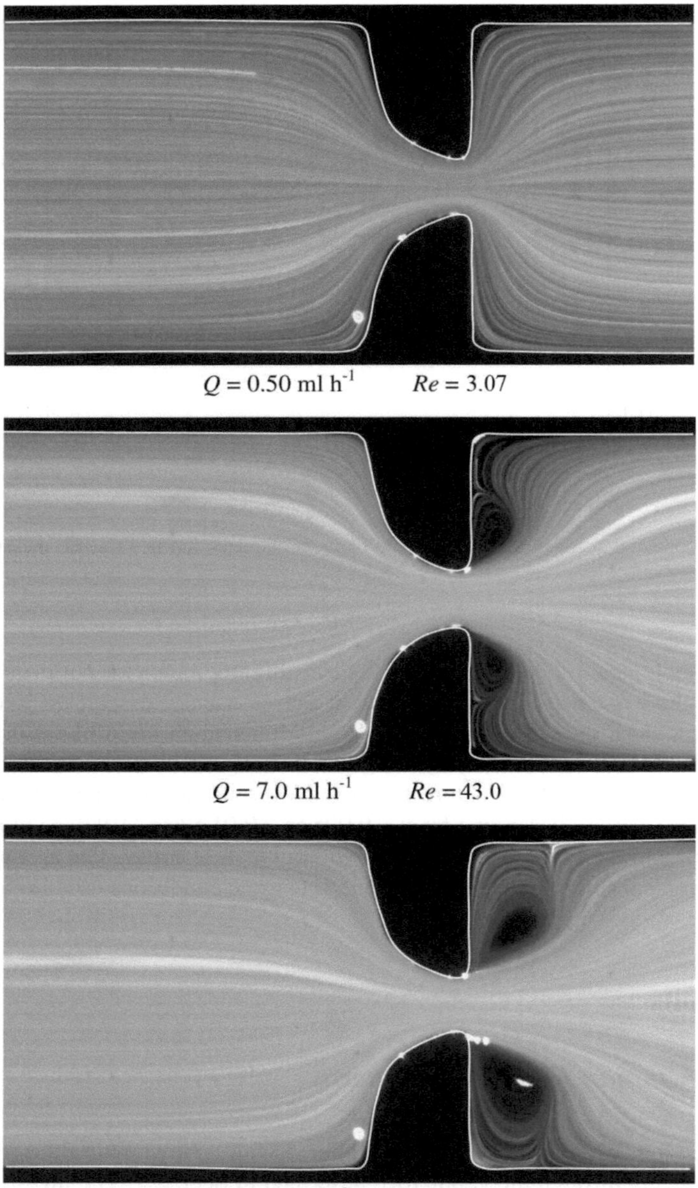

Fig. 4 Newtonian fluid flow patterns through the microchannel S_2, for different flow rates (or *Re*)

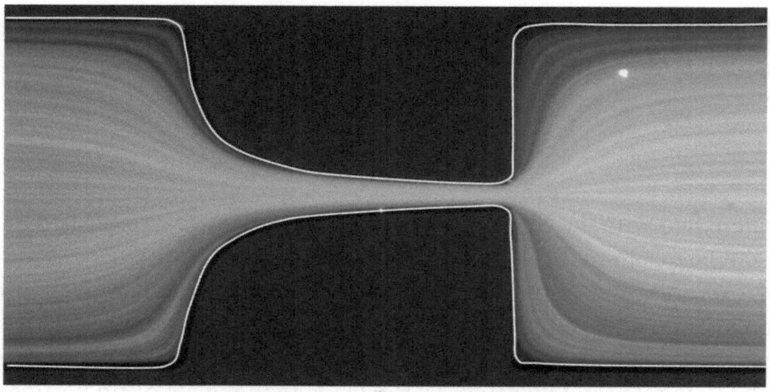

$Q = 1.0$ ml h^{-1} $Re = 6.28$

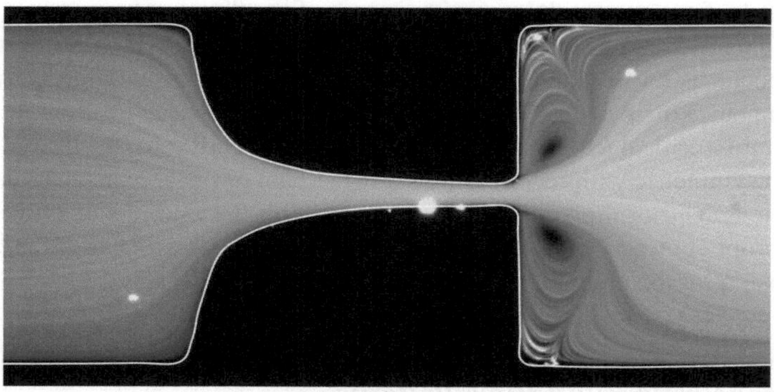

$Q = 3.0$ ml h^{-1} $Re = 18.9$

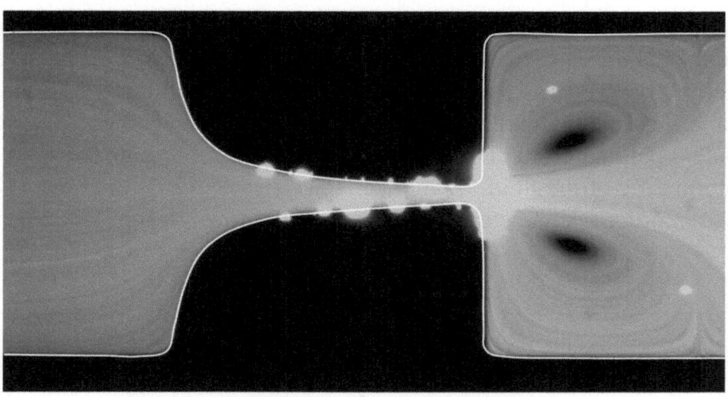

$Q = 6.0$ ml h^{-1} $Re = 37.7$

Fig. 5 Newtonian fluid flow patterns through the microchannel S_3, for different flow rates (or *Re*) where ρ is the density of the fluid and V_2 is the average velocity in the region of the contraction with width D_2. The shear viscosity is evaluated at a characteristic shear rate:

$$\dot{\gamma} = \frac{V_2}{D_2/2} \tag{8}$$

and was calculated with the MPTT model using the parameters described in Sect. 2.3 for the viscoelastics fluid. For the Newtonian fluid the viscosity is constant.

For low *Re*, the fluid is pushed towards the centerline as it moves through the contraction and the flow remains attached to the wall downstream of the expansion, except near the far corner where a small weak separated flow region exists. An increase in the flow rate (and therefore in *Re*) leads to the onset of lip vortices close to the re-entrant corners downstream of the expansion plane. These vortices eventually enlarge to the far corner with increasing inertia of the flow.

For higher Hencky-strain geometries, the value of *Re* at which the onset of lip vortices occurs is lower than for lower Hencky strains and the existing vortices tend to be elongated. Increasing inertia further, causes the vortices to grow in size and strength until a critical *Re* is reached. At these critical conditions, the flow eventually becomes asymmetric with recirculations downstream of the expansion plane having different lengths (not illustrated), in agreement with the findings of Oliveira et al. [9] for abrupt contractions followed by abrupt expansions and Cherdron et al. [3] for expansions at the end of a channel.

3.2 Viscoelastic Fluid Flow Patterns

In Figs. 6 and 7 we show pathline images of the xanthan gum solution flowing through contraction-expansion geometries S_2 and S_3, respectively. The flow patterns observed for the viscoelastic fluid are qualitatively similar for all microgeometries studied, and only selected images are shown here. The following dimensionless parameter, the Deborah number, which represents the ratio between the relaxation time of the fluid, λ, and a characteristic time of the flow, $(D_2/2)/V_2$, is also used in order to characterize the viscoelastic flow (cf. Fig. 1):

$$De = \frac{\lambda V_2}{D_2/2}. \tag{9}$$

At very low flow rates (and *De*), the flow patterns are Newtonian-like and are not shown here for conciseness. Then, on increasing the flow rate, symmetric vortices develop upstream of the hyperbolic contraction due to the elasticity of the fluid. Increasing the Deborah number even further leads to an increase of the vortex size due to the enhancement of elastic effects. The formation of vortices close to the far corner upstream of the contraction has also been discussed by McKinley et al. [7] for flows of a 0.3 wt% PEO solution in a hyperbolic contraction followed by an abrupt expansion similar to the geometry used in this study.

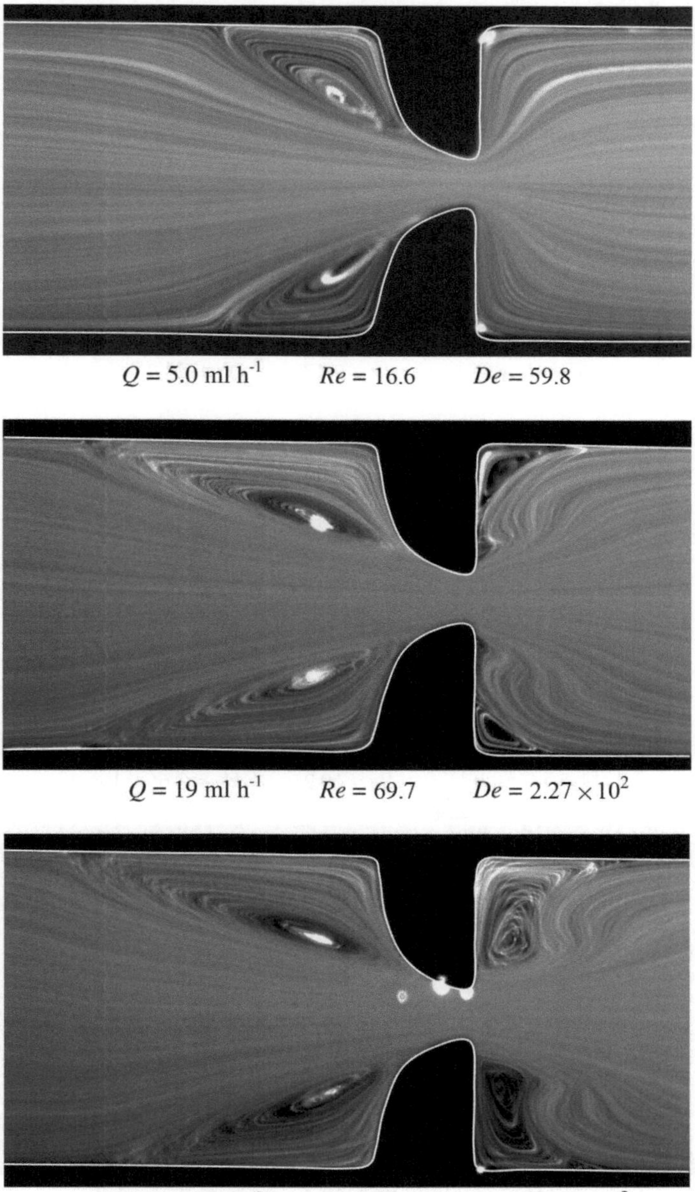

$Q = 5.0$ ml h^{-1} $Re = 16.6$ $De = 59.8$

$Q = 19$ ml h^{-1} $Re = 69.7$ $De = 2.27 \times 10^2$

$Q = 25$ ml h^{-1} $Re = 93.0$ $De = 2.99 \times 10^2$

Fig. 6 Flow patterns of the xanthan gum solution in microchannel S_2

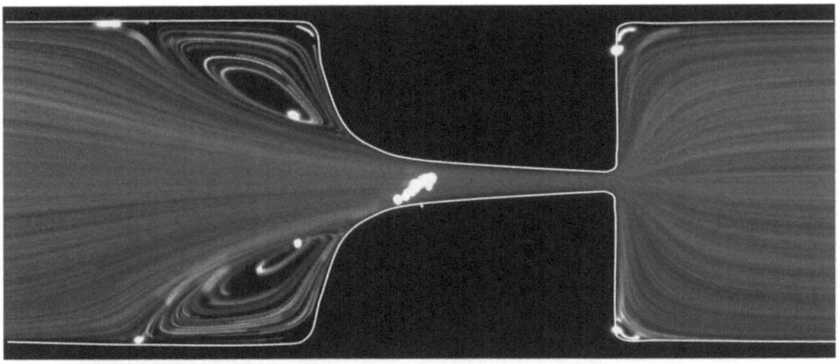

$Q = 1.0$ ml h^{-1} $Re = 3.47$ $De = 73.2$

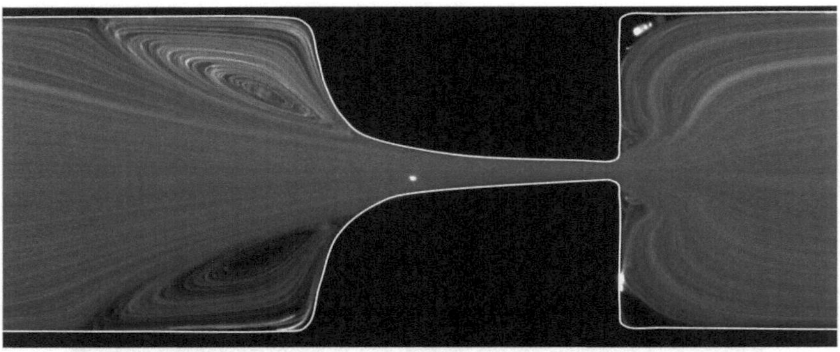

$Q = 5.0$ ml h^{-1} $Re = 19.2$ $De = 3.66 \times 10^2$

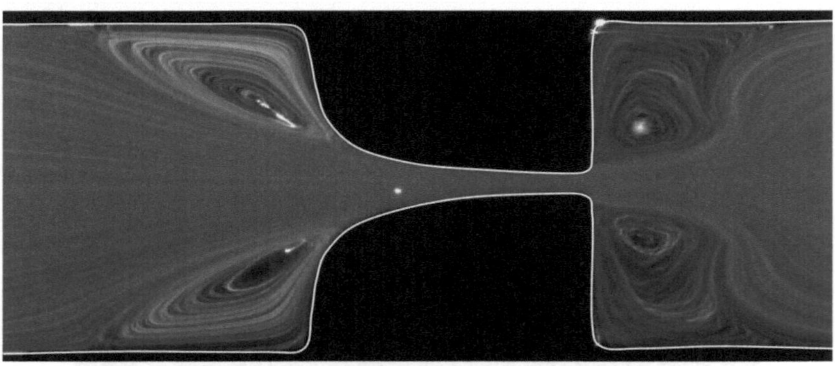

$Q = 10$ ml h^{-1} $Re = 39.4$ $De = 7.32 \times 10^2$

Fig. 7 Flow patterns of the xanthan gum solution in microchannel S_3

When the flow rate is increased even further, competing elastic and inertial effects are present and a lip vortex emerges downstream of the expansion plane as was observed for the Newtonian fluid flow when inertial effects become important. However, as a consequence of the relevance of elastic forces, in this case the inertia-driven downstream vortices are weaker than those observed for the Newtonian fluid at the same *Re*, since elasticity is responsible for the development of normal stresses in shear which are known to lead to jet swelling and consequently to a reduction of the size of downstream recirculations [12].

The small vortex at the far corner of the expansion also exists as for Newtonian fluids but again it is a rather weak entity. As the flow rate is further increased, the two recirculations downstream of the expansion merge into a single vortex that increases in size with the flow rate. Simultaneously, inertial effects start to predominate upstream, leading also to a decrease of the vortices located upstream of the hyperbolic contraction. At even higher flow rates, the flow becomes unstable with the upstream vortices varying in size asymmetrically along time. These results demonstrate that the blood analogue fluid used in this study shows viscoelastic behavior at the microscale, in spite of the small relaxation time. This enhancement of the viscoelastic behavior is particularly important at the microscale, and illustrates that whole human blood can possibly show important elastic effects when the characteristic dimension of the vessels decreases, as occurs in the microcirculation and even without considering the two-phase nature of blood. In the future, we expect to carry out similar experiments using real blood samples flowing in the microfluidic geometries used in this work, to probe whether blood indeed presents these viscoelastic flow features at the microscale.

Figure 8 summarizes our findings by mapping the flow patterns on the two-dimensional $\varepsilon_H - De$ parameter space. With this map, it is possible to foresee the different flow phenomena in the flow of a viscoelastic blood analogue solution through a constriction with different Hencky strains and Deborah numbers (notice the important presence of plane walls bounding the geometry): at low *De*, symmetric vortices develop upstream of the contraction and on increasing flow rate, there is growth of the upstream vortices and the appearance of downstream corner vortices followed then by the appearance of downstream lip vortices and corner vortices growth. Then, merging of the downstream lip and corner vortices occurs and finally unstable flow is observed at even higher flow rates.

4 Conclusions

The flow of a viscoelastic blood analogue solution through microgeometries with a hyperbolic contraction followed by an abrupt expansion exhibits significantly different characteristics from those observed with a Newtonian fluid. In the latter, inertia promotes the appearance of vortices downstream of the abrupt expansion, while in the former complex flow patterns brought about by the elastic nature of the polymeric solution are observed. In particular, symmetric vortices appear upstream of the contraction due to elastic effects and when the flow rate is increased, inertial

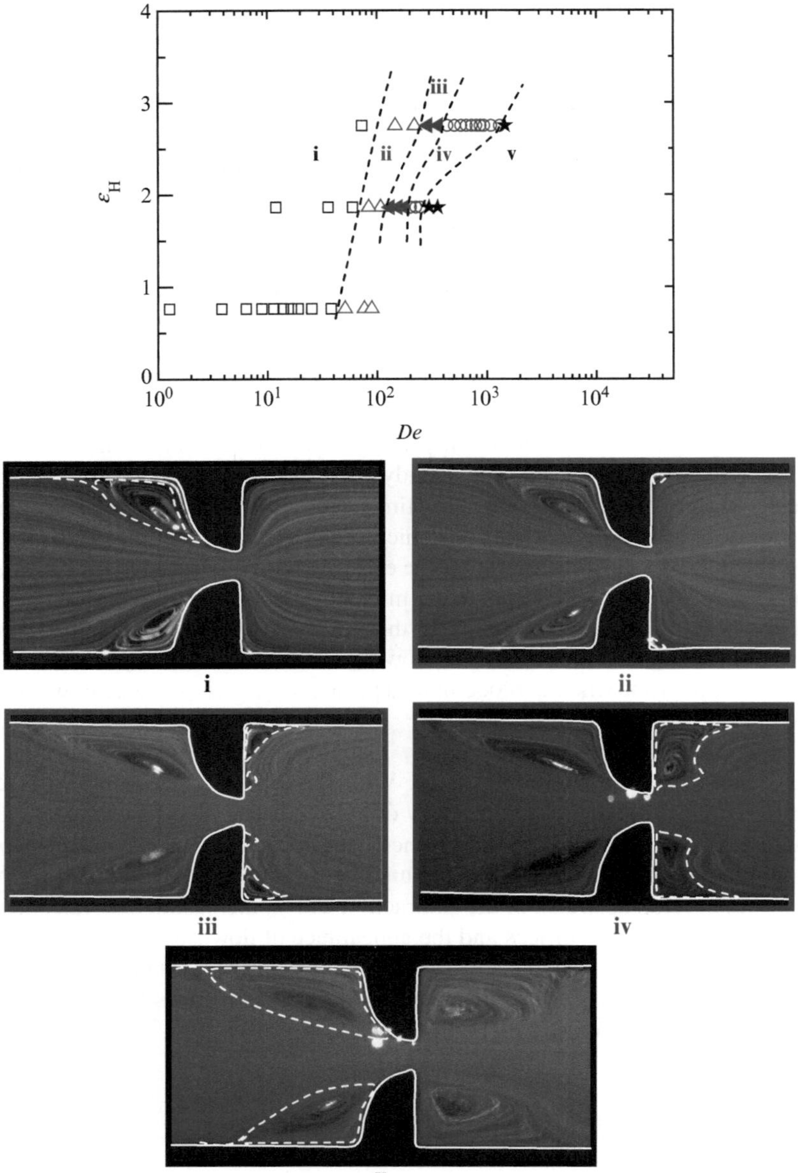

Fig. 8 Flow pattern map: (i) upstream symmetric vortices (□); (ii) downstream corner vortices (△); (iii) downstream lip and corner vortices (◀); (iv) merging of downstream lip and corner vortices (◯); (v) unstable (asymmetric) flow (★)

effects lead to a decrease of the upstream vortices and the appearance and growth of downstream vortices. In addition, elasticity decreases the downstream vortices. These distinct behaviors clearly show that consideration of blood as a Newtonian fluid is a severe over-simplification that can prevent a correct prediction of blood flow behavior, especially in small sized vessels.

Acknowledgements The authors gratefully acknowledge funding by FCT via projects PTDC/EQU-FTT/71800/2006, REEQ/262/EME/2005, REEQ/928/EME/2005, PTDC/EME-MFE/099109/2008 and PTDC/EQU-FTT/70727/2006. In addition, PCS and ISP acknowledge the financial support of scholarships SFRH/BD/28846/2006 and CEFT/BII/2008/01.

References

1. Bird, R.B., Armstrong, R.C., Hassager O.: Dynamics of Polymeric Liquids. Volume 1: Fluid Dynamics Wiley, New York (1987)
2. Caro, C.G., Pedley, T.G., Seed, W.A.: Mechanics of the Circulation. Medical and Technical Publishers, London (1974)
3. Cherdron, W., Durst, F., Whitelaw, J.H.: Asymmetric flows and instabilities in symmetric ducts with sudden expansions. J Fluid Mech **84**, 13–31 (1978)
4. Entov, V.M., Hinch, E.J.: Effect of a spectrum of relaxation times on the capillary thinning of a filament of elastic liquid. J Non-Newt Fluid Mech **72**, 31–54 (1997)
5. Ku, D.N.: Blood flow in arteries. Annual Rev Fluid Mech **29**, 399–434 (1997)
6. McDonald, J.C., Duffy, D.C., Anderson, J.R., et al.: Fabrication of microfluidic systems in poly(dimethylsiloxane). Electrophoresis **21**, 27–40 (2000)
7. McKinley, G.H., Rodd, L.E., Oliveira, M.S.N., et al.: Extensional flows of polymeric solutions in microfluidic converging/diverging geometries. J Cent South Univ Technol **14**, 6–9 (2007)
8. Oliveira, M.S.N., Alves, M.A., Pinho, F.T., et al.: Viscous flow through microfabricated hyperbolic contractions. Exp Fluids **43**, 437–451 (2007)
9. Oliveira, M.S.N., Rodd, L.E., McKinley, G.H., et al.: Simulations of extensional flow in microrheometric devices. Microfluid Nanofluid **5**, 809–826 (2008)
10. Owens, R.J.: A new microstructure-based constitutive model for human blood. J Non-Newt Fluid Mech **140**, 57–70 (2006)
11. Phan-Thien, N., Tanner, R.I.: A new constitutive equation derived from network theory. J Non-Newt Fluid Mech **2**, 353–365 (1977)
12. Poole, R.J., Pinho, F.T., Alves, M.A., et al: The effect of expansion ratio for creeping expansion flows of UCM fluids. J Non-Newt Fluid Mech **163**, 35–44 (2009)
13. Sdougos, H.P., Bussolari, S.R., Dewey, C.F.: Secondary flow and turbulence in a cone-and-plate device. J Fluid Mech **138**, 379–404 (1984)
14. Thurston, G.B.: Viscoelastic properties of blood and blood analogs. Adv Hemodyn Hemorheol **1**, 1–30 (1996)
15. Turitto, V.T.: Blood viscosity mass transport and thrombogenesis. Prog Hemost Thrombog **6**, 139–177 (1982)
16. Vlastos, G., Lerche, D., Koch, B., et al.: The effect of parallel combined steady and oscillatory shear flows on blood and polymer solutions. Rheol Acta **36**, 160–172 (1997)
17. Waite, L., Fine, J.: Applied Biofluid Mechanics. McGraw-Hill, New York (2007)
18. Xue, S.-C., Phan-Thien, N., Tanner, R.I. Numerical study of secondary flows of viscoelastic fluid in straight pipes by an implicit finite volume method. J Non-Newt Fluid Mech **59**, 191–213 (1995)
19. Yilmaz, F., Gundogdu, M.Y.: A critical review on blood flow in large arteries; relevance to blood rheology, viscosity models, and physiologic conditions. Korea-Aust Rheol J **20**, 197–211 (2008)

Molecular Imaging of Hypoxia Using Genetic Biosensors

Pablo Iglesias and J.A. Costoya

Abstract In the last years, the need for visualization of tumoral processes has become a high-top priority in molecular imaging. This is especially true for those methods dedicated to functional imaging that focus on revealing phenomena associated with biological processes such as hypoxia to cancer. Among them, optical imaging methods such as fluorescence are provided with a broad range of proteins and dyes used to visualize many types of these biological processes widely used in cell biology studies. Although the most popular of these proteins is the green fluorescent protein (GFP), autofluorescence due to the absorption of the exciting radiation by endogenous fluorophores and signal dispersion raises doubts about its suitability as an *in vivo* tracer. In the last years a number of groups have developed several NIR fluorescent proteins that enables real-time imaging to take place without interference from autofluorescence events allowing at the same time to take a deep view into the tissues. With all of this in mind, we devised a novel fluorescence-bioluminescence genetically encoded biosensor activated by the neoangiogenesis-related transcription factor HIF-1α, which appears upregulated in growing tumors. At the same time, by fusing a NIR emitting flurochrome (mCherry) and the firefly luciferase together we obtained a bioluminescence resonance energy transfer (BRET) phenomenon turning this fusion protein into a new class of hypoxia-sensing genetically encoded biosensor.

Keywords BRET · Biosensors

P. Iglesias and J.A. Costoya (✉)
Molecular Oncology Laboratory, Departamento de Fisioloxía, Facultade de Medicina, Universidade de Santiago de Compostela, 15782 Galicia, Spain
e-mail: josea.costoya@usc.es

J.M.R.S. Tavares and R.M.N. Jorge (eds.), *Computational Vision and Medical Image Processing: Recent Trends*, Computational Methods in Applied Sciences 19,
DOI 10.1007/978-94-007-0011-6_16,

1 Introduction

1.1 Optical Methods in Molecular Imaging

Visualization of tumoral processes, either for basic research or clinical and prognosis purposes, has been recently experiencing a dramatic gain in popularity and development for obvious reasons, especially functional imaging that focuses on revealing certain activity associated to a biological process [3, 6, 31]. In the case of cancer research, the follow-up of processes such as metastasis or hypoxia, or other events intimately related to cancer biology, is clearly one of the main goals of imaging research. For this purpose, one of the most promising working alternatives to the classical diagnostic imaging techniques, such as PET (Positron Emission Tomography), MRI (Magnetic Resonance Imaging) or X-ray computed tomography (CT) to cite a just a few, is the use of optical methods that involve the emission of visible light. These optical methods, being fluorescence and bioluminescence the most prominent, unlike the former ones do not display the harming effects of ionizing radiations on living organisms or require high-budget equipments to monitor the overall process [24].

Recently, fluorescence has come to a new position of prominence in molecular biology thanks to the widespread use of the *Aequoerea victoria* green fluorescent protein (GFP) [14, 21] that as of today remains as a common reporter gene and a milestone in optical imaging. Since then, it has been developed a whole array of new fluorescent proteins with diverse excitation and emission wavelengths that comprises almost the whole visible spectrum, making this technique very adaptable for a wide range of applications [26]. In addition, these novel fluorescent proteins display interesting features such as NIR-shifted emission wavelengths that permit avoiding overlapping parasite emissions from tissue and/or organic compounds [19, 33].

In the same manner, luciferase enzymes are commonly employed as reporter genes in cell and molecular biology [10]. Bioluminescence is produced by luciferases that catalyze 'light-emitting reactions' by oxygenating a substrate molecule, luciferin in our case. This process occurs in a number of living organisms, vertebrates, invertebrates and microorganisms. Unlike fluorescence where electron excitation and subsequent photon emission is mediated by light absorption, bioluminescence chemically produces singlet state species that subsequently decay emitting photons of visible light. Sources of luciferases are insects such as the firefly *Photynus pyralis*, marine invertebrates (*Renilla reniformis*), plants (*Gaussia princeps*) and microorganisms such as several species of vibrionaceae [12]. Although fluorescent light is usually brighter, with better spatial resolution and more suitable for 3D reconstruction, bioluminescent light lacks the problem of cell and tissue auto-luminescence, which results in a better signal to noise ratio for bioluminescent assays. These novel features are advantageous for downstream applications like resonance energy transfer phenomena like FRET (Fluorescence Resonant Energy Transfer) or BRET (Bioluminescence Resonant Energy Transfer) and genetic reporter assays.

This technology is expected to be fully developed in the forthcoming years as a prognostic tool for the clinical environment and more specifically for cancer treatment. In this context, to ensure a full recovery and to minimize the risk of recurrence is required the complete removal of the tumor prior to metastasis occurrence. The presence of cancer cells in regional lymph nodes indicates metastasis and necessitates more aggressive, systemic treatment, such as chemotherapy. In many cancer surgeries, oncologists remove several lymph nodes in the region of the tumor to detect metastasis through the lymphatic system. As of today, several initiatives have been made to translate optical methods to clinical imaging as an intraoperative aid for surgeons, even though they are still in early phases of development. One of these initiatives involves intraoperative near-infrared fluorescence monitoring employing low weight molecular ligands (peptides and small molecules) able to target tumoral cells in their niches. This approach is currently being assessed as a prospective intraoperatory assistance to surgeons [29, 30] with NIR-emitting derivatives of indocyanine green (ICG), a non specific fluorescent contrast agent normally used for the detection of blood vessel abnormalities, which is currently being tested in a Phase I clinical trial (Fox Chase, USA).

1.2 Bioluminescence Resonant Energy Transfer (BRET)

Transference of resonant energy is a well-known phenomenon on which rely proteomic and biochemical procedures such as protein-protein interaction assays [20]. In the case of BRET, it is required a luminescent donor and a fluorescent acceptor. The energy transfer is strictly dependent on the closeness between donor and acceptor, being the optimal distance in the range of 1–10 nm [18]. Although the choice of the donor/acceptor pair is usually determined empirically, one of the most popular pairs is *Renilla* luciferase/GFP since they exhibit an appropriate spectral overlap of donor emission and acceptor excitation, which is one of the critical steps on the overall performance of the system. As mentioned above, other important aspect to consider is the distance between donor and acceptor, and in the particular case of fusion proteins between both proteins, the freedom of movement necessary to allow a suitable spatial orientation for BRET to occur. This orientation and freedom of movement can be empirically tuned by inserting linkers in-between both proteins [22].

1.3 Hypoxia as a Tumoral Aggresivity Marker in Cancer

One of the most recognizable features of a tumoral cell is the disproportionate growth that is intimately related to tumor aggressiveness and invasiveness. As a consequence of this growth, the number of blood vessels supporting the tumor rises exponentially to fulfill the exacerbated need of nutrients and oxygen. Therefore, and attending to histopathological analyses it is not uncommon to find necrotic regions inside the tumoral core, which is densely populated, in highly proliferative tumoral

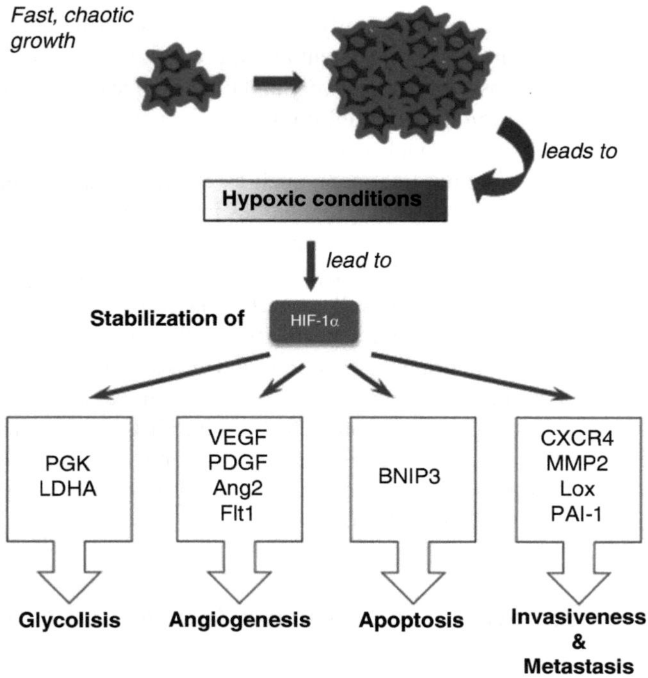

Fig. 1 Different outcomes of the biological functions of the transcription factor HIF-1α. This transcription factor is involved in processes such as glycolisis, cell growth and death, and angiogenesis

phenotypes. In order to alleviate this deficiency, tumoral cells elicit the formation of neovessels by stimulating neoangiogenesis. This angiogenic process is tightly regulated and results in the participation of several transcription factors, being HIF-1α one of the most important. This factor, which appears stabilized in tumors with a high demand of nutrients and oxygen [17], and as Fig. 1 shows, exerts its transcriptional activity on several target genes that intervene in crucial processes for the tumoral phenotype such as glycolysis, apoptosis and metastasis [5], making it a good marker of tumoral aggressiveness and invasion capacity in several types of tumors [7–9, 32].

2 Materials and Methods

2.1 Plasmid Construction

The E-M-H-Luc plasmid (a gift from W. H. Suh) that combines the E-M-H enhancer plus the firefly luciferase was constructed as previously described [16]. The coding sequence for mCherry (a gift from R. Y. Tsien; GenBank accession number

AY678264.1) was amplified by PCR and subsequently cloned into the *Hind*III site of the E-M-H-Luc vector; the *Hind*III site was maintained by inserting compatible overhangs in both primers.

2.2 Cell Culture

Human embryonic kidney HEK 293 cells were cultured in Dulbecco's modified Eagle medium (DMEM) (Sigma) supplemented with 10% of fetal bovine serum (Fischer) and 1% L-glutamine. Cell cultures were maintained at 37 °C and 5% CO_2.

2.3 Transfections

DNA transfections were carried out according to the calcium phosphate transfection method [11]. For the in vitro assay, cells were seeded in 24-well plates at a cellular density of $3.75 \cdot 10^5$ cells/well. Each group was transfected with 0.9 μg of E-M-H-mCherry-Luc and different pcDNA3/pcDNA3-HIF-1α ratios up to 0.15 μg, ranging from 0.01 (lowest concentration) to 0.32 μg of pcDNA3-HIF-1α (highest concentration). For the luciferase assay, cells were seeded in 12-well plates at a cellular density of $7.5 \cdot 10^5$ cells/well. Each group was transfected with 1.8 μg of E-M-H-mCherry-Luc and different pcDNA3/pcDNA3-HIF-1α ratios up to 0.3 μg, ranging from 0.02 to 0.64 μg of pcDNA3-HIF-1α. In addition, 2 μg of CMV-EGFP-Luc were transfected in the control group and 0.4 μg of pCMVβ (carrying the β-galactosidase gene) in all groups as a transfection control. As for the in vivo assay, cells were seeded in 10 cm plates for transfection assays at a cellular density of $3 \cdot 10^6$ cells/plate. Cells were transfected with 7.5 μg of E-M-H-mCherry-Luc along with 0.5 μg of pcDNA3-HIF-1α for the cell population with the 'activated system' described above.

2.4 Luciferase Assay

Cell cultures were lysed 48 h upon transfection with 100 μL of 1X Passive Lysis Buffer (Promega, Spain) for 20 min at room temperature. 50 μL of each cell lysate were mixed with 35 μL of Luciferase Activity Buffer (25 mM Glycilglycine pH 7.8, 15 mM phosphate buffer pH 7.8, 15 mM $MgSO_4$, 4 mM EGTA, 2 mM ATP, 1 mM DTT) and 25 μL of 1 mM solution of the substrate D-luciferin (L9504, Sigma-Aldrich Quimica, Spain). Luciferase activity was measured with a luminometer Lumat LB 9507 (Berthold Technologies). All of these data were normalized with an additional β-galactosidase assay. To this purpose, 50 μL of each cell lysate were mixed with 250 μL of Z buffer (0.06M Na2HPO$_4$ 7H2O, 0.04M NaH_2PO_4 H_2, 0.01M KCl, 0.001M $MgSO_4$, 0.05M 2-mercaptoethanol) and 60 μL of a 4 mg mL^{-1}

solution of *o*-nitrophenyl-ß-D-galactopyranoside (ONPG). Samples were incubated at 37 °C for 1 h and then β-galactosidase activities were measured with a spectrophotometer BioMate 3 (Thermo Spectronic, USA) at 420 nm. Each assay was replicated at least three times for every experimental group.

2.5 Spectrophotometric Profile of the Fusion Protein

λ_{exc} and λ_{em} of mCherry-luciferase were determined in a FluoroMax-3 (ISA Jobin Yvon-Spex, Edison, USA). Measures were obtained from cell lysates from HEK 293 cells transfected as described above.

2.6 Confocal Microscopy

Cells were fixated 48 h upon transfection by incubation in 3.5% paraformaldehyde for 10 min at r.t. and subsequently 5 min at 4 °C. Samples were mounted in Ultra-Cruz Mounting Medium (Santa Cruz, sc-29491). Images were obtained in a Spectral Confocal Microscope Leica TCS-SP2 (Leica, Mannheim, Germany) with a spectral range of detection from 400 to 850 nm.

2.7 Fluorescence–Bioluminescence In Vivo Assays and Animal Care

Upon sedation with isoflurane using the XGI-8 Gas Anesthesia Unit (Caliper Life Sciences, USA) fluorescence and bioluminescence data were registered with an IVIS Spectrum (Caliper Life Sciences, USA) in 30 or 60 s expositions during 30 min. For bioluminescence and BRET assays SCID mice (Charles River Laboratories, USA) were injected intraperitoneally with a single dose of D-Luciferin (L9504, Sigma-Aldrich Quimica, Spain) dissolved in sterile PBS. Mice were housed in specific pathogen-free (SPF) conditions, following FELASA (Federation of European Laboratory Animal Science Associations) guidelines for animal housing and according to the USC Bioethic Board regulation, passed on September 23, 2003.

3 Results

3.1 Outline of the Hypoxia Genetically Encoded Biosensor

Although the development of an inducible genetic biosensor is not a novelty in the field [13,23,28], we describe the design, construction and characterization of a novel hypoxia genetic biosensor that comprises a dual fluorescence-bioluminescence

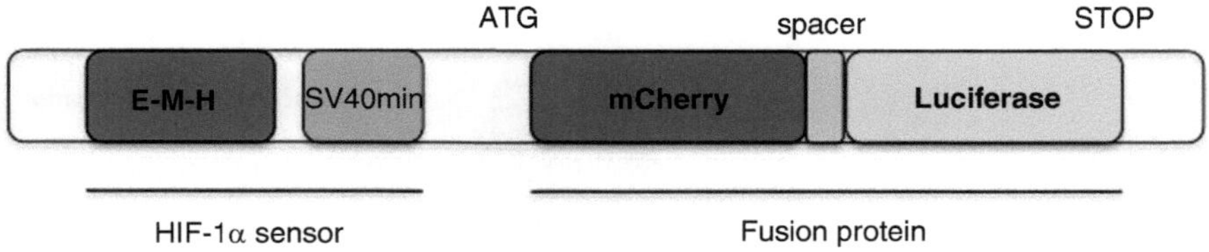

Fig. 2 The scheme shows the design of the genetically encoded biosensor: a regulatory module formed by the E-M-H enhancer and the SV40 minimal promoter, and the tracer module comprised by the fusion protein formed by the mCherry fluorophore and the firefly luciferase

tracer capable of BRET-mediated fluorochrome excitation, overcoming the need for an external excitation source. All of these data has been recently published [15].

Our biosensor comprises two moieties that play different roles as shows Fig. 2. The first of them acts as a transcriptional regulator formed by an enhancer able to bind the alpha subunit of the HIF-1 transcription factor, and the second one is dual tracer formed by a fusion protein of a NIR fluorophore and the firefly luciferase. Several fluorescent proteins were considered on the basis of their excitation and emission wavelengths. Although initially mPlum were tested as prospective fluorochromes, it was eventually discarded due to its low brightness (data not shown; [25]). On the other hand, mCherry presents an excitation wavelength of 585 nm, which makes this fluorochrome an ideal acceptor of bioluminescent light (575 nm), as well as its near NIR-emission avoids autofluorescence phenomena occurring in living tissue.

As for the regulatory moiety of the construct, we chose a chimeric enhancer as HIF-1alpha sensor over the canonical hypoxia response element (HRE). This chimeric enhancer comprises the (Egr-1)-binding site (EBS) from the Egr-1 gene, the metal-response element (MRE) from the metallothionein gene, and the hypoxia-response element (HRE) from the phosphoglycerate kinase 1 gene. This enhancer has been described to trigger a transcriptional response to a greater extent and increases hypoxia responsiveness than to that of the hypoxia-response element (HRE) alone [16]. A SV40 minimal promoter is located downstream of the chimeric enhacer E-M-H.

3.2 *Spectrophotometric Characterization of the Fusion Protein*

We next wanted to assess the fluorescent and bioluminescent activity of the fusion protein. The integrity of the aminoacidic environment of the fluorescent proteins is crucial in order to maintain its activity [1, 4, 27]. Accordingly, we registered the spectrophotometric profiles of mCherry and the firefly luciferase. Figure 3 shows that mCherry retains the same wavelengths of excitation and emission that the ones reported before [26], indicating that fusing the luciferase and mCherry together did not affect the performance of the fluorescent protein *in vitro* and both emission (and excitation, in mCherry) peaks remained unaltered.

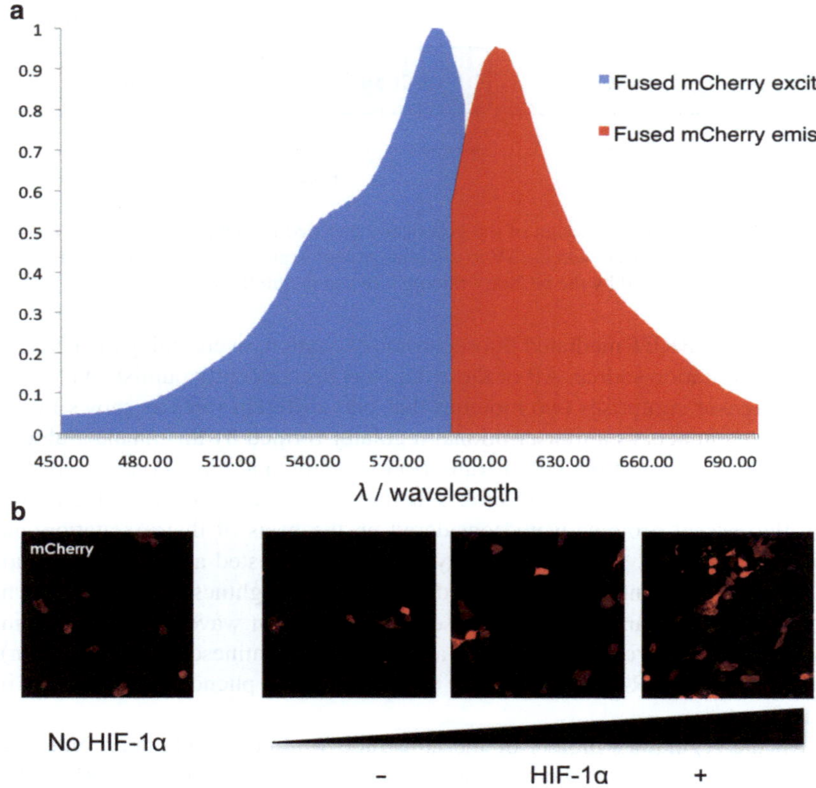

Fig. 3 (**a**) Spectrophotometric profile of mCherry in the fusion protein. Solid line represents mCherry excitation while dashed line represents mCherry emission; (**b**) fluorescence images of the mCherry protein

3.3 In Vitro Inducible Response of the Biosensor to HIF-1α

Upon determining that the fusion protein retained its optical properties, we wanted to corroborate these data by testing the functionality of the cloned fluorescent protein. As Fig. 3 shows, we transfected our construction along with increasing amounts of the HIF-1α transcription factor into the HEK 293 cell line. As expected, our data indicate that the system is proportionally responsive to the amount of transcription factor transfected in each case. Curiously, although the basal induction (i.e. induction by endogenous levels of HIF-1α) proved to be higher than the lowest amount of HIF-1α, the luciferase assay indicates that the response elicited in both cases is similar, thus hinting that the threshold of detection corresponds to the amount of HIF-1α transfected in this case.

Similarly, the luciferase activity of the genetically encoded biosensor, shown in Fig. 4, appears to be increasingly higher as the concentration of the transcription factor rises. The empty vector that lacks the fluorescent protein, included as a

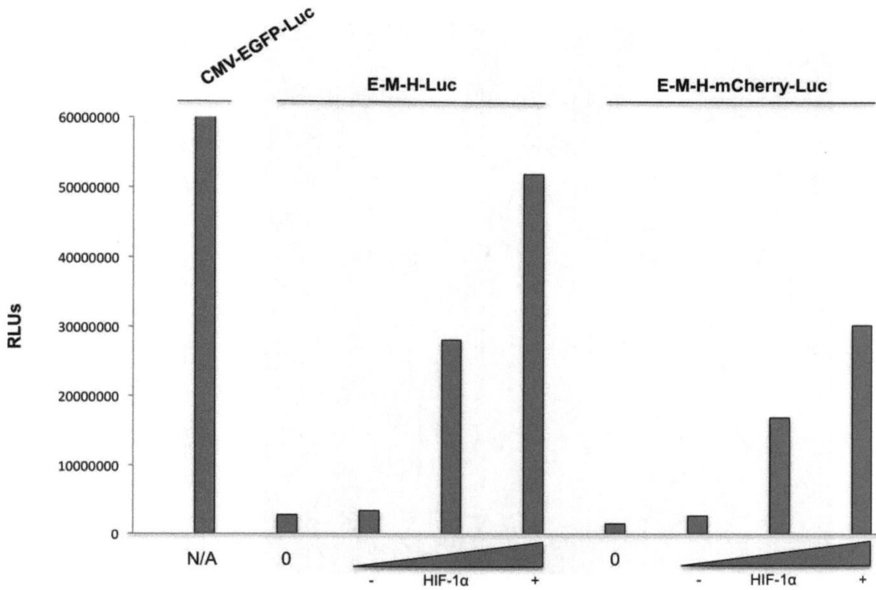

Fig. 4 Luciferase activity of the fusion protein for E-M-H-Luciferase and E-M-H-mCherry-Luciferase

control, shows a similar proportional response but with a significantly higher maximum value than to that of the biosensor. As means of transfection normalization and to rule out discrepancies on transfection efficiency in the different experimental groups, these data were normalized against the β-galactosidase activity of each group, as described in the Sect. 2.

As a whole, these data show that the transcription factor HIF-1α binds efficiently to the response elements located in the chimeric enhancer of the biosensor and elicits the transcription of the fusion protein mCherry-luciferase. Also, the fusion protein retains the fluorescent properties and the luciferase activity although its bioluminescent intensity in this case seems to be lower than to that of the vector containing only the response element and the luciferase (E-M-H-Luc). This difference will be further investigated to determine whether it is caused by a phenomenon of transference of resonant energy between the luciferase and the fluorescent protein, or by a non-expected hindrance of the luciferase catalytic site, originated by the nearby mCherry, that has as a consequence a lower ability to catalyze the bioluminescent reaction.

3.4 In Vivo Inducible Response of the Biosensor to HIF-1α

Subsequently, we investigated whether or not the in vitro performance of the system could be replicated and registered also in an in vivo environment. To test

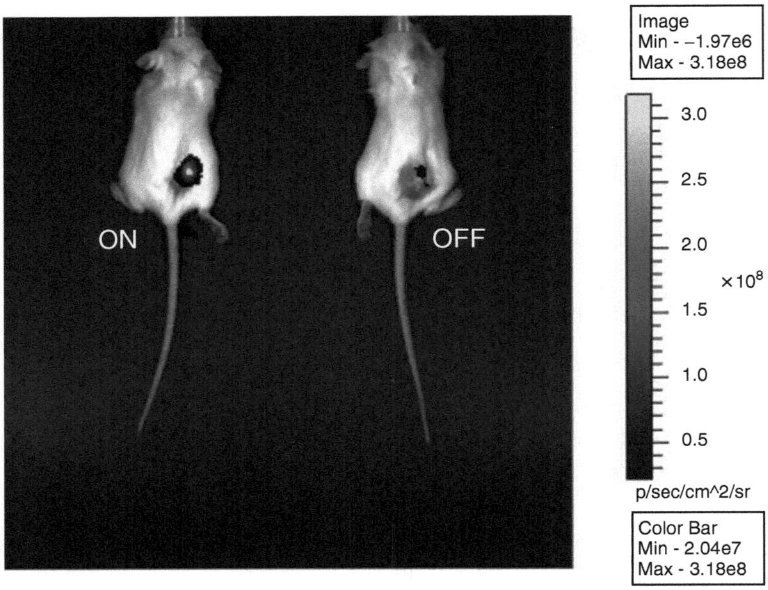

Fig. 5 In vivo fluorescence measure in a xenograft implanted subcutaneously in SCID mice: mCherry fluorescence in the 'activated system' (ON) in HEK 293 cells transfected with E-M-H-mCherry-Luciferase and pcDNA3-HIF-1α and 'non-activated' system (OFF) in cells transfected with E-M-H-mCherry-Luciferase and pcDNA3

this hypothesis, we co-transfected HEK 293 cells with our biosensor and either pcDNA3-HIF-1α, or pcDNA3 alone as a transfection control. Thus, we obtained two groups of cells that contained either the activated system (biosensor + HIF-1α) or just the biosensor (or 'basal state' cells). Both groups were injected subcutaneously in the hindquarters of immunodeficient SCID mice as Figs. 5 and 6 indicate. Figure 5 shows the fluorescent signal measured in vivo 24 h upon injection of both cell populations. With all of this in mind, we corroborated that the system remains active in HEK 293 cells transfected with our biosensor upon subcutaneous injection, and that its intensity is directly correlated to the quantity of the transcription factor HIF-1α present in those cells, as shown by the signal differences between the 'activated' and the 'non-activated' cells.

Likewise, luciferase activity was also registered in vivo (Fig. 6). Upon administration of luciferin, we observed a similar situation as with fluorescence where both cell populations displayed bioluminescent signals but again a higher intensity in the case of cells with the activated system. Taken together, these data demonstrate that our hypoxia biosensor is able to proportionally induce the transcription of the mCherry-luciferase tracer when the concentration of HIF-1α is high enough to bind the response elements upstream the fusion protein coding sequence. Moreover, a similar response was observed both in vitro, in HEK 293 cells transfected with increasing concentrations of HIF-1α, and in vivo xenografts of these transfected cells, as shown in Figs. 5 and 6.

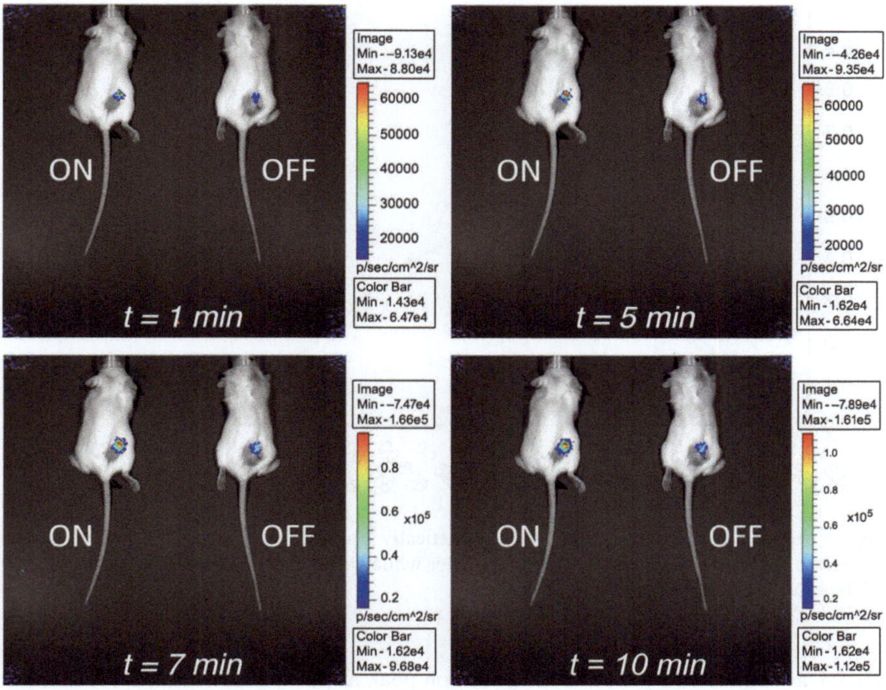

Fig. 6 In vivo luciferase activity in SCID mice, 'ON' denotes the 'activated system', cells transfected with both E-M-H-mCherry-Luciferase and pcDNA3-HIF-1α, and 'OFF' the 'non-activated' system

3.5 In Vivo Bloluminiscence Resonance Energy Transfer Assessment

As discussed above, it was observed a fall in the luciferase activity of the system when compared to the vector that only contains the response element and the luciferase, E-M-H-Luc (Fig. 4). We wanted to prove whether this difference can be attributed to a BRET-mediated mCherry excitation in the absence of an external source, or as we mentioned before it is the result of a hindered and defective luciferase moiety. Consequently, we first tested whether or not this transference was taking place in vitro by comparing the spectrophotometric profiles of the luciferase of the parental vector (E-M-H-Luc) with whole system (E-M-H-mCherry-Luc). As Fig. 7 shows, the luciferase alone displays a maximum value at the expected wavelength of 575 nm. However, although the fusion protein displays a peak at this wavelength, it also displays a lower second peak at a wavelength corresponding with the mCherry emission peak. In addition, the decrease of the bioluminescent activity was also observed in this case and that would be consistent with the existence of

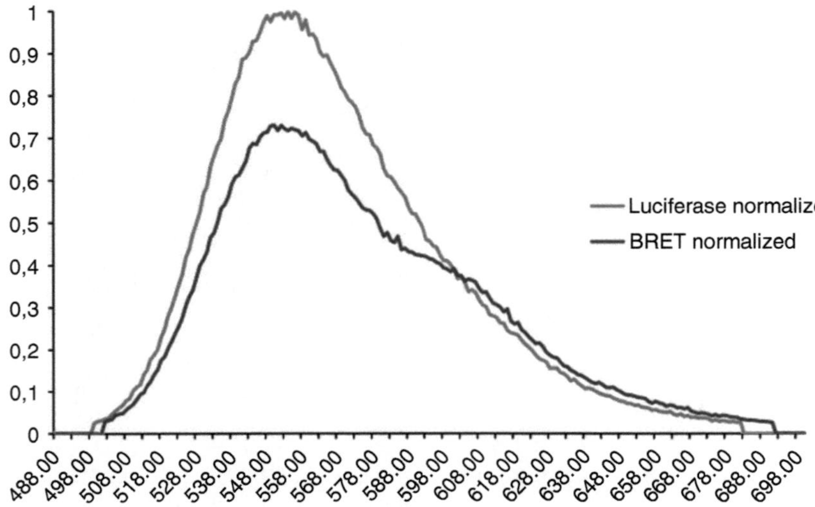

Fig. 7 In vitro BRET performance of the genetically encoded biosensor. Solid line represents luciferase activity of the E-M-H-Luciferase vector while dashed line represents luciferase activity of the E-M-H-mCherry-Luciferase vector

BRET as suggested by the second emission peak as part of the bioluminescent light would be absorbed by the fluorochrome rather than registered by the spectrofluorometer detector.

Finally, we investigated whether this BRET transference could be also detected in vivo. For that purpose, we tried to register the emission of the activated system upon intraperitoneal administration of luciferin and blocking the excitation filter in order to avoid the interference of any external excitation source. Since this process critically depends on the light emitted by the reaction catalyzed by the luciferase, we registered the fluorescence emission upon the injection of the luciferase substrate for a long period of time. Figure 8 shows the most representative points of the series including the peak emission of BRET in SCID mice, reached at 30 min upon luciferin injection.

4 Discussion and Conclusions

In conclusion we have described the designing and development of a hypoxia-sensing system with both NIR fluorescent and bioluminescent properties. This genetically encoded biosensor is induced by the hypoxia transcription factor HIF-1α, which appears up-regulated in tumors with a high demand of nutrients and oxygen. We have demonstrated that when our biosensor is present, this factor binds to the response element located in the regulatory module of the construction

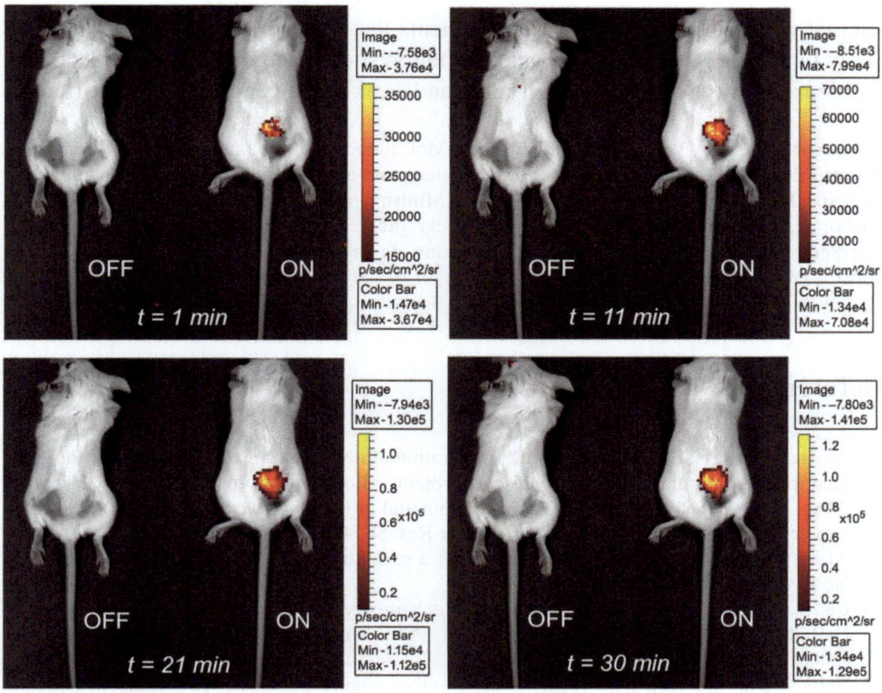

Fig. 8 In vivo BRET performance of the system

inducing the transcription of the fusion protein, and displays a proportional response to the quantity of HIF-1α within the cells that contain the biosensor. The HIF-1α specificity also poses another advantage when compared to other constructs harboring entire promoter regions of target genes regulated by this transcription factor such as VEGF, whose outcomes affect multiple processes [2].

The fluorescent protein mCherry, developed from the red fluorescent protein (RFP) by Roger Tsien and collaborators [25], is one of the latest additions to the fluorescent protein spectrum being its intensity, stability and near infrared emission peak some of its most remarkable characteristics. Its NIR emission enables deeper tissue penetrability, allowing at the same time a low invasiveness-real time visualization of the monitored process. In our biosensor, we have described the HIF-1α induced transcription of the dual tracer and characterized its fluorescent and bioluminescent properties both in vitro and in vivo. At the same time, we have observed a BRET phenomenon occurring between the firefly luciferase (donor) and the mCherry protein (acceptor). Thus, the firefly luciferase acts both as a light emitting source and excitation source for the fluorescence, since it does rely on an external source of excitation as the fluorescence but a chemical reaction.

Although the development of an inducible biosensor is not a novelty in the field [13, 23, 28] the combination of NIR fluorescence and bioluminescence is and alternative approach for future developments that take advantage of BRET, especially in scenarios where an internal excitation source helps to overcome technical problems such as tissue autofluorescence and weak tissue penetration of wavelength.

Acknowledgements We thank the members of Molecular Oncology Lab for helpful discussions. We also thank M.E. Vazquez for helpful discussions and assistance with the spectrophotometric analysis. This study was supported by Spanish Ministry of Science and Innovation, (SAF2005-00306; SAF2008-00543) and Xunta de Galicia grants (PGIDIT05PXIB20801PR); Grupos emerxentes 2007/064) (J.A.C.), and by Fundacion de Investigacion Medica Mutua Madrileña (J.A.C., P.I.).

References

1. Ai, H., Shaner, N.C., Cheng, Z., et al.: Exploration of new chromophore structures leads to the identification of improved blue fluorescent proteins. Biochemistry **46**, 5904–5910 (2007)
2. Akagi, Y., et al.: Regulation of vascular endothelial growth factor expression in human colon cancer by insulin-like growth factor-I. Cancer Res. **58**, 4008–4014 (1998)
3. Alavi, A., Lakhani, P., Mavi, A., et al.: PET: a revolution in medical Imaging. Radiol. Clin. North Am. **42**, 983–1001 (2004)
4. Baird, G.S., Zacharias, D.A., Tsien, R.Y.: Biochemistry, mutagenesis, and oligomerization of DsRed, a red fluorescent protein from coral. Proc. Natl. Acad. Sci. USA **97**, 11984–11989 (2000)
5. Bárdos, J.I., Ashcroft, M.: Negative and positive regulation of HIF-1: a complex network. BioEssays **26**, 262–269 (2004)
6. Dunn, A.K., Bolay, T., Moskowitz, M.A., Boas, D.A.: Dynamic imaging of cerebral blood flow using laser speckle. J. Cereb. Blood Flow Metab. **2**, 195–201 (2001)
7. Evans, S.M., Judy, K.D., Dunphy, I., et al.: Hypoxia is important in the biology and aggression of human glial brain tumors. Clin. Cancer Res. **10**, 8177–8184 (2004)
8. Furlan, D., Sahnane, N., Carnevali, I., et al.: Regulation and stabilization of HIF-1alpha in colorectal carcinomas. Surg. Oncol. **16**, S25–S27 (2007)
9. Gordan, J.D., Simon, M.C.: Hypoxia-inducible factors: central regulators of the tumor phenotype. Curr. Opin. Genet. Dev. **17**, 71–77 (2007)
10. Gould, S.J., Subramani, S.: Firefly luciferase as a tool in molecular and cell biology. Anal. Biochem. **175**, 5–13 (1988)
11. Graham, F.L., van der Eb, E.J.: A new technique for the assay of infectivity of human adenovirus 5 DNA. J. Virol. **52**, 456–467 (1973)
12. Hastings, J.W.: Biological diversity, chemical mechanisms, and the evolutionary origins of bioluminescent systems. J. Mol. Evol. **19**, 309–321 (1983)
13. Hoffman, R.M.: Imaging tumor angiogenesis with fluorescent proteins. APMIS **112**, 441–449 (2004)
14. Hoffman, R.M.: Recent advances on in vivo imaging with fluorescent proteins. Nat. Rev. Cancer **5**, 796–806 (2005)
15. Iglesias, P., Costoya, J.A.: A novel BRET-based genetically encoded biosensor for functional imaging of hypoxia. Biosens. Bioelec. 10:3126–30 (2009)
16. Lee, J.Y., Lee, Y.S., Kim, K.L., et al.: A novel chimeric promoter that is highly responsive to hypoxia and metals. Gene Therapy **13**, 857–868 (2006)
17. Maxwell, P.H., Wiesener, M.S., Chang, G.W., et al.: The tumour suppressor protein VHL targets hypoxia-inducible factors for oxygen-dependent proteolysis. Nature **399**, 271–275 (1999)
18. Michelini, E., Mirasoli, M., Karp, M., et al.: Development of a bioluminescence resonance energy-transfer assay for estrogen-like compound in vivo monitoring. Anal. Chem. **76**, 7069–7076 (2004)

19. Ntziachristos, V., Bremer, C., Weissleder, R.: Fluorescence imaging with near-infrared light: new technological advances that enable in vivo molecular imaging. Eur. Radiol. **13**, 195–208 (2003)
20. Pfleger, K.D.G., Eidne, K.: Illuminating insights into protein-protein interactions using bioluminescence resonance energy transfer (BRET). Nat. Methods **3**, 165–173 (2006)
21. Prasher, D.C., Eckenrodeb, V.K., Wardc, W.W., et al.: Primary structure of the Aequorea victoria green-fluorescent protein. Gene **111**, 229–233 (1992)
22. Prinz, A., Diskar, M., Herberg, F.W.: Application of bioluminescence resonance energy transfer (BRET) for biomolecular interaction studies. Chembiochemistry **7**, 1007–1012 (2006)
23. Safran, M., Kim, W.Y., O'Connell, F., et al.: Mouse model for noninvasive imaging of HIF prolyl hydroxylase activity: assessment of an oral agent that stimulates erythropoietin production. Proc. Natl. Acad. Sci. USA **103**, 105–110 (2006)
24. Sampath, L., Wang, W., Sevick-Muraca, E.M.: Near infrared fluorescent optical imaging for nodal staging. J. Biomed. Opt. **13**, 041312 (2008)
25. Shaner, N.C., Campbell, R.E., Steinbach, P.A., et al.: Improved monomeric red, orange and yellow fluorescent proteins derived from Discosoma sp. red fluorescent protein. Nat. Biotechnol. **22**, 1567–1572 (2004)
26. Shaner, N.C., Steinbach, P.A., Tsien, R.Y.: A guide to choosing fluorescent proteins. Nature **2**, 905–909 (2005)
27. Shu, X., Shaner, N.C., Yarbrough, C.A., et al.: Novel chromophores and buried charges control color in mFruits. Biochemistry **45**, 9639–9647 (2006)
28. So, M.K., Xu, C., Loening, A.M.: Self-illuminating quantum dot conjugates for in vivo imaging. Nat. Biotechnol. **24**, 339–343 (2006)
29. Soltesz, E.G., Kim, S., Kim, S.W., et al.: Sentinel lymph node mapping of the gastrointestinal tract by using invisible light. Ann. Surg. Oncol. **13**, 386–96 (2006)
30. Tanaka, E., Choi, H.S., Fujii, H., et al.: Image-guided oncologic surgery using invisible light: Completed pre-clinical development for sentinel lymph node mapping. Ann. Surg. Oncol. **13**, 1671–81 (2006)
31. Torigian, D.A., Huang, S.S., Houseini, M.: Functional imaging of cancer with emphasis on molecular techniques. CA Cancer J. Clin. **57**, 206–224 (2007)
32. Victor, N., Ivy, A., Jiang, B.H., Agani, F.H.: Involvement of HIF-1 in invasion of Mum2B uveal melanoma cells. Clin. Exp. Metastasis **23**, 87–96 (2006)
33. Weissleder, R., Ntziachristos, V.: Shedding light onto live molecular targets. Nat. Medicine **9**, 123–128 (2003)

Microscale Flow Dynamics of Red Blood Cells in Microchannels: An Experimental and Numerical Analysis

R. Lima, C.S. Fernandes, R. Dias, T. Ishikawa, Y. Imai, and T. Yamaguchi

Abstract The blood flow dynamics in microcirculation depends strongly on the microvascular networks composed with short irregular vessel segments which are linked by numerous bifurcations. This paper presents the application of a confocal micro-PTV system to track RBCs through a rectangular polydimethysiloxane (PDMS) microchannel with a bifurcation. By using a confocal micro-PTV system, we have measured the effect of bifurcation on the flow behaviour of both fluorescent particles diluted in pure water and RBCs in concentrated suspensions. After performing simulations with the commercial finite element software package POLYFLOW®, some experimental results were compared with the numerical results and the limitations of these simulations were outlined.

Keywords Blood flow · Microvascular networks · Bifurcation · Microchannel

---

R. Lima (✉) and R. Dias
ESTiG, IPB, C. Sta. Apolonia, 5301-857 Braganca, Portugal
e-mail: ruimec@ipb.pt; ricardod@ipb.pt
and
CEFT, FEUP, R. Dr. Roberto Frias, 4200-465 Porto, Portugal

C.S. Fernandes
ESTiG, IPB, C. Sta. Apolonia, 5301-857 Braganca, Portugal
e-mail: cveiga@ipb.pt

T. Ishikawa and Y. Imai
Department of Bioengineering & Robotics, Graduate School of Engineering, Tohoku University, 6-6-01 Aoba, 980-8579 Sendai, Japan
e-mail: ishikawa@pfsl.mech.tohoku.ac.jp; yimai@pfsl.mech.tohoku.ac.jp

T. Yamaguchi
Department of Biomedical Engineering, Graduate School of Engineering, Tohoku University, 6-6-01 Aoba, 980-8579 Sendai, Japan
e-mail: takami@pfsl.mech.tohoku.ac.jp

J.M.R.S. Tavares and R.M.N. Jorge (eds.), *Computational Vision and Medical Image Processing: Recent Trends*, Computational Methods in Applied Sciences 19,
DOI 10.1007/978-94-007-0011-6_17,

1 Introduction

The phenomena of blood flow in microvessels (diameters less than 300 μm) are crucial in maintaining healthy organs and tissues. Although these phenomena have been studied for many years it still remains incompletely understood [25]. It is therefore important to investigate the behaviour of blood flow occurring at microvessels in order to better understand the role of blood cells in the process of delivering oxygen and materials to the organs and tissues.

The complexity to control and obtain reliable measurements of the blood flow behaviour through the in vivo microvascular system has led several researchers to perform their studies by using narrow glass tubes with simple geometries. By using in vitro models it allows a more precise control over the experimental variables of interest and extracts detailed information of the flow behaviour of individual blood cells. In fact, much of the understanding of the haemodynamics phenomena observed in microcirculation was obtained from studies on the both macro and microrheology properties of blood flowing through glass microtubes [3, 11, 13, 16, 17, 25].

Although glass microchannels present certain similarities to in vivo microcirculation, it is also clear that these kind of in vitro experiments differ from microvessels in several respects, such as: elasticity of microvessels, effect of the endothelial surface layer and microvascular networks composed with short irregular vessel segments which are linked by numerous bifurcations. Thus it was not surprising that several studies on blood flow in glass microtubes and in microvessels have yielded conflicting results with respect to blood viscosity [20] and flow resistance [27]. Hence, the rheological properties of blood should not be only interpreted from measurements in viscometers and microtubes with simple geometries.

In vivo microvascular networks are composed of many divergent microvascular bifurcations which likely influence the blood flow behaviour in the microcirculation. In the present work, a confocal micro-PTV system is used to measure the blood flow through a symmetric PDMS bifurcation fabricated by soft lithography. Moreover, the experimental data were compared numerically by using the commercial finite element software package POLYFLOW®. By using this combination we expect to gain understanding about several important parameters that affect the blood flow through a diverging microvessel bifurcation.

2 Materials and Methods

2.1 Fabrication of the Microchannels

The microchannels will be manufactured in polydimethylsiloxane (PDMS) due to their advantageous properties, including good optical transparency and biocompatibility, easily reversible sealing to glass, elasticity, replication of fine and complex

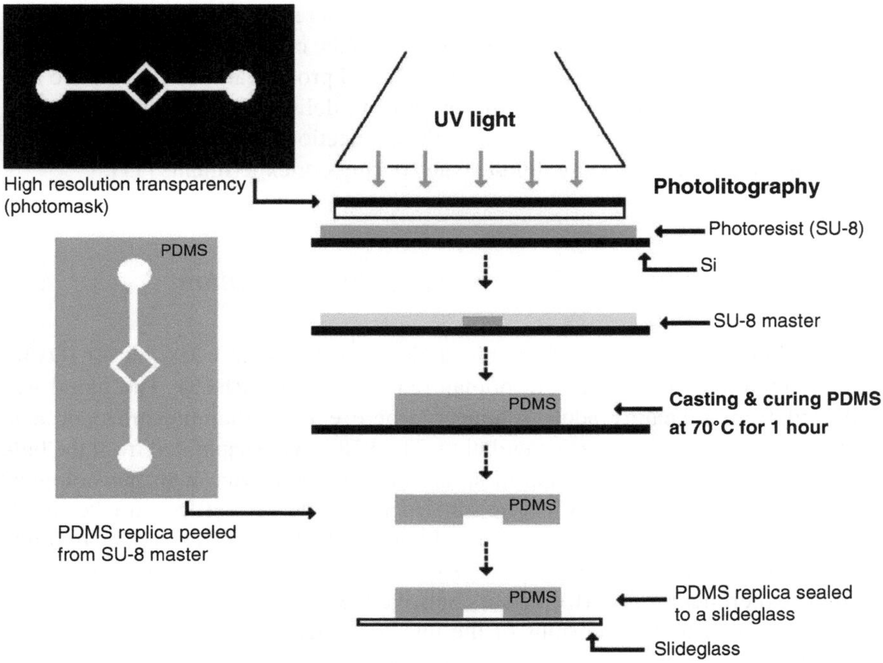

Fig. 1 Main steps of the soft lithographic technique to manufacture a microchannel with a symmetrical bifurcation geometry

geometries, and high gas permeability which is suitable for culturing cells inside the microchannels [17]. The procedure to manufacture the PDMS microchannel with a symmetric bifurcation is illustrated in Fig. 1. Briefly, the microchannel geometry was designed using a CAD system, and a high resolution (25,400 dpi) photomask was printed on plastic (polyester) transparencies at CAD/Art Services, Inc. (Bandon, USA). By applying a photolithographic technique (see Fig. 1), a solid master was fabricated on a silicon (Si) wafer with an ultrathick photoresist (SU-8). In this process, by using a spin-coating technique, a thin layer of SU-8 photoresist was coated on Si wafer and then patterned by UV exposure through the photomask. Using a SU-8 developer, it was possible to obtain the desired mold master. Then, metal wire posts were placed on the SU-8 mold master to create the connection channels to the input/output ports. The PDMS was made by mixing a base and curing agent (Silpot 184; Dow Corning, USA) at a weight ratio of 10:1. After removing the bubbles created during mixing, the PDMS was poured over the mold master and baked on a hot plate for about 1 h at 70 °C. Both master and PDMS were then cooled to room temperature and the PDMS design and embedded metal wire posts were removed from the SU-8 master and PDMS, respectively. Finally, the three-dimensional PDMS microchannel structure was cleaned with ethanol and brought into contact with a clean slide glass, where a reversible seal was formed spontaneously. The input/output ports were made by means of a 200 μl micro-pipette tip. This tip was inserted tightly into the connection channels where it exerts pressure on the PDMS and provides a liquid proof seal. Top tubes were also fitted tightly into the micro-pipette tip in order to deliver the working fluids from the syringe pump. Due to the elasticity of the connection tubes and conical shape of the tip, we did not observe any fluid leakage during our experiments [17].

2.2 *Working Fluids and Geometry of the Bifurcation*

Two working fluids were used in this study: pure water and dextran 40 (Dx40) containing about 14% (14Hct) of human red blood cells (RBCs). The blood was collected from a healthy adult volunteer, where ethylenediaminetetraacetic acid (EDTA) was added to prevent coagulation. The RBCs were separated from the bulk blood by centrifugation and aspiration and then washed twice with physiological saline (PS). The washed RBCs were labeled with a fluorescent cell tracker (CM-Dil, C-7000, Molecular Probes) and then diluted with Dx40 to make up the required RBCs concentration by volume. All blood samples were stored hermetical at 4 °C until the experiment was performed at controlled temperature of about 37 °C [13].

The geometry and dimensions of the microchannel bifurcation is illustrated in Fig. 2. In the present study we decided to use the following dimensions: 150 μm wide for parent vessel (W_0); 75 μm wide for daughter vessel ($W_1 = W_2 = 1/2W_0$) and 50 μm deep.

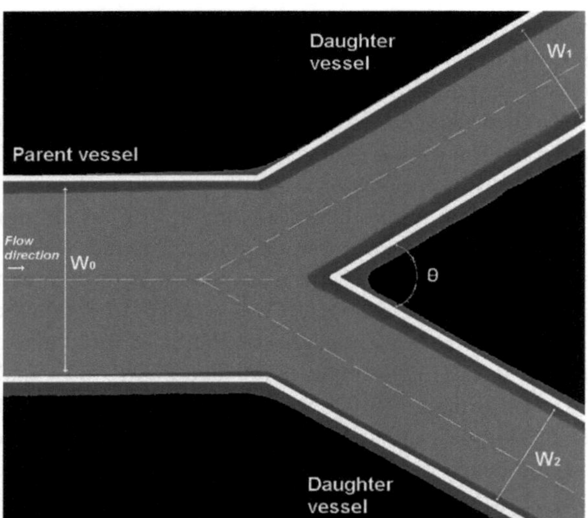

Fig. 2 Symmetrical bifurcation geometry used in this study: $W_0 = 150\,\mu m$, $W_1 = W_2 = 75\,\mu m$, $\theta = 60°$, depth $= 50\,\mu m$

Table 1 Experimental parameters used to calculate the Re

Density (kg/m^3)	1,046
Mean velocity (m/s)	3.8×10^{-4}
Hydraulic diameter (m)	7.5×10^{-5}
Viscosity of Dx-40 (Ns/m^2)	4.5×10^{-3}
Re	0.007

2.3 Confocal Micro-PTV Experimental Set-Up

The confocal micro-PTV system used in our experiment consists of an inverted microscope (IX71, Olympus, Japan) combined with a confocal scanning unit (CSU22, Yokogawa) and a diode-pumped solid state (DPSS) laser (Laser Quantum Ltd) with an excitation wavelength of 532 nm. Moreover, a high-speed camera (Phantom v7.1) was connected into the outlet port of the CSU22. The microchannel was placed on the stage of the inverted microscope where the flow rate of the working fluids was kept constant (Re = 0.007) by means of a syringe pump (KD Scientific Inc.). The Reynolds number (Re) and associated experimental parameters are summarized in Table 1. A thermo plate controller (Tokai Hit) was set to 37 °C. All the confocal images were captured in the middle of the microchannels with a resolution of 640 × 480 pixels, at a rate of 100 frames/s with an exposure time of 9.4 ms. The recorded images were transferred to the computer and then evaluated in the Image J (NIH) [1] by using the manual tracking MtrackJ [21] plugin. As a result it was possible to track single RBCs through the middle plane of the microchannel (Fig. 3).

2.4 Simulation Method

The numerical calculations for the laminar isothermal flow of pure water were performed using the finite-element computational fluid dynamics (CFD) program POLYFLOW®. The simulations were carried out in a 3D geometry representing the microchannel (see Fig. 4). The mesh used in the simulations was mainly constituted by quadrilateral elements, the discretization of the walls of the channel being presented in Fig. 4. The size of the elements was fixed after a grid independence test. The grids were successively refined and the velocity obtained with the different meshes were compared, the results being considered independent of the mesh when a difference bellow 1% was achieved [4, 8–10].

The equations solved were the conservation of mass and momentum equations for laminar incompressible flow of water. The problem is a non-linear problem, so it was necessary to use an iterative method to solve the referred equations. In order to evaluate the convergence of this process; a test based on the relative error in the velocity field was performed. For the velocity field, the modification on each node between two consecutive iterations is compared to the value of the velocity at the current iteration. In the present work, the convergence value was set to 10^{-4}, since this value is appropriate for the studied problem [5, 8–10].

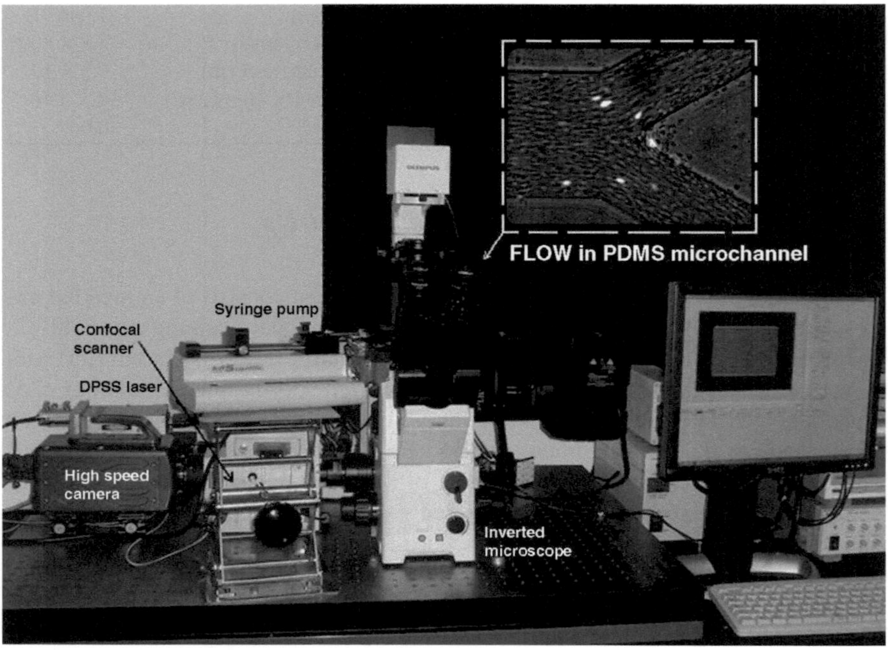

Fig. 3 Experimental set-up

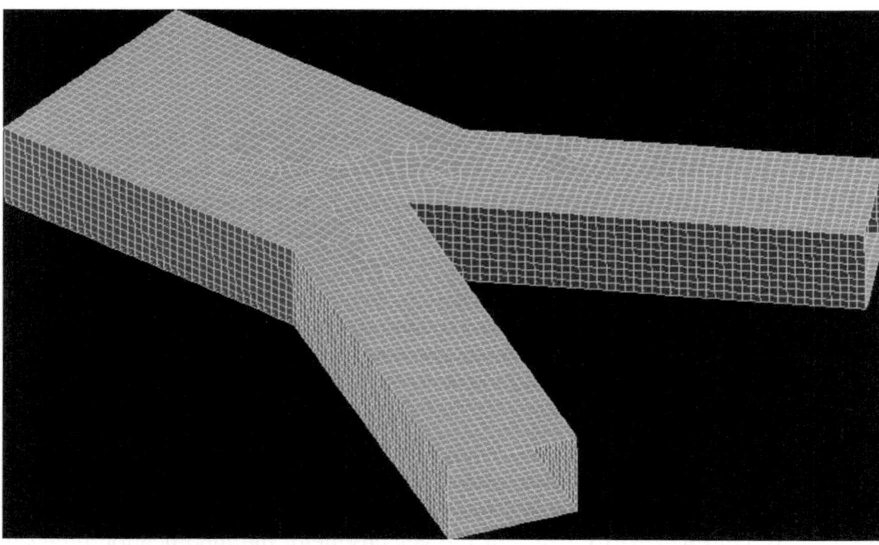

Fig. 4 Computational domain and mesh used

Table 2 Rheological parameters of blood [12]

Rheological model	η(Pa.s)	$K(-)$	$n(-)$	λ(s)	η_∞(Pa.s)	η_0(Pa.s)
Newtonian	0.00345	–	–	–	–	–
Power law model	–	0.035	0.6	–	–	–
Carreau model	–	–	0.3568	3.313	0.00345	0.056

The boundary conditions were established in order to reproduce the experimental conditions. The geometry of the bifurcation was idealized and close to the original dimensions of the photomask. Additionally, the mean velocity at the inlet of the microchannel was 3.8×10^{-4} m/s and slip at the walls of the channel was assumed to be non-existent. The referred velocity was imposed considering a constant flow rate on the referred boundary.

In the numerical study, blood was considered a Newtonian and non-Newtonian fluid In the last case, the rheology of the blood was described by two different constitutive models – power law model and the Carreau model [12] – which are, respectively, traduced mathematically by the equations:

$$\eta = K\dot{\gamma}^{n-1}, \tag{1}$$

$$\eta = \eta_\infty + (\eta_0 - \eta_\infty)\left[1 + (\lambda\dot{\gamma})^2\right]^{(n-1)/2}, \tag{2}$$

where η is the viscosity of the fluid, K the consistency index, n the flow index behavior, $\dot{\gamma}$ the shear rate, η_∞ the viscosity for high shear rates, η_0 the viscosity for low shear rates and λ the natural time. For the blood, the rheological parameters present in the above equations are reported in Table 2.

3 Results and Discussion

The confocal micro-PIV system was first evaluated by comparing the experimental results not only with a well established analytical solution for steady flow in a rectangular microchannel [15] but also with a reliable numerical method that was used in past investigations to study the flow behaviour of Newtonian or non-Newtonian fluids at low Reynolds numbers [9, 10].

The numerical, experimental and analytical results of the present work were obtained for the middle plane (25 μm height) of the rectangular microchannel. The averaged velocity data obtained from the confocal micro-PTV measurements, analytical solution and numerical simulation were in good agreement. A more detail description of these results can be found elsewhere [22].

By using a confocal micro-PTV system it was possible to obtain series of successive images at the middle of the bifurcation. Figures 5a and 6 show images with both fluorescent particles and labeled RBCs (laser-emitted light) flowing through a symmetric bifurcation, together with the correspondent time position tracking of both

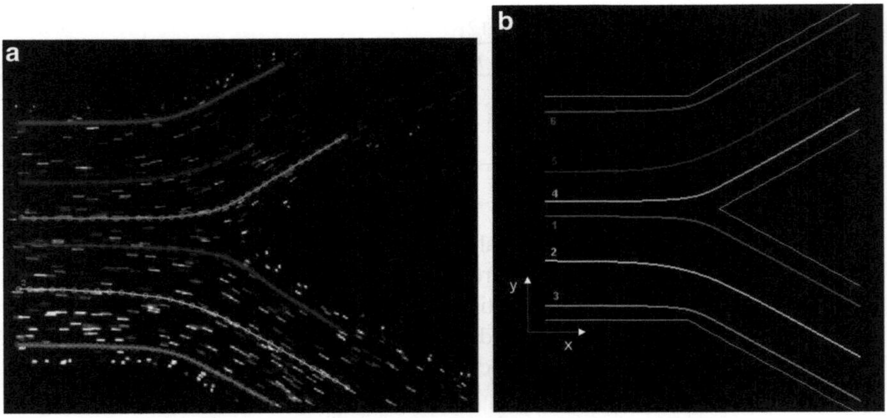

Fig. 5 (**a**) Paths displacement of fluorescent particles flowing in pure water; (**b**) Numerical trajectories using pure water

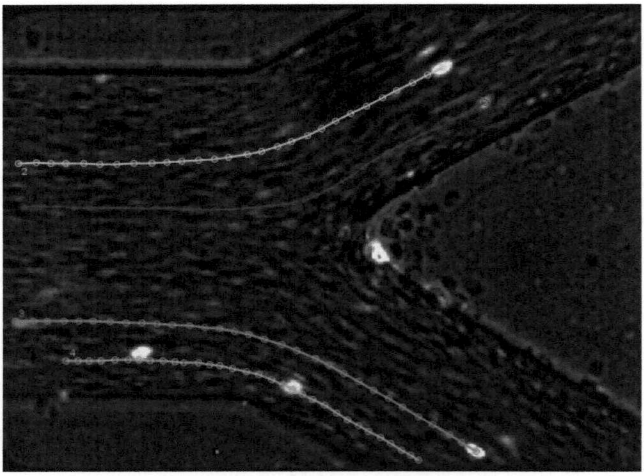

Fig. 6 Paths displacement of labeled RBCs (*bright spots*) flowing in physiological fluid with 14% Hct (32×)

particles and individual RBCs. Qualitative comparison between the experimental data from pure water (see Fig. 5a) and the numerical simulation (see Fig. 5b), shows that in both cases the trajectories do not exhibit any appreciable deviations in the transversal (*yy* axis) direction.

In addition by comparing qualitatively the experimental data from both pure water and in vitro blood (14% Hct) it is possible to observe that some RBC paths seems

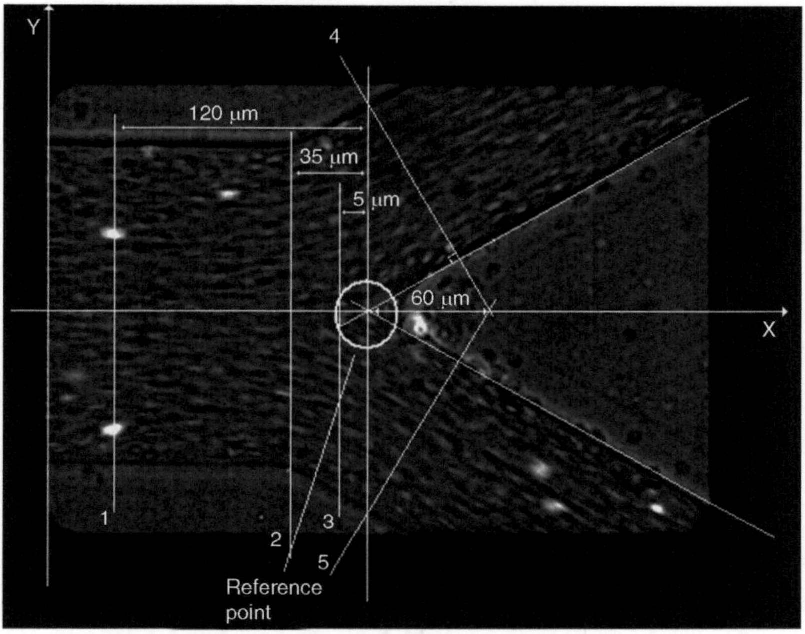

Fig. 7 Regions where the velocity profiles of the numerical and experimental results were compared

to suffer small deviations from the streamlines of the plasma flow probably due to flow perturbations caused by cell interactions in the neighbourhood of the apex of bifurcation.

Moreover numerical simulations of non-Newtonian models were performed around the bifurcation at the regions 1–5 (see Fig. 7).

Figures 8 and 9 show the velocity profiles for both computational and experimental results before and after the bifurcation, respectively.

Figures 8 and 9 suggest that the RBCs velocities close to the microchannel wall are higher than that obtained with the numerical models since slip at the walls of the channel was assumed to be non-existent in the latter case. It is well know, in microcirculation and other areas [4, 5, 13, 20, 28, 32], that RCBs, macromolecules, colloids, etc., are excluded from the region of the channel with low velocity and this may explain the observed differences.

Moreover, Figs. 8 and 9 confirm [35] that the velocity profiles obtained with the power law model ($n = 0.6$) are more flat than the ones obtained with the Newtonian model ($n = 1$). For infinite pseudoplasticity ($n = 0$) a plug flow should be obtained [35]. It is important to note that in Figs. 8 and 9 the average velocity obtained with the different constitutive equations was the same.

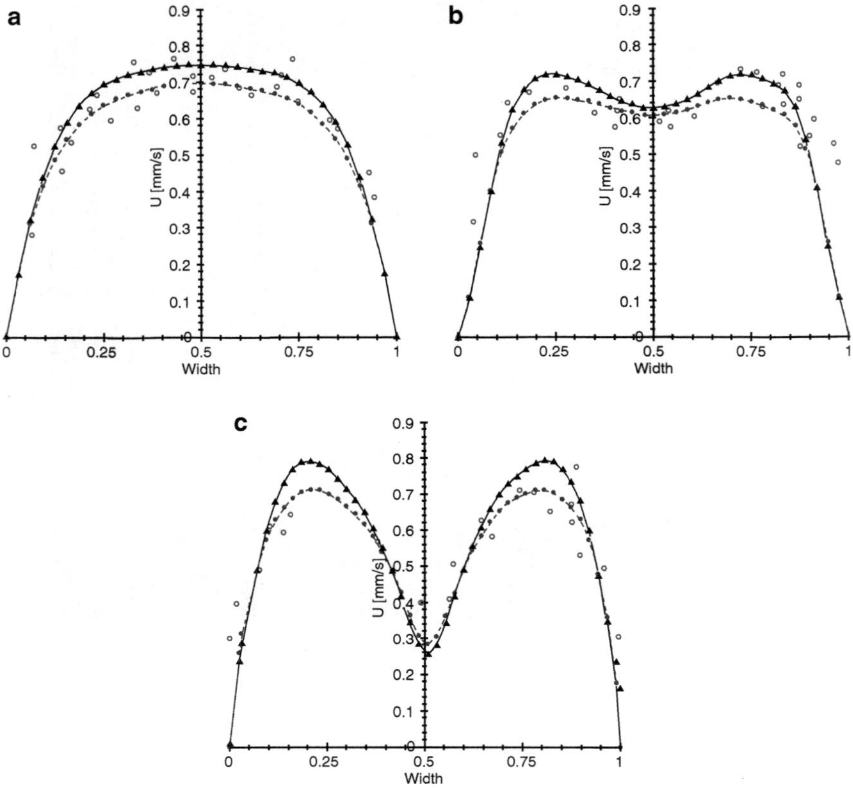

Fig. 8 Velocity profiles for both computational and experimental results before the bifurcation: (**a**) region 1; (**b**) region 2; (**c**) region 3. (—) Newtonian; (–•–) Power Law; (▲) Carreau Model; (○) Confocal micro-PTV RBC velocities

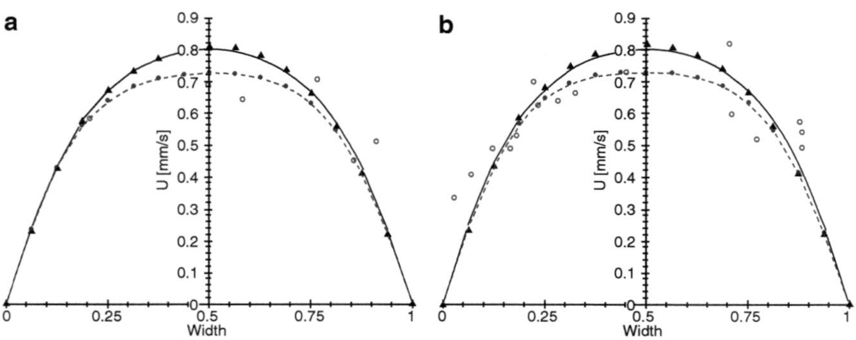

Fig. 9 Velocity profiles for both computational and experimental results after the bifurcation: (**a**) region 4; (**b**) region 5. (—) Newtonian; (–•–) Power Law; (▲) Carreau Model; (○) Confocal micro-PTV RBC velocities

4 Limitations and Future Directions

The primary goal of the present work is to provide new insights on the rheological properties of blood in microvascular network models. To accomplish it experimental flow studies was performed with a confocal micro-PTV system complemented with the most recent advances in microfabricated technologies. However, the soft-litography quality is strongly dependent not only on the photolitography methodology but also on the photomask resolution and its fidelity to the original design. In the present work we used a plastic photomask and according to our preliminary results we found small discrepancies between the tested in vitro model and the original design. Although these discrepancies were not taken into account in the present study we are aware about the possible influence of them on the results shown. Hence, in the future we are planning to carry on the current research by taking into account such discrepancies.

In vitro experimentation has the potential to provide a more realistic information on the flow properties of blood when compared with numerical simulations. However, once validated the numerical models can be a valuable tool to obtain more detailed insights about the blood rhelogical properties in microvascular networks. Generally, there are two major approaches to model of the non-Newtonian nature of blood [33]. One is based on the conventional continuum approach, in which a blood constitutive equation is assumed such as the casson model and the power-law model [36]. A more complex and realistic approach is based on a multiphase approach, in which the blood is considered as a multiphase suspension of deformable particles and where levels of submodeling for the behaviour of blood components are introduced. Some examples for this type of approach are the boundary element method [23, 26, 34], the immersed boundary method [2, 7, 24, 31], the lattice Boltzmann method [6, 29] and the moving particle semi-implicit (MPS) method [19, 30]). Recent reviews on these numerical methods can be found in Liu et al. [18], Yamaguchi et al. [33] and Lima et al. [14]. Although the multiphase flow approach is a very promising method it requires massive computational power. Hence, only recently this latter approach is being actively pursued due to the advances of the computational techniques and the computing power.

In the current study we have only performed simulations by using a continuum computational approach to model of the non-Newtonian nature of blood. However for the size of the microcahnnel used in presented work we can not neglect the effect of the suspension of deformable cells on its flow behaviour. Hence, we expect in a near future to compare the obtained experimental results with multi-phase numerical models.

5 Conclusions

A confocal micro-PTV system for the analysis of the complex phenomena happening at bifurcations was proposed. The system was complemented by a soft-litography technique to fabricate the in vitro models and by a continuum computational model approach to study the non-Newtonian nature of the working fluids.

Qualitative experimental observations suggested that RBC paths around the bifurcation apex seems to suffer small deviations from the streamlines of the plasma flow probably due to cell interactions enhanced by the high local Hct originated at this region.

The simulations performed with a finite-element computational fluid dynamics (CFD) program POLYFLOW emphasized the need of developing a multiphase approach.

Acknowledgements This study was supported in part by the following grants: Grant-in-Aid for Science and Technology (BII/UNI/0532/EME/2008, PTDC/SAU-BEB/108728/2008, PTDC/SAU-BEB/105650/2008 and PTDC/EME-MFE/099109/2008) from the Science and Technology Foundation (FCT) and COMPETE, Portugal and Grant-in-Aid for Scientific Research (S) from the Japan Society for the Promotion of Science (JSPS; No.19100008). We also acknowledge the support from the 2007 Global COE Program "Global Nano-Biomedical Engineering Education and Research Network". The authors would like also to thank Dr. C. Balsa for his valuable assistance and support for the MATLAB numerical calculations and Ms. B. Oliveira, Ms. D. Cidre and Mr. M. Lagoela for their valuable technical assistance in this research work.

References

1. Abramoff, M., Magelhaes, P., Ram, S.: Image processing with image J. Biophotonics Int. **11**, 36–42 (2004)
2. Bagchi, P.: Mesoscale simulation of blood flow in small vessels. Biophys. J. **92**, 1858–1877 (2007)
3. Chien, S., Usami, S., Skalak, R.: Blood flow in small tubes In: Renkins, M., Michel, C.C. (eds.) Handbook of Physiology–The Cardiovascular System IV, pp. 217–249. American Physiological Society, Bethesda (1984)
4. Dias, R.P.: Size fractionation by slalom chromatography and hydrodynamic chromatography. Recent Patents Eng. **2**, 95–103 (2008)
5. Dias, R.P., Fernandes, C.S., et al.: Starch analysis using hydrodynamic chromatography with a mixed-bed particle column, Carbohydr. Polym. **74**, 852–857 (2008)
6. Dupin, M.M., Halliday, I., et al.: Modeling the flow of dense suspensions of deformable particles in three dimensions. Phys. Rev. E. **75**, 066707 (2007)
7. Eggleton, C.D., Popel, A.S.: Large deformation of red blood cell ghosts in a simple shear flow. Phys. Fluids. **10**, 1834–1845 (1998)
8. Fernandes, C.S., Dias, R.P., et al.: Simulation of stirred yoghurt processing in plate heat exchangers. J. Food Eng. **69**, 281–290 (2005)
9. Fernandes, C.S., Dias, R.P., et al.: Laminar flow in chevron-type plate heat exchangers: CFD analysis of tortuosity, shape factor and friction factor. Chem. Eng. Process.: Process Intensif. **46**, 825–833 (2007)
10. Fernandes, C.S., Dias, R.P., et al.: Friction factors of power-law fluids in plate heat exchangers. J. Food Eng. **89**, 441–447 (2008)
11. Goldsmith, H., Turitto, V.: Rheological aspects of thrombosis and haemostasis: Basic principles and applications. ICTH-Report-Subcommittee on Rheology of the International Committee on Thrombosis and Haemostasis. Thromb. Haemost. **55**, 415–435 (1986)
12. Johnston, B.M., Johnston, P.R., et al.: Non-Newtonian blood flow in human right coronary arteries: Steady state simulations. J. Biomech. **37**, 709–720 (2004)
13. Lima, R., Ishikawa, T., et al.: Measurement of individual red blood cell motions under high hematocrit conditions using a confocal micro-PTV system. Ann. Biomed. Eng. **37**, 1546–1559 (2009)

14. Lima, R., Ishikawa, T., et al.: Blood flow behavior in microchannels: Advances and future trends. In: Single and Two-Phase Flows on Chemical and Biomedical Engineering. Bentham (in press) (2011)
15. Lima, R., Wada, S., et al.: Confocal micro-PIV measurements of three dimensional profiles of cell suspension flow in a square microchannel. Meas. Sci. Tech. **17**, 797–808 (2006)
16. Lima, R., Wada, S., et al.: In vitro confocal micro-PIV measurements of blood flow in a square microchannel: The effect of the haematocrit on instantaneous velocity profiles. J. Biomech. **40**, 2752–2757 (2007)
17. Lima, R., Wada, S., et al.: In vitro blood flow in a rectangular PDMS microchannel: Experimental observations using a confocal micro-PIV system. Biomed. Microdevices **2**(10), 153–167 (2008)
18. Liu, W.K., Liu, Y., et al.: Immersed finite element method and its applications to biological systems. Comput. Methods Appl. Eng. **195**, 1722–1749 (2006)
19. Kondo, H., Imai, Y., et al.: Hemodynamic analysis of microcirculation in malaria infection. Ann. Biomed. Eng. **37**, 702–709 (2009)
20. Maeda, N.: Erythrocyte rheology in microcirculation. Jpn. J. Physiol. **46**, 1–14 (1996)
21. Meijering, E., Smal, I., Danuser, G.: Tracking in molecular bioimaging. IEEE Signal Process. Mag. **3**(23), 46–53 (2006)
22. Oliveira, B., Lagoela, M., et al.: Analyses of the blood flow in a microchannel with a bifurcation. In: Proceedings of 3° Congresso Nacional de Biomecânica, Bragança, Portugal (2009)
23. Omori, T., Ishikawa, T. et al.: Behavior of a red blood cell in a simple shear flow simulated by a boundary element method, In: Proceedings of Bioengineering 08, London, UK (2008)
24. Peskin, C.S.: Numerical analysis of blood flow in the heart. J. Comput. Phys. **25**, 220–233 (1977)
25. Popel, A., Johnson, P.: Microcirculation and hemorheology. Annu. Rev. Fluid Mech. **37**, 43–69 (2005)
26. Pozrikidis, C.: Numerical simulation of the flow-induced deformation of red blood cells. Ann. Biomed. Eng. **31**, 1194–1205 (2003)
27. Pries, A., Secomb, T., et al.: Resistance to blood flow in microvessels in vivo. Circ. Res. **75**, 904–915 (1994)
28. Small, H.: Hydrodynamic chromatography a technique for size analysis of colloidal particles. J. Colloid. Interface Sci. **48**, 147–161 (1974)
29. Succi, S.: The Lattice Boltzmann Equation for Fluid Mechanics and Beyond, Clarendon Press, Oxford (2001)
30. Tsubota, K., et al.: Particle method for computer simulation of red blood cell motion in blood flow. Comp. Methods Programs Biomed. **83**, 139–146 (2006)
31. Univerdi, S.O., Tryggvason, G.: A front-tracking method for viscous, incompressible multi-fluid flows. J. Comput. Phys. **100**, 25–37 (1992)
32. Venema, E., Kraak, J.C., et al.: Packed-column hydrodynamic chromatography using 1-μm non-porous silica particles. J. Chromatogr. A **740**, 159–167 (1996)
33. Yamaguchi, T., Ishikawa, T., et al.: Computational blood flow analysis – new trends and methods. J. Biomech. Sci. Eng. **1**, 29–50 (2006)
34. Youngren, G.K., Acrivos, A.: Stokes flow past a particle of arbitrary shape: A numerical method of solution. J. Fluid Mech. **69**, 377–403 (1975)
35. Wilkinson, W.L.: Non-Newtonian fluids: Fluid mechanics, mixing and heat transfer, pp. 61–63. Pergamon Press, London (1960)
36. Zhang, J.B., Kuang, Z.B.: Study on blood constitutive parameters in different blood constitutive equations. J. Biomech. **33**, 355–360 (2000)

Two Approaches for Automatic Nuclei Cell Counting in Low Resolution Fluorescence Images

Thierry Brouard and Aurélie Chantôme

Abstract This paper deals with the problem of counting nuclei in low-resolution fluorescence images. The low resolution is a consequence of the usage of a large field of view, this to reduce the number of experiments, implying time saving and money saving. But the small size of nuclei increases the risk of error in counting. In this work we used some image processing operators in order to extract potential shapes. These shapes are then characterized (size, shape, edges) to decide if they are noise or not. Two approaches are presented for this: the first one correspond to a translation of some basic knowledge used by practitioners; the second one uses a supervised classification technique where it is the computer who discovers the knowledge by the analysis of a database of cases. This leads to a fast technique which gives very good results, validated by cell biology experts.

Keywords Image processing · Classification · SVM · Cell counting

1 Introduction

The biological background of this work is the cell migration. This is one of the crucial steps in the metastatic cascade which is in part responsible for death in cancer. A better understanding of this cascade is a requisite before to develop new therapies against their development. Since a few years, there is accumulating evidences that ion channels and particularly potassium channel are involved in the oncogenic process [20]. Among these channels it was reported that SK3 channel (a calcium-activated potassium channel sensitive to apamin) is expressed in a highly

T. Brouard (✉)
Laboratoire d'Informatique, Université François Rabelais, EA2101,
64 av. J.Portalis, 37200, Tours, France
e-mail: brouard@univ-tours.fr

A. Chantôme
INSERM U921, Nutrition, Croissance & Cancer 10, Bld Tonnellé 37032, Tours, France
e-mail: chanto_a@med.univ-tours.fr

J.M.R.S. Tavares and R.M.N. Jorge (eds.), *Computational Vision and Medical Image Processing: Recent Trends*, Computational Methods in Applied Sciences 19,
DOI 10.1007/978-94-007-0011-6_18,

metastasizing cancerous cell line, MDA-MB-435s, where it is involved in cell migration but not in cell proliferation [14].

The Fig. 1 represents a typical picture we worked on. It shows nuclei cell colored by fluorescence. The major problem with such images is that they are disturbed by out-of-focus light mostly due to the thickness of the specimen. This can lead to some overlapping areas between several nuclei since they are not on the same focal plane. Other problems may be encountered: uneven illumination, lighting artifacts, apoptotic bodies. In this one, cells are programmed to die. When it arrives, the nucleus is fragmented into several parts. In this case, the software must count one nucleus, not *n* fragments of the same nucleus (see Fig. 2).

In the remaining of this paper, the Sect. 2 presents the related work while the Sect. 3 describes our contribution. The results are presented and discussed in Sect. 4.3 and Sect. 5 concludes the paper.

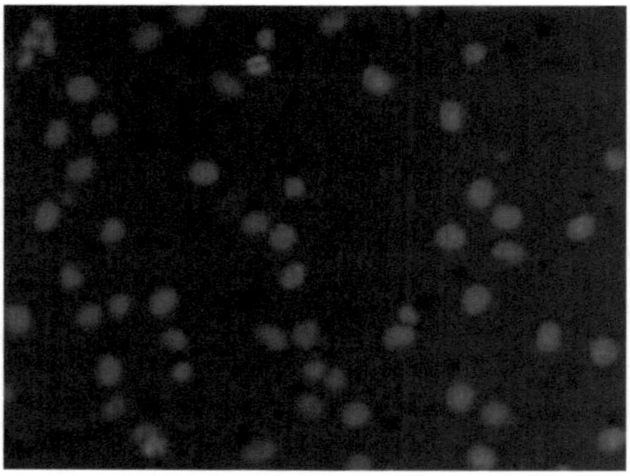

Fig. 1 A sample (about 1/6th) of an input picture. Cell nuclei are colored by fluorescence. An input picture contains from 200 to 800 nuclei. The size of the picture is about 680 × 512 pixels and weights about 40 KB (RGB, JPEG)

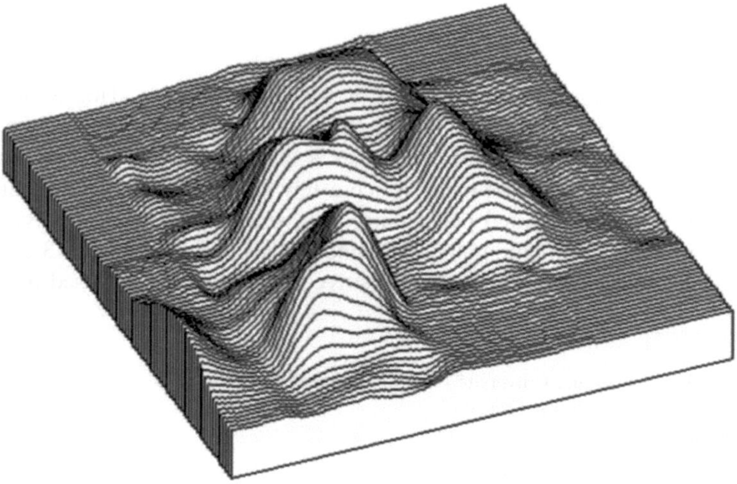

Fig. 2 3D representation of one apoptotic body (elevation represents grey level intensities). In this case the software must count only one nucleus instead of four

2 Related Work

Counting objects in an image can lead to three different but not necessarily mutually incompatible problems. These are not specific to our context and are widely encountered in the image analysis community. The first one is based on a two steps image processing to extract shapes from the image, then a processing applied to shapes themselves gave the result. The image processing corrects the problems of illumination, deformation, noise whereas the shape processing merge close forms or, in contrast, separate what appears to be a group. We can notice in the literature [4] (cell counting without fluorescence) where a normalization of the picture is applied to help a binarization algorithm to extract shapes and where morphological operators ended the work on shapes. Authors announce a global performance rate about 90% on medium resolution pictures (2 mega pixels). In [18] a theoretical framework was developed to count blood cells. The problem takes place in the field of granulometry: the goal is to separate all the cells into several classes (a classification problem) and then to compute the cardinality of each set (a counting problem). In this work, the two steps are performed simultaneously, based on the theory developed applied to pattern spectrums obtained by morphological erosions. The error was evaluated to 10%.

In the first approach, the ability of image processing for separating shapes from the rest of the image is assumed. If not, a second approach involving classification is required. After locating all potential shapes, a set of features is extracted for each shape (area, circularity, length of edges, skeleton...). This set is sometimes simplified (by a PCA for example) and then divided into as many classes there are categories of shapes. Then all the founded shapes could be counted. In [8, 9], the presented work deals with a methodology to extract, select and then classify sets of features. Features are extracted form RGB and HSV color spaces. A PCA is used to optimize the use of features before classification. Some classifiers are compared: neural networks, support vector machine, bayesian classifiers. This work is applied to FISH images. In [11] features such as TAS, LBP and Haralick coefficients are used to train neural networks or SVMs to classify cell phenotype images. Good results are obtained using large feature vectors, implying large shapes representing nuclei. In all works, a detection step is therefore needed to locate cells before classification.

The third approach consists in the separation of the shapes in a challenging environment. It is then a problem of segmentation. We mainly see two approaches: a region-based one vs. an edge-based one. In [3] a watershed is used to split overlapping or aggregating nuclei cells. A right set of markers is chosen to initialize the watershed process in order to correctly separates overlapping or aggregating nuclei (25% of the nuclei contained in the picture). This process in not applicable in our case because of the lighting conditions and the resolution of the picture. Tests report a mean error about 13.5%. In [15] the edges of the shapes are analyzed using an iterative voting process leading to approximate the position of the center of mass for each shape. This let the authors to initialize a watershed process. Authors say that good results are obtained on high resolution pictures, but did not quantify them. In [1] a watershed is used to split the aggregates on high-resolution pictures too. A rules-based process is then used to merge closer shapes, avoiding over-segmentation. A rate of 95% of good segmentation is reported on pictures containing about 20 cells, this obtained after 80 seconds of processing time. A graph-based approach is presented in [21]. This works like a region-growth algorithm which operates in a space of graphs. A 92% of good segmentation was reported on high resolution pictures of nuclei (natural lighting).

Our work falls into the first or the second category, depending of the studied kind of cell. In some cases, statistics computed over the shapes are sufficient to build a rules-based classifier. In other cases, a features vector is computed for each shape. A classifier is used to label each unknown shape. A training phase is needed to parametrize the classifier.

3 The Proposed System

Three stages could be seen (see Fig. 3): a preprocessing step which extracts, prepares and adjusts the information used to perform the counting, a segmentation step for

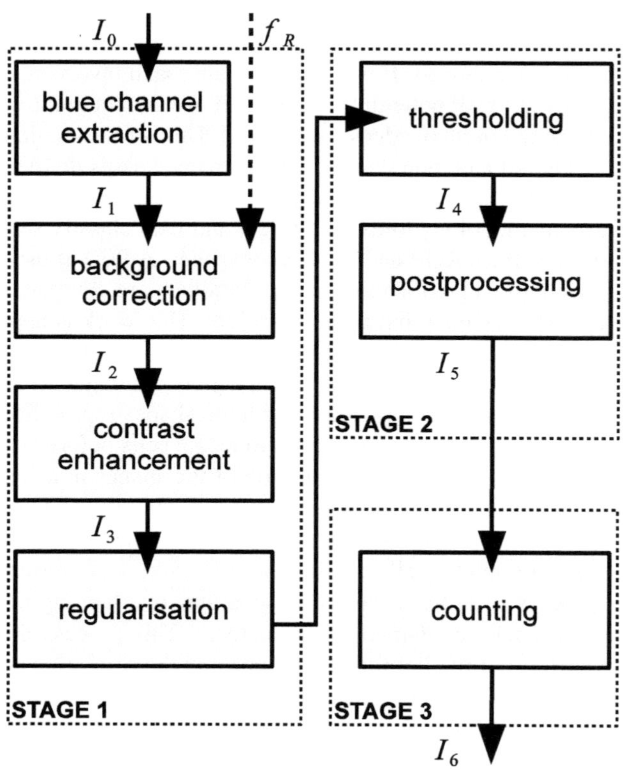

Fig. 3 Global view of the processing chain designed for the counting. The first stage prepares the picture while the second one extract the shapes. The last one is dedicated to counting (two techniques have been used: basic rules for the easiest cases, classification based system otherwise)

extracting the patterns and finally a counting step which produces the final results. Next paragraphs are dealing with these three stages.

3.1 Acquisition

The 680×512 pixels wide, RGB-encoded, pictures are given by an Olympus system: a IX51 Olympus microscope equipped with a fluorescent illuminator (Olympus U-RFL-T) and Olympus DP70 camera. The acquisition software was the rev. 3.2 of the Olympus DP-soft. For the moment, the pictures are saved onto a hard drive in JPEG format.

3.2 Preprocessing

This section describes the first stage shown on Fig. 3. Some illustrating pictures taken at different steps of the process are shown on Fig. 8.

The input picture I_0 taken by the camera is split into red, green and blue channels. Only the blue one is kept, resulting a 8 bits grayscale image denoted I_1. Several experiments were conducted with other color spaces (see Fig. 4). We finally retained the channel B of the RGB space. The L channel from HSL space was also a good candidate, it seems visually more contrasted, but final results are almost identical. Some adjustments are needed: its histogram usually takes place in the first 30% of the grayscale range, the background illumination is not homogeneous (see Fig. 5) and globally, the picture is low-contrasted.

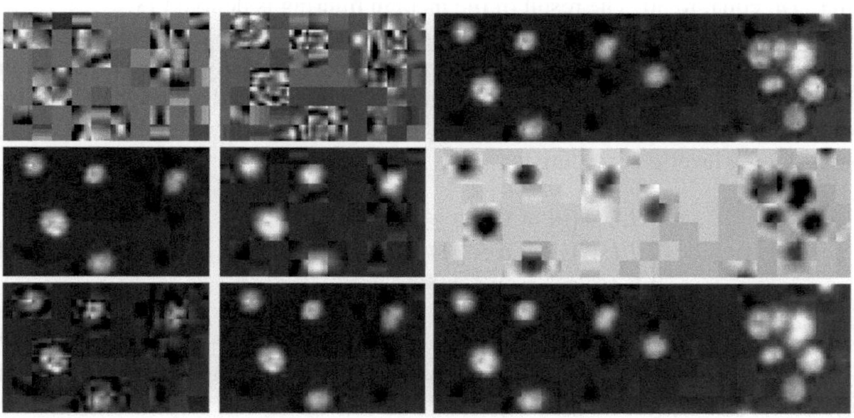

Fig. 4 Some examples of the pictures obtained in different color spaces (from *top left* to *down right* – x/y means x compound extracted from y representation): H/HSL, S/HSL, L/HSL, Y/YCbCr, Cb/YCbCr, Cr/YCbCr, R/RGB, G/RGB, B/RGB. On some of these we can easily distinguish the effect of the JPEG compression

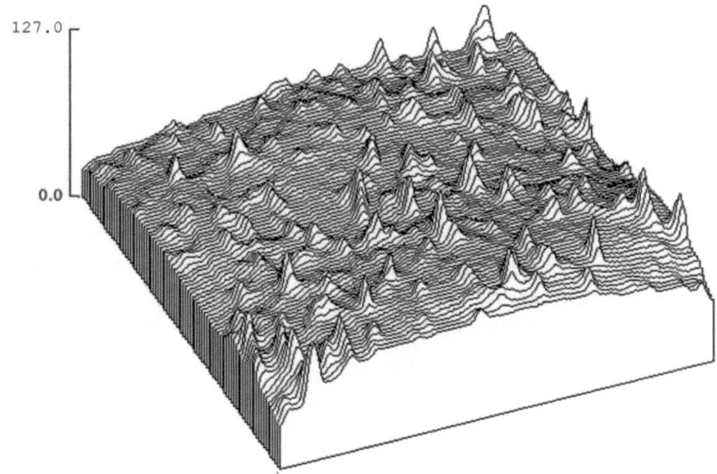

Fig. 5 3D view of an image background model computed by the median filter. The vignetting effect is clearly visible in the corners where the values are smaller than in the middle

A model of the background is made using a median filter. Denoted I_B, this picture is then subtracted from I_1. The size of the filter is a parameter to set. A partial answer is given by the context. Considering that a large field of view is required to have significant results after the counting and that aggregates does not implies a large number of cells (5-6 seems to be a maximum) an upper bound could be computed for the size of a cell nucleus. The worst situation would be where the nuclei were arranged like the filter. In this case, this aggregates would have a radius lower than three times the radius of one nucleus. So, we choose to set the radius of the filter, f_R, equal to 30. The result of the median filtering is denoted I_2.

A typical histogram of I_2 is shown Fig. 6. More than 60% of the pixels belongs to the background. Some nuclei are not well lighted, especially in the corners of the picture (see Fig. 7, left). Log of the histogram is approximated with 3 lines. The two points of intersection defines two bounds B_{inf} and B_{sup}. So we compute $LUT[g]$ for each grey level g according to:

$$\begin{cases} LUT[g] = 0, \forall g \leq B_{inf} \\ LUT[g] = \alpha \times g + \beta, \forall g \in]B_{inf}, B_{sup}[\\ LUT[g] = 255, \forall g \geq B_{sup} \end{cases} \tag{1}$$

where $\alpha = \frac{255}{B_{sup} - B_{inf}}$ and $\beta = -\alpha \times B_{inf}$. After applying the LUT to I_2 we obtain I_3 ($I_3(x, y) = LUT[I_2(x, y)]$). A low-pass filter is finally applied to regularize the signal before the segmentation step.

Figure 8 shows the evolution of the same scene during stage 1 (I_0 to I_3), stage 2 (I_4 and I_5) and stage 3 (I_6).

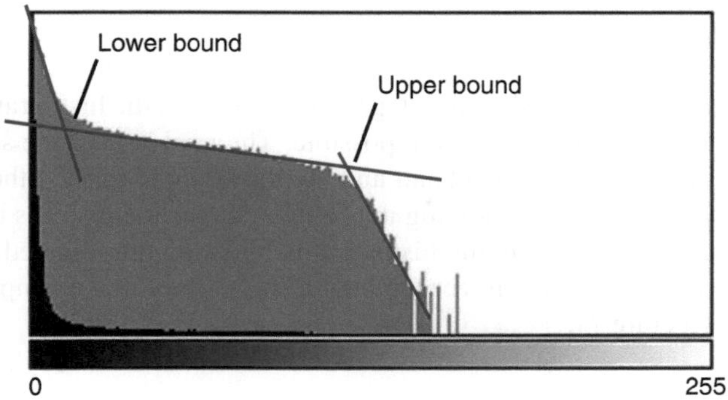

Fig. 6 Histogram of a picture at step I_2 before stretching: the histogram is drawn in black and the log of the histogram is drawn in grey. Intersections of the three red lines define the two bounds used to stretch the histogram ($\bar{g} = 9.06, \sigma_g = 22.7, mode = 0$)

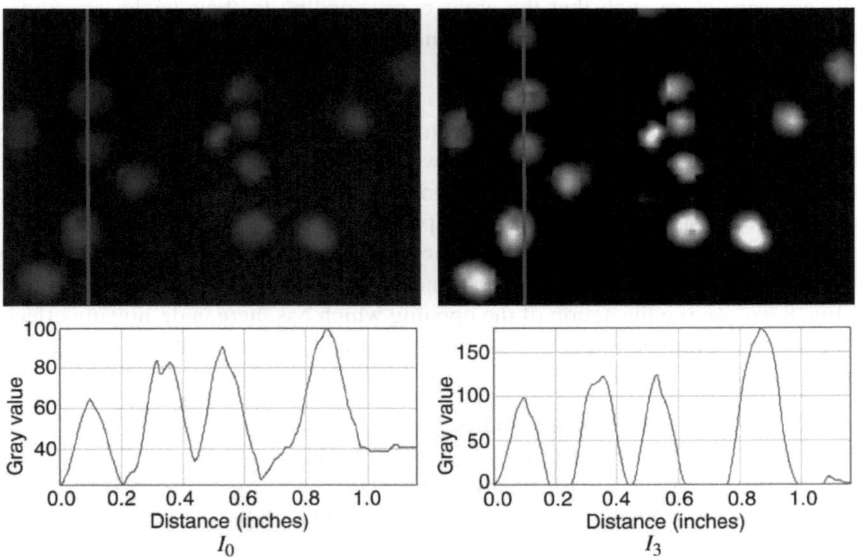

Fig. 7 The same scene taken in I_1 (*left*) and I_3 (*right*). The vertical line shows the area where the profile is plotted (below each picture). On the *left* profile, 4 nuclei are represented, the mean grey level of the background is about 40. On the *right* profile, the separation of the nuclei is better (there is much space between them), the contrast is better (the mean of the highest values on the *left* is about 80 than it is about 130 in the *right*) and the background is neutralized (its mean grey level is about 0)

3.3 Segmentation

The next step is the segmentation. It is divided into two steps: the thresholding to make the picture binary and the post processing to clean the picture.

3.3.1 Thresholding

The transformation performed by the stage 1 operations on the histogram makes the use of a global thresholding algorithm possible. The goal is here the separation of the patterns – the nuclei – in one hand and the background in the other hand. We can find a good survey of thresholding in [16]. Our experiments leads us to use the Otsu technique [12]. Assuming the histogram is bimodal, the founded threshold is optimal in the way that it maximizes the interclass variance. An example of picture is given Fig. 8, picture I_4.

3.3.2 Post Processing

Some defaults may remains after thresholding. Because of lighting, the holes of the porous membrane on which the cells are cultivated are sometimes visible. Some cells are very close such that the areas corresponding to their nuclei are joined. We have already talk about apoptosis: one nucleus could be fragmented into several smaller parts. To perform an efficient counting, these three situations should be corrected.

A watershed is first applied on the picture I_4. This to separate the nuclei. Sometimes, the nuclei are so close that the watershed did not separate them. This is corrected during the counting process. On the picture I_5 Fig. 8 we can see the action of the watershed process which has splitted some aggregates into single nuclei. Then, an opening using a 3-pixels diameter disc as structuring element removes small artifacts due to the porous membrane and smoothes the edges. On the picture I_5 Fig. 8 we can see the action of the opening which has, here, a de-noising effect.

A connex component labeling is then performed. For each area founded some information is computed:

1. A, the area (a positive integer, in pixels).
2. C, the circularity (a real from 0 – line to 1 – circle).
3. c_x, c_y the coordinates of the centre of mass.
4. n, the number of nuclei inside the area, initialized with 0.

All these informations are used during the counting process.

3.4 Nuclei Counting

We used two different systems to count nuclei, depending of the studied kind of cell. The easiest situations are solved using a classifier based on rules which deals with statistics computed over shapes. This is described in Sect. 3.4.1. In more difficult cases, we use a SVM-based classifier to label features vectors associated to shapes. This is described in Sect. 3.4.2.

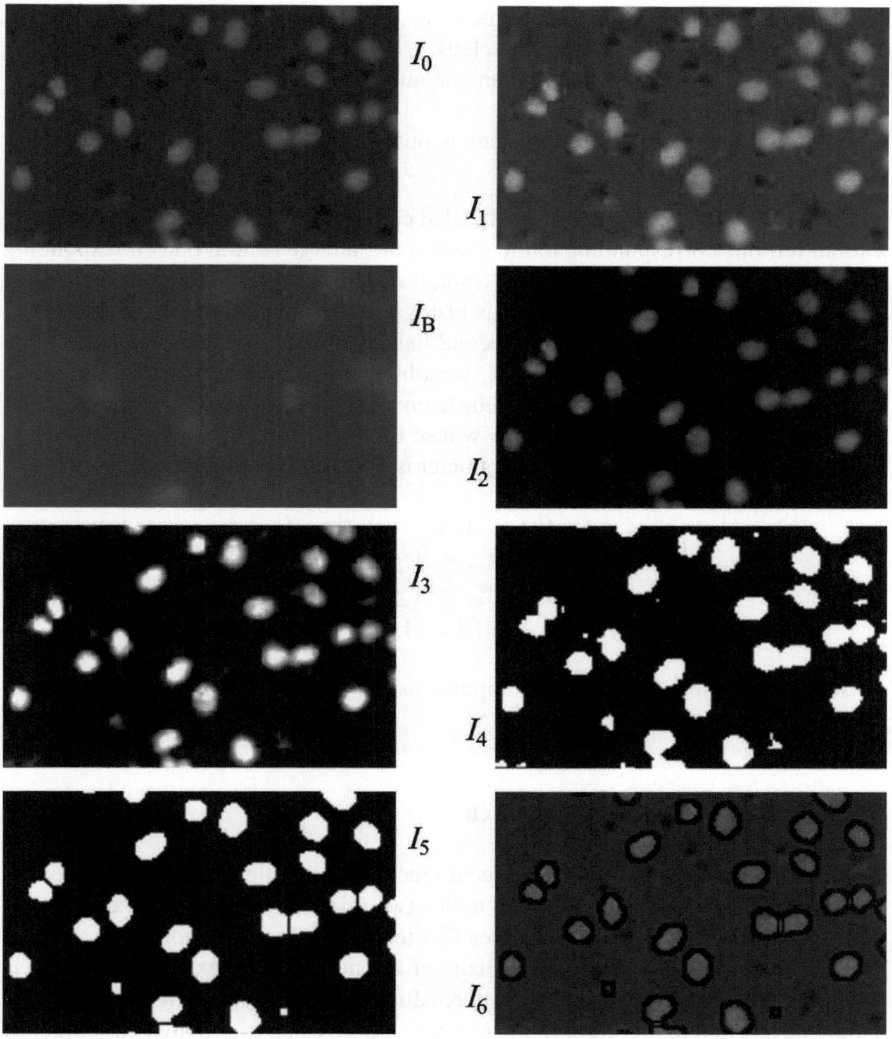

Fig. 8 Detail of a picture to process (I_0), the corresponding blue channel (I_1), the background model computed with median filtering (I_B), the picture obtained after subtracting the background (I_2) and after enhancing the contrast (I_3), the binary picture obtained (I_4), the same after post processing (I_5) and the final image (I_6) where the nuclei are highlighted

3.4.1 A First Approach, Based on Rules

The approach based on rules is used to compute how many nuclei are associated to each component. The rules simply translate the ones used by practitioners when they manually perform the counting:

1. All the nuclei have slightly the same area.
2. A too small area could not be a nucleus.
3. A too large area contains more than one nucleus.
4. A nucleus is rather circular.
5. When the major part of the nucleus is outside the field of view we see only a small area.

The histogram of the areas of the labeled component analysis shows three parts: a small left one corresponding to the small areas; a large central one corresponding to the standard size of a nucleus and a small right one corresponding to the largest areas. Considering the first-half of this histogram, the Otsu algorithm gives us A_m. Applying the same technique, the second-half of the histogram let us to compute A_M. Considering the rule number 4, we obtain by the same way C_m the lower circularity index to separate one nucleus from an aggregate. We then compute $\bar{A}$ the mean area of labeled components for whose $C \geq C_m$ and $A_m \leq A \leq A_M$. Then, for each labeled component the n parameter is updated according to:

$$\begin{cases} n = 0, \{\forall A | A < A_m\} \\ n = 0, \{\forall A, C | A_m \leq A \leq A_M \wedge C < C_m\} \\ n = 1, \{\forall A, C | A_m \leq A \leq A_M \wedge C \geq C_m\} \\ n = \lceil A/\bar{A} \rceil, \{\forall A | A > A_M\} \end{cases} \tag{2}$$

The total number of nuclei is computed as the sum over all the labeled components of the parameter n.

3.4.2 The SVM Classifier Approach

Results obtained (see Table 1) with technique based on rules are very good for the cell line MDA-MB-435s. But we can notice two things: (i) some nuclei are not correctly labeled, (ii) with other cell lines this technique does not work very well. In the first case, errors are due to the shape of the nucleus. For example, this one is deformed when it passes through the pores during migration (see Fig. 9d). So, rules should be adapted to this case. In the second case we can notice a high variability of the nuclei shapes. Here we need more complex rules to distinguish good shapes (nuclei) from the bad ones (noise) if we want the same software to count all kind of cell.

Table 1 Results of the counting (rules-based classifier), validated by an expert (mean recall $\bar{r}$, mean precision $\bar{p}$, mean error $\bar{e}$, standard deviation of the error σ_e)

	$\bar{r}$	$\bar{p}$	$\bar{e}$	σ_e
R_1	96.5%	99.6%	2.2%	0.011
R_2	97.0%	99.1%	3.3%	0.017

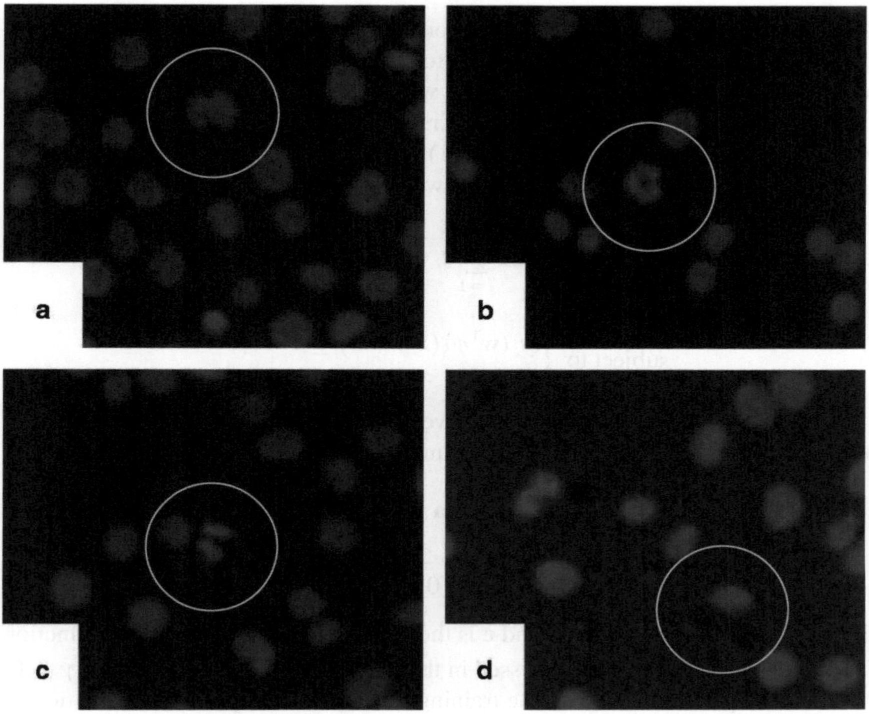

Fig. 9 Some examples of the shape variety encountered in the pictures: (**a**) two nuclei after cell division, (**b**) apoptotic body, (**c**) noise due to the substance used to color the nuclei, and (**d**) *rice grain* form of the nucleus after the cell migration through a pore. Cases (**b, d**) and sometimes (**c**) are difficult for the rules based approach. For example, by adapting the rules to count correctly the nuclei like (**d**) the number of errors due to the noise shown in picture (**c**) increases

Many techniques are available in the field of classification in order to produce the rules. Considering we always have an expert to state if that particular area is a noise or a nucleus, we choose a supervised technique (support vector machine, neural nets, hidden Markov models...) Considering too that the description of the shape is always possible, we do not use techniques dealing with uncertainty (like Bayesian networks for example). Finally, according to the information we can compute on shapes and other projects we realized in the past [7, 10, 19], we choose support vector machine (SVM).

Basic Principles

SVM [13, 17] is used here as a classification technique. A classification task usually involves with training and testing data which consist of some data instances.

Each instance in the training set contains one *target value* (class labels) and several *attributes* (features). The goal of SVM is to produce a model which predicts target value of data instances in the testing set which are given only the attributes. So, given a training set of k instance-label pairs $(\mathbf{x}_i, y_i), i = 1, ..., k$ where the feature vectors $\mathbf{x}_i \in \mathbb{R}^n$ and the label $y_i \in (1, -1)^k$, the support vector machine separates the training vectors in a ϕ-mapped space, with an error cost $C > 0$:

$$\min_{\mathbf{w},b,,} \frac{1}{2}\mathbf{w}^{\mathrm{T}}\mathbf{w} + C \sum_{i=1}^{k} \xi_i$$
$$\text{subject to} \begin{cases} y_i(\mathbf{w}^{\mathrm{T}}\phi((x_i) + b) \geq 1 - \xi_i, \\ \xi_i \geq 0, i = 1, ..., k. \end{cases} \tag{3}$$

Due to the high dimensionality of the vector variable $\mathbf{w}$, this problem is usually solved through its Lagrangian dual problem:

$$\min_{\mathbf{a}} F(\mathbf{a}) = \frac{1}{2}\mathbf{a}^{\mathrm{T}} Q\mathbf{a} - \mathbf{e}^{\mathrm{T}}\mathbf{a}$$
$$\text{subject to} \begin{cases} 0 \leq a_i \leq C, i = 1, ..., k, \\ \mathbf{y}^{\mathrm{T}}\mathbf{a} = 0 \end{cases} \tag{4}$$

where $Q_{ij} \equiv y_i y_j \phi(\mathbf{x}_i)^{\mathrm{T}}\phi(\mathbf{x}_j)$ and $\mathbf{e}$ is the vector of all ones. The kernel function $K(\mathbf{x}_i, \mathbf{x}_j) \equiv \phi(\mathbf{x}_i)^{\mathrm{T}}\phi(\mathbf{x}_j)$ is expressed in the RBF case by $e^{-\gamma(\mathbf{x}_i - \mathbf{x}_j)^2}$ with $\gamma > 0$. So, when using the RBF kernel, the training of the model requires the definition of C and γ.

Features Extraction

In the training set, each class of input data is represented by several instances. An instance is defined by a set of attributes extracted from the connex components (CC) founded in picture I_5.

We use the following features:

1. The area a of the CC, in pixels ($a \in \mathbb{N}^+$). This information let us to know if the CC is rather small or rather big.
2. The circularity c of the CC, ($c \in [0..1]$). This information can indicate whether the component is more round or more elongated.
3. The normalized histogram $\mathbf{H}$ of the Freeman code of the edge of the component: we first compute the Freeman code of the CC to obtain a string describing how the edge of the CC evolves. The histogram $\mathbf{h}$ of this string is then computed to obtain a vector of 8 components (these steps are shown on Fig. 11). The histogram $\mathbf{h}$ is then normalized by dividing all its components by $\sum_k h_k$ to obtain $\mathbf{H}$.

These features are arranged for the instance i as a vector $\mathbf{x}_i = (a, c, \mathbf{H})$.

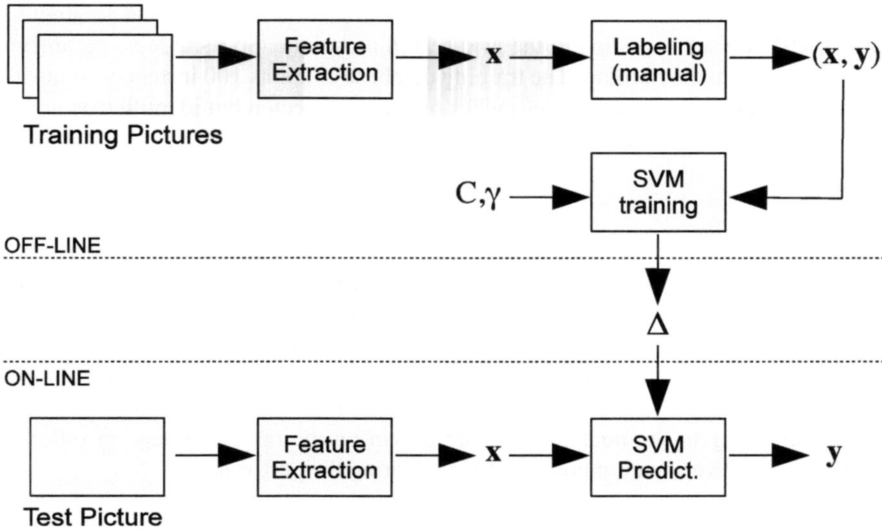

Fig. 10 Block scheme of the use of support vector machine. An off-line process let us to get a model Δ minimizing the classification error of an instance database $(\mathbf{x}, \mathbf{y})$. This model is used during an on-line process to label ($\mathbf{y}$ is the result) all the shapes (described by $\mathbf{x}$) embedded in a test picture

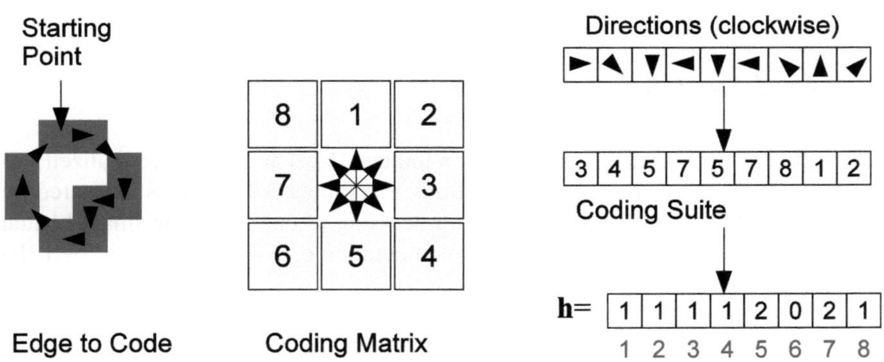

Fig. 11 The Freeman code of the connex component: (*left*) an example of an edge with a starting point and a direction consider each point; (*middle*) the Freeman matrix showing how each direction is coded; (*right*) the list of directions corresponding to the used edge (*top*), the coding of these directions according to the Freeman matrix (*middle*) and the histogram $\mathbf{h}$ before normalization

Training the SVM (See Fig. 10)

In order to create the training set we need to label (i.e., to set y_i) many samples ($\mathbf{x}_i$). The kernel function used to map the input data is the radial basis one (RBF, which can handle non-linear relations). The training algorithm implemented in LIBSVM is

SMO [5]. The training is made using a five-fold cross validation and the parameters of the RBF are set according to the grid search technique. So there is no parameter to set to perform the training. The training database contains 100 instances of nuclei (alone or in aggregates) and 50 instances of shapes detected but identified as noise. The overall performance computed over this database was 99.4%.

Final Evaluation

The labels provided by the classifier are used to highlight the connex components founded in the picture. Then, the same process as the one used for the other counting approach is applied. A statistical analysis was conducted over the shapes to find a correct range for one nucleus size. This information is then use to correct the number of nuclei forming an aggregate. The edges and the number of nuclei found for each shape belonging to the nucleus class are drawn on the original image in order to make a manual verification possible for evaluating the performance.

4 Implementation and Tests

We now present the implementation, some information about computation time, the test protocol and the obtained results.

4.1 Implementation

The software was written as a script for ImageJ [6]. The tests were realized under Mac OS X environment, on a MacBook Pro (about 3.95 GFlops measured by XBench [22]). In classification task, the processing of one picture in ImageJ batch mode needs about 2.3 seconds. The implementation of SVM is provided by LIBSVM [2].

4.2 Test Protocol

Pictures were acquired at two magnifications: $R_1 = \times 100$ and $R_2 = \times 200$. Each input picture is processed in order to produce an output picture in which nuclei are highlighted. Then, a manual verification is made. Two experts count, on each output picture: (i) N_1 the number of nuclei correctly counted, (ii) N_2 the number of nuclei forgotten, and (iii) N_3 the things wrongly counted as nuclei. The result given by the software is $N_1 + N_3$. The correct value is $N_1 + N_2$. We evaluate the performance of the counting by: the recall: $r = N_1/(N_1 + N_2)$; the precision: $p = N_1/(N_1 + N_3)$ and the global error: $e = (N_2 + N_3)/(N_1 + N_3)$. The results presented in Table 2 concern the counting of 10738 cell nuclei (R_1) and 4017 cell nuclei (R_2).

Table 2 Results of the counting (SVM classifier), validated by an expert (mean recall $\bar{r}$, mean precision $\bar{p}$, mean error $\bar{e}$, standard deviation of the error σ_e)

	$\bar{r}$	$\bar{p}$	$\bar{e}$	σ_e
R_1	96.9%	98.2%	3.1%	0.018
R_2	98.4%	99.3%	2.4%	0.023

4.3 Results

The approach based on rules gave better results at the lower resolution. The circularity criteria is responsible of that: at better resolution it is too restrictive for some cell nuclei whose are deformed when the cells pass through the porous membrane. The count is accurate, but a small fraction of nuclei are poorly identified and counted as noise. Various experiments have shown that the error was stable and did not depend on the configuration of the image.

The approach using the SVM classifier seems to use the best the information in the image made at the resolution R2. The accuracy is comparable to the other approach and is slightly better in the case of SVM classifier. Again the error is stable.

5 Conclusion

This paper has presented a process of counting cell nuclei in images obtained by optical microscopy in fluorescent light. In particular, it describes the different steps of image processing followed by two techniques used for counting nuclei. While the first technique is based on a translation of business knowledge, the second uses a supervised classifier trained in advance on a database of cases. The results obtained are very good, especially for the approach based on the classifier, which is more universal.

Acknowledgements The authors wish to thank C. Vandier and A. Girault (both belonging to the INSERM U921, Nutrition, Croissance & Cancer Lab.) for their advice and assistance in carrying out this work.

References

1. Adiga, P., Chaudhuri, B.: An efficient method based on watershed and rule-based merging for segmentation of 3-d histo-pathological images. Pattern Recogn. **34**, 1449–1458 (2001)
2. Chang, C.-C., Lin C.-J.: LIBSVM: a library for support vector machines (2001) http://www.csie.ntu.edu.tw/~cjlin/libsvm

3. Cloppet, F., Boucher, A.: Segmentation of overlapping/aggregating nuclei cells in biological images. In: 19th International Conference on Pattern Recognition (ICPR), Tampa, FL, USA (2008)
4. Dill, D., Scholz, A., Gül, M., Wolf, B.: Methods for counting cells supported by digital image processing. In: Heidelberg, S.B. (ed.) 14th Nordic-Baltic Conference on Biomedical Engineering and Medical Physics. In: IFMBE Proceedings, vol. 20, pp. 493–496. Riga, Latvia (2008)
5. Fan, R.-E., Chen, P.-H., Lin, C.-J.: Working set selection using second order information for training SVM. J. Mac. Learn. Res. **6**, 1889–1918 (2005)
6. Imagej: Image processing and analysis in java. http://rsb.info.nih.gov/ij/
7. Kuba, H., Hotta, K., Takahashi, H.: Automatic Particle Detection and Counting by One-Class SVM from Microscope Image. LNCS 5507/2009, pp. 361–368 (2009) doi: 10.1007/978-3-642-03040-6_44
8. Lerner, B., Clocksin, W., Dhanjal, S., Hulten, M., and Bishop, C.: Feature representation and signal classification in fluorescence in-situ hybridization image analysis. IEEE Trans. Syst. Man Cybern. Part A Syst. Humans **31**(6), 655–665 (2001)
9. Lerner, B.: Bayesian fluorescence in situ hybridisation signal classification. Artif. Intelli. Med. **30**(3), 301–316 (2004)
10. Markiewicz, T., Osowski, S., Mariańska, B.: White Blood Cell Automatic Counting System Based on Support Vector Machine. LNCS 4432/2007, pp. 318–326 (2007) doi: 10.1007/978-3-540-71629-7_36
11. Nanni, L., Lumini, A.: A reliable method for cell phenotype image classification. Artif. Intell. Med. **43**(2), 87–97 (2008)
12. Otsu, N.: A threshold selection method from gray-level histograms. IEEE Trans. Syst. Man Cybern. Part A Syst. Humans **9**(1), 62–66 (1979)
13. Pedroso, J.-P., Murata, N.: Support vector machines with different norms: motivation, formulations and results. *Pattern Recogn. Lett.* **22**(12), 1263–1272 (2001)
14. Potier, M., Joulin, V., Roger, S., Besson, P., Jourdan, M.-L., Leguennec, J.-Y., Bougnoux, P., Vandier, C.: Identification of sk3 channel as a new mediator of breast cancer cell migration. Mol. Cancer Ther. **5**(11), 2946–2953 (2006)
15. Schmitt, O., Hasse, M.: Radial symmetries based decomposition of cell clusters in binary and grey level images. Pattern Recogn. **41**, 1905–1923 (2008)
16. Sezgin, M., Sankur, B.: Survey over image thresholding techniques and quantitative performance evaluation. J. Electron. Imag. **13**(1), 146–168 (2004)
17. Shawe-Taylor, J., Cristianini, N.: Support Vector Machines and other kernel-based learning methods. Cambridge University Press (2000)
18. Theera-Umpon, N., Dougherty, E., Gader, P.: Non-homothetic granulometric mixing theory with application to blood cell counting. Pattern Recogn. **34**, 2547–2560 (2001)
19. Ushizima, D.M., Lorena, A.C., de Carvalho, A.C.P.: Support Vector Machines Applied to White Blood Recognition. In: 5th International Conference Hybrid Intelligent Systems, Rio de Janeiro, pp. 234–237. Rio de Janeiro, Brazil (2005)
20. Villalonga, N., Ferreres, J.-C., Argilés, J.-M., Condom, E., Felipe, A.: Potassium channels are a new target field in anticancer drug design. Recent Pat. Anticancer Drug Discov. **2**(3), 212–223 (2007)
21. Ta, V.-T., Lézoray, O., Elmoataz, A., Schüpp, S.: Graph-based tools for microscopic cellular image segmentation. Pattern Recogn. **42**, 1113–1125 (2009)
22. Xbench homepage. http://xbench.com/

Cerebral Aneurysms: A Patient-Specific and Image-Based Management Pipeline

M.C. Villa-Uriol, I. Larrabide, J.M. Pozo, M. Kim, M. De Craene, O. Camara, C. Zhang, A.J. Geers, H. Bogunović, H. Morales, and A.F. Frangi

Abstract This work presents an image- and biomechanics-based data processing pipeline able to build patient-specific models of cerebral aneurysms. The pipeline also contemplates the virtual modeling and release of endovascular devices such as stents and coils. As a result of the morphological, morphodynamic, hemodynamic and structural analyses, a set of complex descriptors relevant for aneurysm's diagnosis and prognosis is derived. On the one hand these will bring an insight into the processes behind aneurysm genesis, growth and rupture. On the other one, the inclusion of virtual devices enables the *in silico* personalized evaluation of alternative treatment scenarios before intervention and constitutes a valuable tool for the industrial design of more effective devices. Several of its components have been evaluated in terms of robustness and accuracy. The next step should comprehensively assess the complete pipeline, also proving its clinical value. This pipeline illustrates some of the ideas behind the Virtual Physiological Human (VPH) and the integration of complex data for a better understanding of human physiology in health, disease and its treatment.

M.C. Villa-Uriol (✉), J.M. Pozo, M. Kim, M. De Craene, O. Camara, C. Zhang, A.J. Geers, H. Bogunović, and H. Morales
Center for Computational Imaging & Simulation Technologies in Biomedicine (CISTIB), Universitat Pompeu Fabra, Networking Research Center on Bioengineering, Biomaterials and Nanomedicine (CIBER-BBN), c/ Tanger 122–140, E08018, Barcelona, Spain
e-mail: cruz.villa@upf.edu; jose.pozo@upf.edu; minsuok.kim@upf.edu; mathieu.decraene@upf.edu; oscar.camara@upf.edu; chong.zhang@upf.edu; arjan.geers@upf.edu; hrvoje.bogunovic@upf.edu; hernan.morales@upf.edu

I. Larrabide
Networking Research Center on Bioengineering, Biomaterials and Nanomedicine (CIBER-BBN), Center for Computational Imaging & Simulation Technologies in Biomedicine (CISTIB), Universitat Pompeu Fabra, c/ Tanger 122–140, E08018, Barcelona, Spain
e-mail: ignacio.larrabide@upf.edu

A.F. Frangi
Center for Computational Imaging & Simulation Technologies in Biomedicine (CISTIB), Universitat Pompeu Fabra, Networking Research Center on Bioengineering, Biomaterials and Nanomedicine (CIBER-BBN), Institució Catalana de Recerca i Estudis Avançats (ICREA), c/ Tanger 122–140, E08018, Barcelona, Spain
e-mail: alejandro.frangi@upf.edu

J.M.R.S. Tavares and R.M.N. Jorge (eds.), *Computational Vision and Medical Image Processing: Recent Trends*, Computational Methods in Applied Sciences 19,
DOI 10.1007/978-94-007-0011-6_19, © Springer Science+Business Media B.V. 2011

Keywords Cerebral aneurysms · Image segmentation · Image processing · Morphology · Morphodynamics · Haemodynamics · Computational physiology · Structural mechanics · Virtual treatment · Virtual physiological human

1 Introduction

Saccular cerebral aneurysms are abnormal focal dilatations of the vessel lumen commonly arising from arterial bifurcation points. Once an aneurysm ruptures, subarachnoid hemorrhage usually follows producing high morbidity and mortality rates [10, 76]. The wide availability of diagnostic and interventional imaging techniques as well as the emergence of sophisticated therapeutic devices, has significantly transformed during the last decade the understanding and management of cerebral aneurysms. Despite this, the knowledge about aneurysm genesis, growth and rupture is still limited [66]. On the one hand, structural defects in the vascular wall causing a localized weakness have been confirmed by histologic findings [40]. On the other hand, the combination of these with hemodynamic factors are thought to play a significant role in their pathogenesis and thrombosis [38, 41]. Consequently, treatment seeks their exclusion from the circulation while returning the blood flow in the parent vessel to normal physiological conditions. Among the multiple techniques pursuing this objective, coiling [31] and stenting [11, 50] have become the preferred options over the traditional surgical clipping. In the recent years, computational models have also been developed [36, 69] to better understand these mechanisms from the anatomical and biomechanical points of view. Nevertheless, these models need to be exhaustively evaluated before they become part of the standard clinical practice and several existing open computational problems are circumvented [72].

In this context, this chapter presents a data processing pipeline primarily focusing on the extraction of diagnostic and prognostic indices from medical images and from patient-specific biomechanical models. We are interested in providing a personalized assessment of aneurysm growth and rupture, particularly associating it to image-based computational characterization of intra-aneurysmal flow [14, 22, 30] as well as to mechanical and morphodynamical features of cerebral aneurysms [5, 6, 8, 19, 20, 32, 52, 58, 77, 78]. This is combined with the development of techniques for the virtual simulation of treatment using medical devices like stents and coils [25, 42, 47, 53, 61]. The aim is to optimize not only the device design process, but also its selection during an aneurysm embolization procedure.

One of the main motivations for this approach is the Virtual Physiological Human (VPH) concept [24, 70]. This initiative is endeavored with the development of patient specific computational models for human biology in health and disease as well as for its treatment. The present pipeline can been seen as a comprehensive approach for aneurysm management in this context.

2 Patient-Specific and Image-Based Data Processing Pipeline

Our image-based processing pipeline streamlines the creation of anatomic, structural and hemodynamic models to derive robust and reliable quantitative descriptors for patient-specific assessment and treatment planning. These models are built using two-dimensional (2D) and three-dimensional (3D) medical images from the patient. Two-dimensional X-ray angiographic imaging techniques have been heavily used for diagnosis, interventional guidance and follow-up. In particular, digital subtraction angiography (DSA) provides sequences of 2D projections showing the vessel lumen as the contrast medium is gradually injected. Three-dimensional rotational angiography (3DRA), computed tomography angiography (CTA) and magnetic resonance angiography (MRA) are able to obtain volumetric reconstructions of the cerebral vasculature. Among them, 3DRA provides the highest spatial resolution and is the first option during endovascular treatment. Given the less invasive nature of CTA and MRA, they are used in standard clinical practice at early diagnostic stages as well as for patient screening and monitoring [10]. Information about hemodynamic variables such as blood flow velocities can be obtained from MRA, while measuring pressure requires the use of intravascular probes.

Figure 1 provides an overview of the proposed pipeline and the methodologies involved in the creation of such models and how it exploits the above-mentioned medical imaging techniques. The first step in personalized vascular modeling consists of obtaining the geometrical representation of the patient's own anatomy. This requires the use of image segmentation and surface correction techniques. The accuracy of this step is crucial for the following steps. Complete 3D morphological

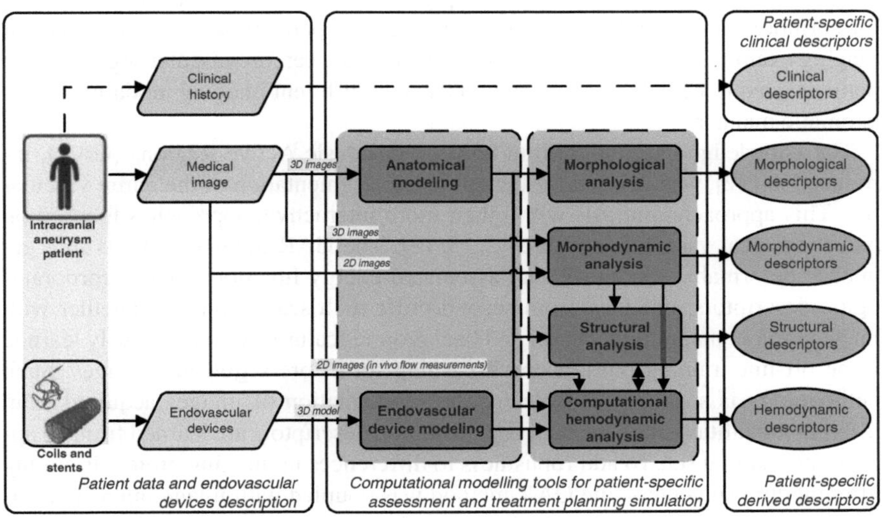

Fig. 1 Data processing pipeline for patient-specific assessment and treatment planning

descriptors can be obtained directly from the vascular models, which can be linked with aneurysm growth or rupture. Incorporating the temporal component at different time-scales allows to recover the aneurysm wall morphodynamics at patient follow-up or during a cardiac cycle. The former facilitates evaluating the evolution of treatment between follow ups, while the latter is essential to estimate the structural properties of the aneurysm wall indicating potential areas of weakness. Computational Hemodynamics (CHD) simulations [14] are able to provide a description of patient-specific hemodynamic variables with high spatial and temporal detail. Additionally, computational models have been developed to represent the virtual implantation of endovascular devices (stents and coils). Finally, the proposed pipeline, by combining all these techniques provides a mean to scientifically support the verification of clinical hypothesis as well as assessing a priori patient evolution with the aid of computer models. This will allow a switch in the treatment paradigm from reactive and conservative to proactive and patient-specific.

3 Anatomical Modeling: From Medical Images to Anatomical Models

The presented processing pipeline relies on the availability of accurate patient-specific vascular models, in the form of a polygon mesh, extracted from medical images. The process used to extract such models should ensure operator-independence, accuracy and high repeatability to minimize variability and its propagation to other steps of the pipeline. This task is challenging and heavily influenced by the underlying image quality as well as the complexity of the vascular geometry at hand. Furthermore, throughout their management cycle, patients undergo a variety of imaging examinations with various modalities. Thus, cerebrovascular segmentation methods need to be able to cope coherently with different imaging modalities in an automatic manner.

The knowledge-based algorithm built on Geodesic Active Regions (GAR), introduced in [32], was devised for the automatic segmentation of the entire vascular tree. This approach contrasts with other, more interactive, approaches focused on extracting local vascular segments [2, 13, 18]. The GAR method consists in a geometric deformable model with an associated energy functional that incorporates region descriptors, obtained from second-order multiscale features, together with image gradient magnitude. Vessel and background features were previously learned in the off-line training phase using a training set of pre-segmented images. Such methodology is specially suitable for the segmentation of images acquired from different modalities since for each one the region descriptors are learned from an appropriate training set. To add robustness to differences in imaging protocols among different clinical centers, the GAR method was coupled with image intensity standardization (IIS) method [8], which standardizes intensity ranges of tissue classes.

IIS is integrated as a pre-processing step to the segmentation and is applied to all the images used as a training set and to each image that undergoes the segmentation process. The resulting segmentation algorithm is fully automatic, operator independent and its computational cost is in the order of 15 min for a 256^3 voxels volume using a commodity personal computer. The extracted vascular models have been recently compared and validated against a gold standard built from manual measurements performed by clinicians. Preliminary results indicate that average absolute differences for 3DRA and MRA with respect to the gold standard were 0.2 and 0.3 mm respectively, values which were comparable to the ones of manual measurements and were below the corresponding image spatial resolutions.

On the extracted vascular model, a sequence of global and local operations are typically applied to improve the mesh quality and to correct for geometrical and topological irregularities. High-frequency noise on the surface mesh is removed by globally applying a volume-preserving smoothing. More pronounced irregularities on the surface as well as problems due to touching and missing vessels effects (Fig. 2a) are locally corrected using a combination of mesh element removal and hole filling, followed by an additional smoothing operation. Throughout the stages of the mesh processing, the vascular models need to be visually compared with 3D visualizations of the medical images to reduce the impact of the discrepancies introduced by this manual editing of the surface mesh.

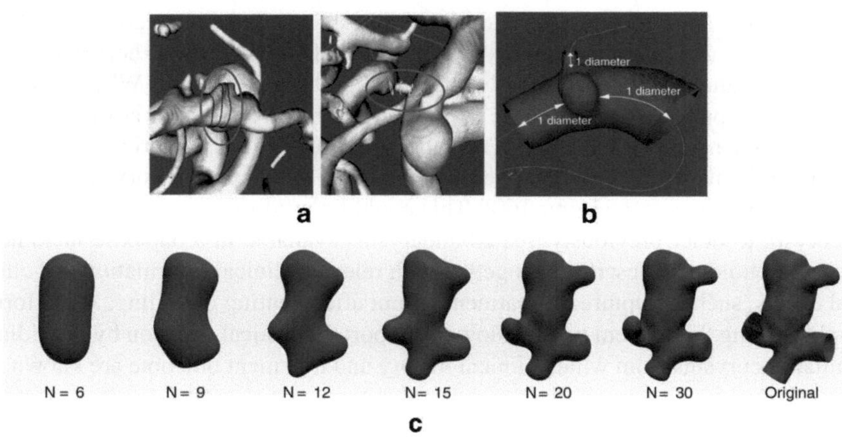

Fig. 2 Details of the anatomical modeling and morphological analysis stages. (**a**) Examples of topological problems introduced during the segmentation: touching vessels (*left*) and missing vessel (*right*) sections. (**b**) Aneurysm isolation for the morphological characterization (including one diameter for each adjacent vessel). (**c**) Reconstruction of the aneurysm geometry from 3D Zernike moments up to order N. The higher the order the more detailed information contained in the moments

4 Morphological Analysis: From Anatomical Models to Shape Descriptors

Aneurysm location, size and morphology are among the main criteria used by interventional neuroradiologists for treatment decision and selection. Several clinical works [51, 62, 64, 73] support the hypothesis that these geometrical descriptors have an influence on the risk of aneurysm rupture and have a link to rupture events.

Most of the proposed morphological indices are defined from a few linear measurements extracted from projectional imaging. Raghavan et al. [62] defined global 3D indices and evaluated them against the rupture event. In Millan et al. [52], we proposed an efficient methodology to take fully into account cerebral aneurysms tridimensional morphology. This strategy is based on moment invariants and allows to include part of the parent vessel in the aneurysm isolation protocol (Fig. 2b). In this way, information concerning the aneurysm and its vascular surroundings, which is ignored in other proposed indices, is also considered. The robustness and the prediction capacity of two different types of moments were explored: Geometrical Moment Invariants (GMI) [49] and 3D Zernike Moment Invariants (ZMI) [56, 60]. They were computed for a database of 31 ruptured aneurysms and 24 unruptured aneurysms, obtaining the best results with ZMI, for which a correct rupture prediction rate of $\simeq$ 80% was achieved. This contrasted with the 66% rate obtained with the aspect ratio index.

Zernike moments provide a set of morphological descriptors that are complete, meaning that, up to a certain level of detail, the shape can be recovered from their moments Fig. 2c. In addition, they are orthonormal, which makes their Euclidean distance a natural and geometrically meaningful distance measure. When this distance is computed in the space of ZMI, we obtain the additional advantage that the pose dependency is excluded. Thus, the morphological characterization of each aneurysm by its ZMI, provides an efficient method to compare aneurysm morphological similarities in real time [60]. This could be used to compare a new patient aneurysm to other previously treated aneurysms available in a database including their morphological descriptors together with relevant clinical information and clinical events, such as rupture or treatment output after stenting or coiling. A platform implementing this system would allow to support the clinical decision by providing similar aneurysms from which clinical history and treatment outcome are known.

5 Morphodynamic Analysis: Evaluating Temporal Changes in Medical Images

As stated above, quantification of aneurysm morphological changes has clinical relevance at two different time scales: at patient follow-up or during one cardiac cycle. While the first case considers periods of several months or years, the second focuses on a time interval of one second. In the proposed pipeline, we evaluate these temporal changes from clinically available image modalities. In the first case, we assess the evolution of coiled patients using follow-up images. Patients were followed during a period ranging from two months to 2 years to quantify the degree of coil compaction over time. In the second case, the wall motion displacement of a cerebral aneurysm is estimated along one cardiac cycle of the patient. The final objective is determining the biomechanical properties of the vascular wall localizing areas on the tissue that might be prone to rupture.

5.1 Quantification of Volumetric Changes

The quantification of the morphological changes over the months and years following an endovascular intervention is a critical factor to determine the treatment stability. In the case of coiling, up to one third of the treated aneurysms present recanalization [63]. Among the different causes, there is the compaction of the coil inside the aneurysm, the growth of the aneurysm, or the co-occurrence of both phenomena. In the latter scenario, the compacted coil migrates inside the aneurysm dome being pushed by flow-induced forces or blocked by thrombosis. In this perspective, the accurate detection and quantification of local shape changes in the aneurysm is critical for monitoring aneurysm stability and, when required, decide for (re-)treatment.

In clinical practice, the neuroradiologist usually detects and quantifies aneurysm recanalization evaluating the presence of a residual neck in the substracted reconstructions of 3DRA, DSA and MRA. Although the residual neck clearly assesses the reperfusion of the aneurysm, it does not allow to determine if it is due to coil compaction or aneurysm growth. In De Craene et al. [20], we investigated the use of automatic non-rigid image registration methods to produce local deformation maps as quantified by the Jacobian of a non-rigid transformation. State of the art intensity-based non-rigid registration algorithms were applied to produce local volume change maps between sequential images obtained at follow-ups after aneurysm coiling. This strategy not only permits reconstructing volume temporal evolution of coil and aneurysm, but also computing local growth maps showing the relative lengthening of a patch of the aneurysm wall rather than its absolute displacement as performed by [9]. In De Craene et al. [19], we extended the methodology to account for very large deformations in the case of severe aneurysm growth. The evolution of coil and aneurysm volumes along the follow-up period was obtained separately, which allows distinguishing between coil compaction and aneurysm growth. On the four cases studied, aneurysm recanalization was always associated to aneurysm growth, as opposed to strict coil compaction. Figure 3 shows quantification results for one of these cases.

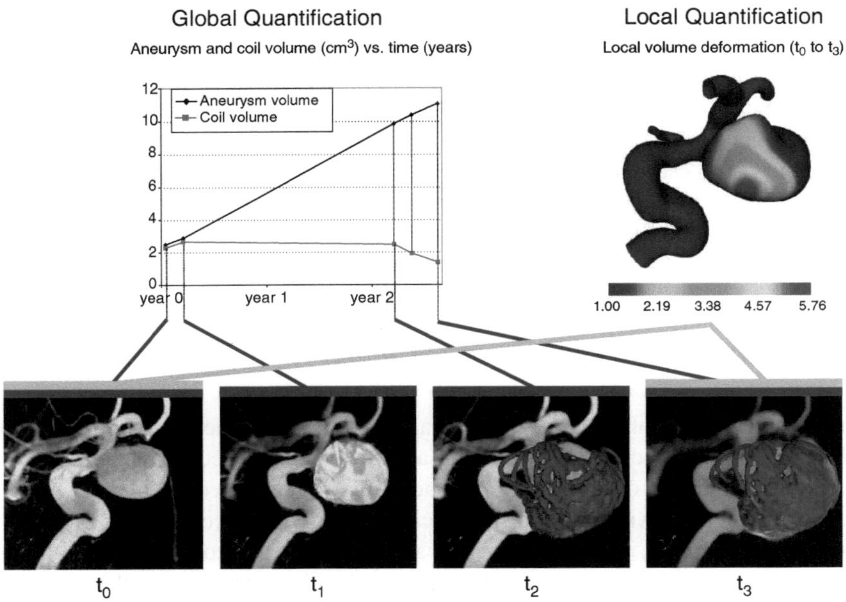

Fig. 3 Example of quantification of aneurysm growth and coil compaction. *Bottom* row shows an aneurysm before coiling and at several follow-ups. Volumetric coil and aneurysm images are used to perform global and local quantification. Global quantification is expressed as coil and aneurysm volume evolution vs. time curves. Local quantification is expressed as a growth map in the aneurysm, where 1 indicates no change, >1 expansion and <1 compression, and is computed between the first (t_0) and last treatment (t_3). In this case, the local aneurysm changes concentrate in one part of the aneurysm dome. Such heterogeneity could later be confronted to aneurysm environment or patient-specific modeling of the interactions between the blood flow and the coil

5.2 Wall Motion Estimation

Analyzing aneurysm wall motion throughout the cardiac cycle is becoming important owing to its potential connection to rupture, and as a way to estimate vascular compliance and to incorporate it in CHD simulations [22]. This allows to study the aneurysm hemodynamics using personalized models considering geometry and boundary conditions which are closer to reality than to rigid models. On the other hand, there are studies suggesting that direct visualization of wall motion may help in the detection of cerebrovascular abnormalities [35, 44]. Therefore, quantifying aneurysm wall motion has the potential of impacting treatment selection and preoperative planning of cerebrovascular diseases. However, since such motion is expected to be in the order of sub-millimeters, it represents a challenging task for most of the current clinical imaging techniques due to their relatively limited spatial resolution.

In [22] and [58], we proposed two motion estimation methods from DSA using 2D non-rigid image registration. The estimated wall motion was then imposed to the

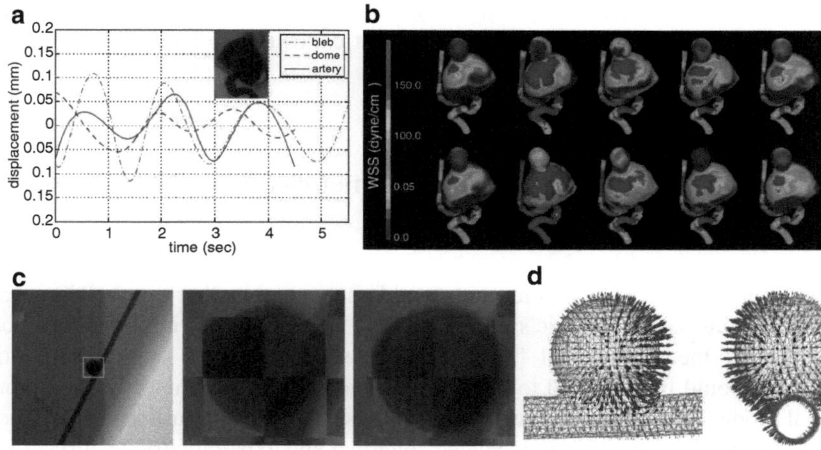

Fig. 4 (**a**) Estimated wall motion for the DSA sequences. (**b**) WSS distributions obtained from CHD simulations, using compliant (*top*) and rigid walls (*bottom*). (**c**) From left to right, an X-ray measured projection image from the physical phantom, checkerboard images of the measured and the forward projection from the reference volume and our estimation using [77], respectively. (**d**) Frontal and lateral views of reconstructed displacement field for a silicone phantom

3D model derived from the medical images to study the effects of wall compliance on the aneurysmal hemodynamics. Figure 4a shows the estimated wall displacement curves within different regions. Visualizations of the Wall Shear Stress (WSS) distributions of CHD simulations at five instants of the cardiac cycle are presented in Fig. 4b, using compliant wall and rigid wall. Since DSA images were captured from a single point of view, motion was only partially recovered.

Recently, we presented two image registration-based algorithms [77, 78] to estimate 3D + t patient-specific aneurysm wall motion from a single 3DRA acquisition. In the first work [78], aneurysm morphology at a given time instant was estimated from its temporal vicinity by registering forward projections of a deformed 3D reference volume to the corresponding reduced set of 2D measured projections in a weighted scheme. In the second work [77], the previously discussed methodology was extended by using a 4D transformation, and a registration between the entire 2D measured projection and the forward projection sequences. We evaluated the performance of these techniques using digital and physical pulsating aneurysm phantom models. Experiments with digital phantoms showed quantitative results of estimation errors below 10% of the maximum pulsation, which in general presented subvoxel wall displacements. Physical phantom experiments allowed to demonstrate the feasibility of pulsation estimation under clinical conditions. The simulated projections from the estimated volume images matched the corresponding measured ones, which was not the case from those of the reference volume (Fig. 4c). In Fig. 4d, two views of the corresponding reconstructed motion field for the silicone phantom in Fig. 4c are shown and evidence the differences in pulsatility among regions on the aneurysm wall.

Finally, the advantage of requiring only a single 3DRA acquisition facilitates its clinical take-up and also eliminates the need of exposing the patient to additional radiation dose.

6 Structural Analysis: Estimating Aneurysm Wall Mechanical Properties

The recovery of aneurysm wall motion should allow among others, embedding wall compliance into hemodynamic simulations [22] as well as deriving biomechanical properties of the vessel wall [5, 6]. For the second case, a data assimilation framework could be designed to estimate the mechanical parameters of a computational model of the cerebral aneurysm wall based on these measurements. Kroon et al. [45] used this strategy on idealized spherical and axisymmetric aneurysm geometries. In Balocco et al. [5,6], we incorporated geometrical information provided by *in vivo* imaging data to study the feasibility of estimating regional mechanical properties of cerebral aneurysms. The deformation field capturing aneurysm wall pulsation was obtained applying a registration technique to a pair of simulated MR images. A parametric biomechanical model generated the modeled aneurysm morphology in systole from: the diastolic morphology segmented from subject-specific images and a set of boundary conditions. The structural mechanics behavior of the model was controlled by regional elasticity parameters, which were initialized with values based on *ex vivo* experiments available in the literature. Subsequently, these parameters were optimized at the inverse problem stage to minimize the difference between the two aneurysm morphologies in systole: the one given by the biomechanical model; and the one generated from applying the deformation field capturing the aneurysm wall pulsation to the diastolic morphology. A local pressure distribution that was estimated with computational fluid-dynamics was introduced into the structural mechanics as an additional constraint.

Several *in silico* experiments tested the robustness of the proposed data assimilation framework. The workflow proved to be robust with respect to several input geometries. Increasing the number of regions with different elasticity in the aneurysm moderately decreased the performance. The choice of the registration configuration had a substantial effect on the recovered stiffness distribution and estimated values depending on the associated number of degrees of freedom.

Finally, according to our *in silico* experiments, 0.1 mm was the minimum image resolution required for the proposed data assimilation framework to distinguish aneurysm regions with different mechanical properties, as illustrated in Fig. 5. These findings were in agreement with results obtained by [78] where we concluded that cerebral aneurysm wall pulsation could be recovered from registration techniques applied on volumes reconstructed from projections having an isotropic spatial resolution of 0.155 mm.

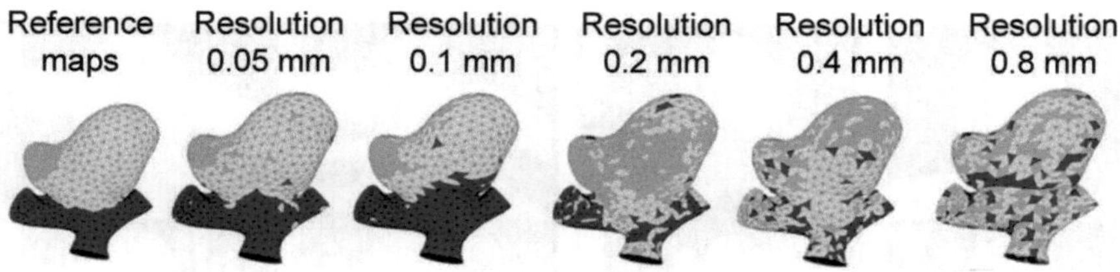

Fig. 5 Stiffness distribution results obtained with different image resolution (from *left* to *right*: reference maps, 0.05, 0.1, 0.2, 0.4, and 0.8 mm). The different clusters correspond to the vessel, the dome, and the bleb regions (respectively in dark grey, light grey and medium grey)

7 Computational Hemodynamic Analysis: From Anatomical Models to Personalized Flow Descriptors

CHD requires proper patient-specific boundary conditions specification in terms of flow rate or pressure to solve the governing equations. These flow boundary conditions can be obtained from phase-contrast magnetic resonance images for the main branches of the circle of Willis. Nevertheless, since patient-specific measurements are seldom available, reference data obtained from normal volunteers [1, 26] or 1D/0D lumped parameter models [7, 57] are often employed instead. To model the blood flow in cerebral aneurysms the assumptions of incompressible, laminar flow and Newtonian/non-Newtonian fluid in the rigid/compliant vessel walls are commonly used and accepted within the community [14].

In order to introduce these techniques into routine clinical practice, validation against ground truth *in vivo* flow measurements is mandatory. Because such data can not possibly be obtained with the technology available nowadays, different alternatives have been proposed. A number of authors have compared simulation results with experimental flow measurements in idealized phantoms [33] and anatomically realistic replicas [27]. Another alternative corresponds to the comparison of simulation results with gross hemodynamical features obtained with routine image modalities. In particular, [15] compared the isovelocity surfaces extracted from the hemodynamic simulation to isointensity surfaces in TOF-MRA images obtained by [65]. They found a good agreement in the aneurysmal inflow region.

In two separate works, Ford et al. [28] and Calamante et al. [12] presented a strategy to simulate the transport of the contrast agent in cerebral vasculature and produced visualizations which reproduce conventional angiography. This technique, named virtual angiography, allows a direct qualitative comparison of simulation results with high frame rate angiographic images routinely acquired during treatment. We believe that the use of such visualization techniques [17, 28] will play an important role in the clinical acceptance of CHD in the clinical practice.

One major strength of the proposed modeling pipeline is its applicability to the variety of image modalities used throughout the patient care cycle. Recently, Geers et al. [30] studied the differences between vascular models derived from 3DRA and CTA and the subsequent differences in the hemodynamic simulations. Four

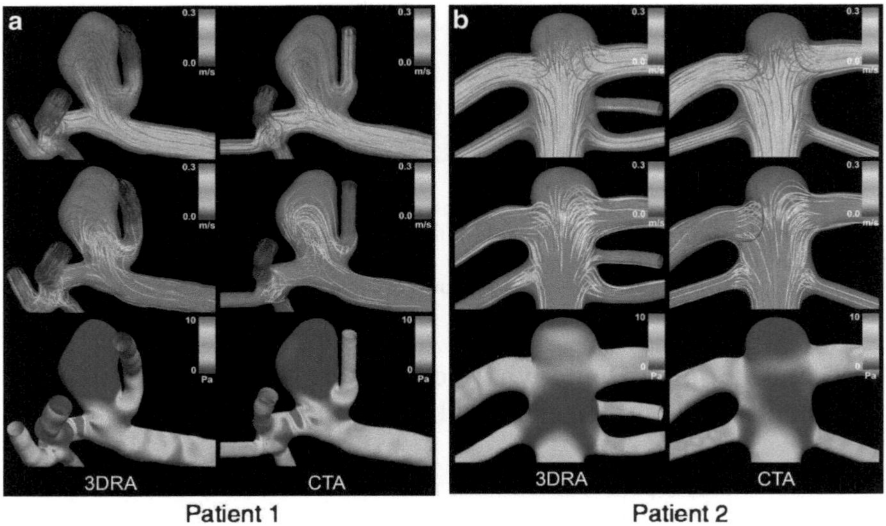

Fig. 6 Two patient-specific vascular models extracted from 3DRA and CTA. Streamlines color-coded by the velocity magnitude visualize the flow field at peak systole and end diastole (*top* and *middle* rows respectively) and the distribution of the time-averaged wall shear stress magnitude is visualized with a contour plot (*bottom* row)

aneurysms on the middle cerebral artery M1-M2 bifurcation (Fig. 6) were imaged within a one-day time interval with both 3DRA and CTA. For both image modalities a hemodynamic model of each aneurysm was created. The lower contrast and spatial resolution of CTA gave rise to differences in the vascular models. On the one hand, the segmentation algorithm had more difficulties to separate vascular structures that were close to each other. As a result, the aneurysm neck appeared to be wider, which altered the flow rate into the aneurysm as well as other hemodynamic variables. On the other hand, contrast values of small vessels of less than 1mm in diameter were more blurred and the segmentation algorithm failed to recognize them. This often produced a higher flow rate in the parent vessel and, therefore, in the aneurysm. Overall, quantitative hemodynamic measurements did give substantially different results (in some cases up to a 40%), but qualitatively the main flow characteristics were found to be well-reproduced between the 3DRA- and CTA-based simulations.

8 Endovascular Device Modeling: From Anatomical Models to Treatment Assessment

The ultimate purpose when treating an aneurysm is to exclude it from the circulation while returning the blood flow in the parent vessel to normal physiological conditions. Among the multiple techniques pursuing this objective, coiling [31] and

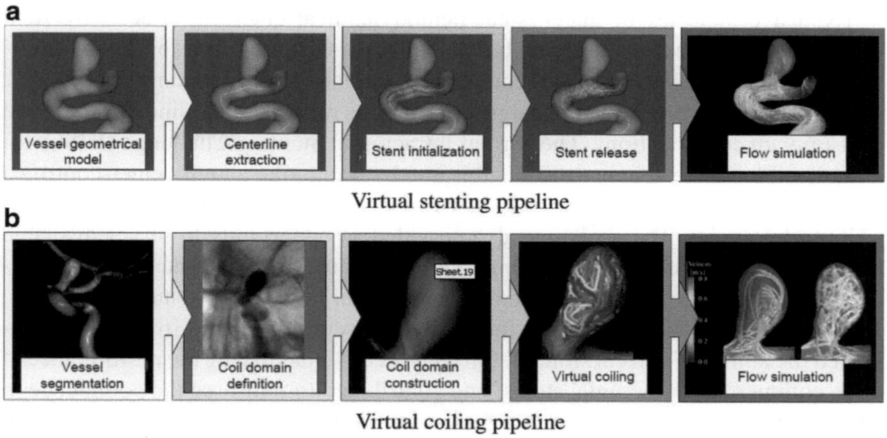

Fig. 7 Endovascular device modeling pipelines to virtually simulate stenting and coiling interventions

stenting [11, 50] have become the preferred options over the traditional surgical clipping. In this section, we propose two methodologies to simulate *in silico* the release of stents (Fig. 7a) and coils (Fig. 7b) during a virtual aneurysm embolization intervention.

8.1 Virtual Stenting

The presence of vascular stents in aneurysmatic vessels has been modeled in the past [16]. Larrabide et al. [46, 47] proposed a methodology for virtual stent deployment based on constrained deformable simplex models called Fast Virtual Stenting (FVS). This work extended the method proposed by Delingette [21]. In this approach, a second order differential equation was used to deform a simplex mesh under the effect of physical constraints such as stent mesh design, size, and radius. These parameters were selected because they are relatively easy to obtain and are sufficient to describe the global stent geometry when the detailed structural behavior of the device is not of interest. This technique effectively embeds the geometrical properties of the stent and achieves favorable execution times in the order of one minute. In the recent work of [25] we developed FVS and Finite Element (FE) models for a commercial stent and compared the results after stent release. A series of parametric vascular models were designed varying stent diameter, vessel and aneurysm neck sizes where the stents where deployed. Results show good agreement between the two methodologies accompanied by a significant reduction (1000:1) in the computational cost of FVS.

Extensive analyses of aneurysmal hemodynamical changes induced by stent deployment have been provided by both in vitro and CHD studies [16]. These observations suggest the importance of considering patient-specific anatomy to assess the performance of a specific stent design and study its relation with clinical events and post-implant complications. The Virtual Intracranial Stenting Challenge (VISC) international initiative sought fulfilling this aim by promoting a multicenter-controled benchmark to analyze differences induced by diverse grid generation methods and CHD technologies. The challenge also provided an opportunity to survey available technologies currently adopted by international teams from both academic and industrial institutions for constructing computational models of stented aneurysms. The results of the 2007 edition of the challenge were reported in [61] and demonstrated the ability of current strategies in consistently quantifying the performance of three commercial intracranial stents, and contributed to reinforce the confidence in CHD simulations, thus taking a step forward towards the introduction of simulation tools to support diagnostics and interventional planning.

Several computational hemodynamic studies have been carried out to clarify the effect of stents on aneurysmal flow [16, 43, 48, 71]. These studies concluded that the flow in an aneurysm treated with stents is influenced by multiple factors of the stent geometry such as strut size, and stent porosity. To study the impact of the stent positioning, we investigated the influence of stenting with various axial orientations on saccular aneurysm hemodynamics [42]. Two commercial stents (stent 1 and stent 2) were modeled in this study: a Neuroform stent (Boston Scientific, Natick, MA) and a Zilver stent (Cook medical Inc., Bloomington, IN). Both stents were virtually released using the FVS algorithm in four different axial orientations to fit into the luminal surface of a patient-specific internal carotid artery model with a lateral aneurysm. Computational hemodynamic analyses were carried out for the unstented and stented aneurysm models (Fig. 8). The intra-aneurysmal flow for stented models show disturbed and complex flow patterns while the flow activity and the forces acting on the aneurysm wall are generally alleviated. The influence of the axial orientation of the stent on the aneurysm hemodynamics is more significant for stent 2 which has a larger strut size compared to stent 1. Interestingly, the flow activity in the aneurysm is rather increased when the intra-luminal scaffolding of the stent is not sufficient.

The combined use of CHD and virtual stenting techniques provides a feasible mean to investigate the stent induced hemodynamic alterations in patient-specific aneurysm models, not only facilitating the personalized selection of an optimal stent before intervention, but also providing tools to medical device companies for exploring new designs.

8.2 Virtual Coiling

Performing CHD analyses for a patient-specific aneurysm treated with coils is not a trivial task, mainly due to the complexity and quasi-random distribution of the coil

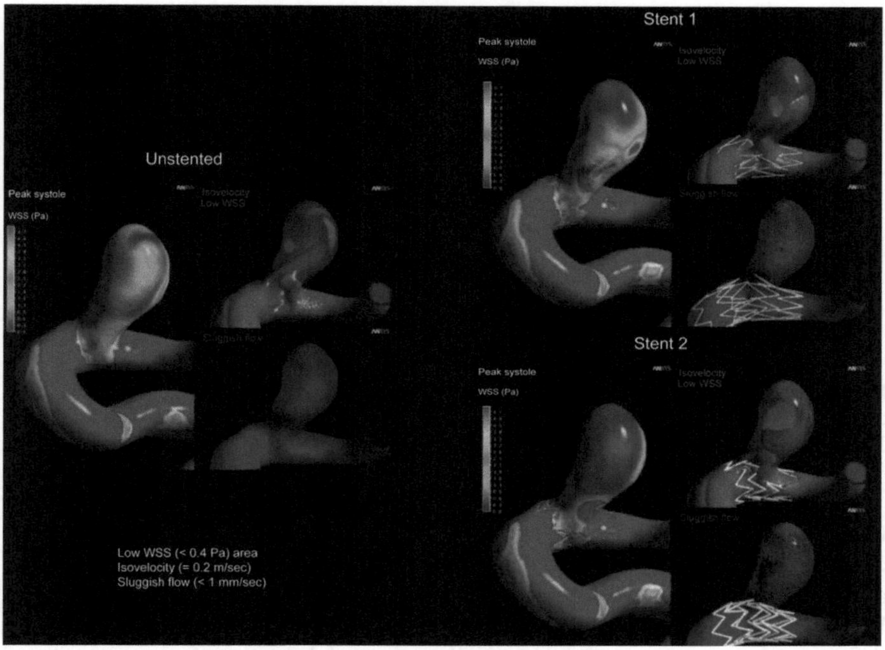

Fig. 8 Influence on WSS, iso-velocity contour (0.2 mm/s), low WSS areas (<0.4 Pa), and sluggish flow (velocity <1 mm/s) at the peak systole. It can be observed that for the unstented geometry, the flow enters much stronger into the aneurysm (iso-velocity) and there are no visible regions of sluggish flow. On the contrary, after the stent is implanted, the flow inside the aneurysm region is drastically changed. For stent 1, it can be observed the flow impingement is located on the lateral side (while it was on the distal side before the implantation of the device). For stent 2, large areas of low WSS are observed together with larger continuous regions of sluggish flow

mesh, as well as the small diameter of the coil wires [75]. Some of these difficulties have been tackled with the assumption of a homogenous and isotropic porous media [37, 39] that models the presence of the devices inside the aneurysm. Other approaches [16, 54] have provided explicit models of the coils but have not been able to achieve realistic coil packing rates [68, 75].

In Morales et al. [53], we proposed a method to create explicit models of endovascular coils using 3D medical images and treatment information able to provide realistic coil configurations and packing rates. The method advances the coil tip while minimizing the influence of a potential energy associated to the vessel wall boundaries and the previously released coils within the aneurysm domain. Additionally, the coil is allowed to retreat and advance in a different direction when a dead-end is found. As a result, the method was able to achieve clinical coil packing rates as performed with bare coils.

The influence of the coil packing rate and coil configuration (distribution and structure of the released coils) was evaluated for an internal carotid aneurysm in terms of its intra-aneurysmal hemodynamics. The model was virtually coiled with

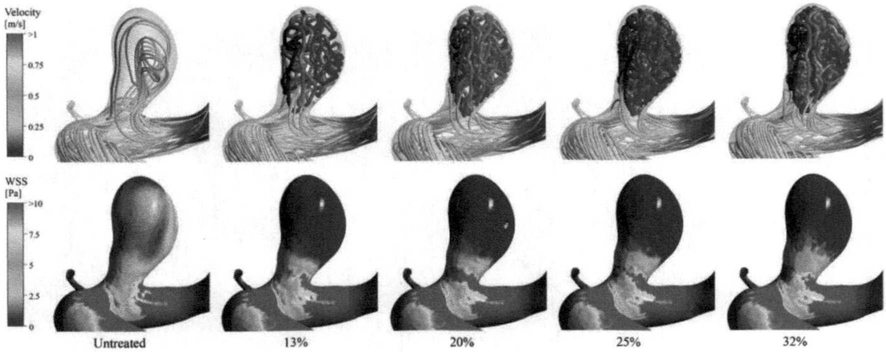

Fig. 9 Virtual release of coils with different packing rates (13, 20, 25, and 32%) vs. the untreated case. The released coils are shown in grey in the *top row* together with the velocity streamlines. The *bottom row* shows the reduction in WSS on the aneurysm dome for each coil packing rate

four packing rates (13, 20, 25, and 32%), each one of them with three different coil configurations. CHD analyses were performed both in the untreated and treated aneurysm models (Fig. 9). The results revealed that aneurysmal flow velocity and WSS were reduced by coiling even for low packing rates. Also, we observed that WSS near the aneurysm ostium drastically increased due to interference introduced by the coils. Finally, we found that the hemodynamic differences due to coil configurations were negligible when the coil packing rate was high (above 20%) which is in agreement with previous clinical findings [59]. Thus, we concluded that the virtual coiling technique has the potential to become a valid tool to *a priori* assess the post-treatment aneurysm hemodynamics.

9 Discussion

This work has proposed an image- and biomechanics-based computational modeling data processing pipeline for the advanced and personalized management of cerebral aneurysms. Patient-specific vascular models are created and used to derive a collection of complex descriptors. These morphological, morphodynamic, hemodynamic and structural descriptors have been selected as key representatives of the physical properties and biomechanical mechanisms thought to play a role in the natural history of cerebral aneurysms. The pipeline integrates them into a single workflow that also includes the modeling and release of virtual devices.

The main strength and contribution of this pipeline is that it provides a compact representation of the multifactorial nature of cerebral aneurysms even in presence of virtual endovascular devices, facilitating the selection of an optimal treatment for a specific patient as well as the design of endovascular devices. In terms of vascular anatomical modeling, this pipeline contributes an automatic and reproducible segmentation technique [8, 32]. The algorithm's accuracy has been evaluated against ground truth measurements performed by clinicians in MRA and 3DRA, and used to evaluate the sensitivity of hemodynamic simulations to the imaging modality (3DRA and CTA) [30]. The @neurIST project [55, 67] selected this method as its segmentation of choice. This project was an European initiative funded within the Sixth Framework Programme Priority 2 of the Information Society Technologies IST [55, 67].

As for the morphological analysis, the real-time morphological characterization of aneurysms using their Zernike moment invariants [52,60] is robust and constitutes a first candidate to be used as a basis for the comparison of aneurysm morphological features to other previously treated aneurysms available in a database. A platform implementing this system would allow to support the clinical decision by providing similar aneurysms from which their clinical history and treatment outcome are known. Extending such similarity searches to include other complex descriptors such as the ones already computed by this pipeline should capture the heterogeneous nature of aneurysms.

Two morphodynamic analyses have been performed to quantify aneurysm morphological changes at two time scales: at patient follow-up or during one cardiac cycle. In the first case, the evolution of untreated and treated aneurysms is possible using images obtained at different patient follow-ups (months to years) by registering them into a common coordinate frame and by quantifying local and global volume changes at the aneurysm level [19, 20]. In the second, since vessel wall weakness is thought to be a surrogate of the risk of rupture, a plausible option has been proposed for the indirect *in vivo* estimation of aneurysm wall mechanical properties. In this direction, wall motion displacements [58, 77, 78] have been estimated from 3DRA and extensively validated with digital and silicone phantoms. The structural analysis uses measurements obtained from simulated MRA images together with flow and pressure measurements to optimize these vessel biomechanical properties using a data assimilation framework [6].

The combined use of CHD analyses with virtual endovascular devices modeling techniques allow to reproduce different treatment situations like the use of different stents [46,47] and coils [53] at low computational cost. Evaluation of the variability in the stent positioning within the vessel [42] have shown to have strong implications in the device design. As demonstrated in the VISC 07 Challenge [61], hemodynamics studies in presence of a stent were reproducible, even when developed by distributed teams. The combination of device models with blood clotting and cellular models capturing the vessel wall physiological behavior, should allow in the future a further assessment of the patient evolution after treatment.

Multiple challenges need to be sorted out in order to integrate this pipeline into a clinical routine workflow, for the diagnosis and prognosis of the disease as well as for the prototyping of more effective medical devices. The most important one is its validation, which needs to be guaranteed at the technical and clinical acceptance levels. Aspects such as repeatability, accuracy, reproducibility, robustness and sensitivity need to be evaluated first for each of the individual components as well as for the complete pipeline. At the clinical level, multi-centric trials should demonstrate sufficient predictive power to justify their adoption. During the design of the present pipeline, a special attention has been paid on the validation of its various components, particularly focusing on assessing the accuracy, the reproducibility and the repeatability of the results where appropriate either by using digital phantoms [6, 77, 78], physical phantoms [77, 78] and/or manual measurements [32, 61]. Some of the components were also evaluated as part of the patient-specific image-based simulation pipeline developed under the umbrella of the @neurIST project [67].

A second challenge is the availability of human and computational resources to perform and exploit the outcomes of these analyses. Creating representative anatomical and physiological models still requires a reduced amount of operator's manual intervention. Decreasing and quantifying the impact of such manipulations should be feasible by establishing operators evaluation metrics, improving their training, increasing the usability and level of automation of the tools to ensure smooth transitions between the analyses. Interpreting the results of this pipeline is not trivial and also demands the presence of highly skilled operators. This is expected to improve in the midterm by the creation of intuitive decision support systems that would automatically trigger alarms when a dangerous combination of clinical events is identified.

Computational costs are still nowadays an issue for some of the stages involved in this pipeline. Currently, efforts are directed towards the better use of computational resources by exploiting GPU computing power in personal computers [79], or by externalizing the computational load to clusters using grid or cloud computing techniques. Once large clinical trials aiming at the validation of such a pipeline are started, massive data storage resources will be needed for images, clinical records and computed derived descriptors. This will require advanced IT infrastructures to provide connectivity to distributed databases enabling the use of data mining techniques to investigate the posed clinical hypotheses.

The presented effort is framed in the context of the Virtual Physiological Human (VPH) Initiative [74]. On the one hand, all our current scientific and technical efforts aim at extending the present pipeline along the lines supporting the VPH vision, which aims at progressing towards a comprehensive and integrated view of human physiology that enables the delivery of sound diagnostic and prognostic decisions in health care management. On the other hand, the VPH initiative provides the framework that allows all these tools to converge, maximizing its impact on industry, as well as on the scientific and clinical communities. The existence of appropriate IT infrastructures should allow collecting data in a rational manner and establishing links with a broader scientific community. The European project @neurIST is an example of this integration, where image-derived morphological, hemodynamical and structural descriptors are also combined and cross-linked with clinical and genetic information underpinned and enabled through advanced IT infrastructures for data sharing and efficient reuse of computational resources [3, 4, 23, 29, 34].

Acknowledgements This work was partially supported by the @neurIST Integrated Project (co-financed by the European Commission through the contract no. IST-027703), the CDTI CENIT-CDTEAM grant funded by the Spanish Ministry of Science and Innovation (MICINN-CDTI) and Philips Healthcare (Best, The Netherlands). The authors would also like to thank the support provided by ANSYS Inc. (Canonsburg, PA, USA).

References

1. Alastruey, J., Parker, K., Peiró, J., Byrd, S., Sherwin, S.: Modelling the circle of Willis to assess the effects of anatomical variations and occlusions on cerebral flows. J. Biomech. **40**(8), 1794–1805 (2007)
2. Antiga, L., Piccinelli, M., Botti, L., Ene-Iordache, B., Remuzzi, A., Steinman, D.: An image-based modeling framework for patient-specific computational hemodynamics. Med. Biol. Eng. Comput. **46**(11), 1097–1112 (2008)
3. Arbona, A., Benkner, S., Engelbrecht, G., Fingberg, J., Hofmann, M., Kumpf, K., Lonsdale, G., Woehrer, A.: A service-oriented grid infrastructure for biomedical data and compute services. IEEE Transactions on NanoBioscience **6**(2), 136–141 (2007)
4. Arbona, A., Benkner, S., Fingberg, J., Frangi, A.F., Hofmann, M., Hose, D.R., Lonsdale, G., Ruefenacht, D., Viceconti, M.: Outlook for grid service technologies within the @neurIST eHealth environment. Stud. Health. Technol. Informat. **120**, 401–404 (2006)
5. Balocco, S., Camara, O., Frangi, A.F.: Towards regional elastography of intracranial aneurysms. In: Medical Image Computing and Computer-Assisted Intervention – MICCAI. Lecture Notes on Computer Science, vol. 5242, pp. 131–138. Springer, Berlin, Heidelberg, New York, USA (2008)
6. Balocco, S., Camara, O., Vivas, E., Sola, T., Guimaraens, L., Gratama van Adel, H., Majoie, C., Pozo, J., Bijnens, B.H., Frangi, A.F.: Feasibility of estimating regional mechanical properties of cerebral aneurysms in vivo. Med. Phys. **37**, 1689–1706 (2010)
7. Blanco, P.J., Feijóo, R.A., Urquiza, S.A.: A unified variational approach for coupling 3D-1D models and its blood flow applications. Comput. Meth. Appl. Math. **196**(41–44), 4391–4410 (2007)
8. Bogunović, H., Radaelli, A., De Craene, M., Delgado, D., Frangi, A.F.: Image intensity standardization in 3D rotational angiography and its application to vascular segmentation. In: SPIE Medical Imaging 2008: Image Processing, vol. 6914, p. 691419 (2008)
9. Boussel, L., Rayz, V., McCulloch, C., Martin, A., Acevedo-Bolton, G., Lawton, M., Higashida, R., Smith, W.S., Young, W.L., Saloner, D.: Aneurysm growth occurs at region of low wall shear stress: Patient-specific correlation of hemodynamics and growth in a longitudinal study. Stroke **39**(11), 2997–3002 (2008)
10. Brisman, J., Song, J., Newell, D.: Medical progress: cerebral aneurysms. New Engl. J. Med. **355**(9), 928–939 (2006)
11. Brisman, J., Song, J., Niimi, Y., Berenstein, A.: Treatment options for wide-necked intracranial aneurysms using a self-expandable hydrophilic coil and a self-expandable stent combination. Am. J. Neuroradiol. **26**(5), 1237–1240 (2005)
12. Calamante, F., Yim, P., Cebral, J.R.: Estimation of bolus dispersion effects in perfusion MRI using image-based computational fluid dynamics. Neuroimage **19**(2), 341–353 (2003)
13. Castro, M.A., Putman, C.M., Cebral, J.R.: Patient-specific computational modeling of cerebral aneurysms with multiple avenues of flow from 3D rotational angiography images. Acad. Radiol. **13**(7), 811–821 (2006)
14. Cebral, J.R., Castro, M.A., Appanaboyina, S., Putman, C.M., Millan, D., Frangi, A.F.: Efficient pipeline for image-based patient-specific analysis of cerebral aneurysm hemodynamics: technique and sensitivity. IEEE Trans. Med. Imag. **24**(4), 457–467 (2005)
15. Cebral, J.R., Castro, M.A., Satoh, T., Burgess, J.: Evaluation of image-based CFD models of cerebral aneurysm using MRI. In: ISMRM Flow Motion Workshop, Zurich, Switzerland, pp. 11–13 (2004)
16. Cebral, J.R., Löhner, R.: Efficient simulation of blood flow past complex endovascular devices using an adaptive embedding technique. IEEE Trans. Med. Imag. **24**(4), 468–476 (2005)
17. Cebral, J.R., Pergolizzi, R., Putman, C.M.: Computational fluid dynamics modeling of intracranial aneurysms: qualitatively comparison with cerebral angiography. Acad. Radiol. **14**(7), 804–813 (2007)
18. Chang, H.H., Duckwiler, G.R., Valentino, D.J., Chu, W.C.: Computer-assisted extraction of intracranial aneurysms on 3D rotational angiograms for computational fluid dynamics modeling. Med. Phys. **36**(12), 5612–5621 (2009)

19. De Craene, M., Camara, O., Bijnens, B.H., Frangi, A.F.: Non-stationary diffeomorphic registration: application to endovascular treatment monitoring. In: SPIE Medical Imaging 2009: Image Processing, vol. 7259, p. 72591F (2009)
20. De Craene, M., Pozo, J.M., Villa-Uriol, M.C., Vivas, E., Sola, T., Guimaraens, L., Blasco, J., Macho, J., Frangi, A.F.: Coil compaction and aneurysm growth: image-based quantification using non-rigid registration. In: SPIE Medical Imaging 2008: Computer-Aided Diagnosis, vol. 6915, p. 69151R (2008)
21. Delingette, H.: General object reconstruction based on simplex meshes. Int. J. Comput. Vis. **32**(2), 111–146 (1999)
22. Dempere-Marco, L., Oubel, E., Castro, M.A., Putman, C.M., Millan, R.D., Frangi, A.F.: CFD analysis incorporating the influence of wall motion: application to intracranial aneurysms. In: Medical Image Computing and Computer-Assisted Intervention – MICCAI, Lecture Notes on Computer Science, vol. 4191, pp. 438–445. Springer, Berlin, Heidelberg, New York, USA (2006)
23. Dunlop, R., Arbona, A., Rajasekaran, H., Lo Iacono, L., Fingberg, J., Summers, P., Benkner, S., Engelbrecht, G., Chiarini, A., Friedrich, C., Moore, B., Bijlenga, P., Iavindrasana, J., Hose, R., Frangi, A.F.: @neurIST – Chronic disease management through integration of heterogeneous data and computer-interpretable guideline services. Stud. Health. Technol. Inform. **138**, 173–177 (2008)
24. Fenner, J., Brook, B., Clapworthy, G., Coveney, P., Feipel, V., Gregersen, H., Hose, D., Kohl, P., Lawford, P., McCormack, K., Pinney, D., Thomas, S., Van Sint Jan, S., Waters, S., Viceconti, M.: The EuroPhysiome, STEP and a roadmap for the virtual physiological human. Proc. R. Soc. A **366**(1878), 2979–2999 (2008)
25. Flore, E., Larrabide, I., Petrini, L., Pennati, G., Frangi, A.F.: Stent deployment in aneurysmatic cerebral vessels: Assessment and quantification of the differences between Fast Virtual Stenting and Finite Element Analysis. In: CI2BM09 – MICCAI Workshop on Cardiovascular Interventional Imaging and Biophysical Modelling, vol. 5242, pp. 790–797, Springer, Berlin, Heidelberg, London (2009)
26. Ford, M.D., Alperin, N., Lee, S., Holdsworth, D., Steinman, D.: Characterization of volumetric flow rate waveforms in the normal internal carotid and vertebral arteries. Physiol. Meas. **26**(4), 477–488 (2005)
27. Ford, M.D., Nikolov, H.N., Milner, J.S., Lownie, S.P., DeMont, E.M., Kalata, W., Loth, F., Holdsworth, D.W., Steinman, D.A.: PIV-measured versus CFD-predicted flow dynamics in anatomically realistic cerebral aneurysm models. J. Biomech. Eng. **130**(2), 021015 (2008)
28. Ford, M.D., Stuhne, G., Nikolov, H., Habets, D., Lownie, S., Holdsworth, D., Steinman, D.: Virtual angiography for visualization and validation of computational models of aneurysm hemodynamics. IEEE Trans. Med. Imag. **24**(12), 1586–1592 (2005)
29. Friedrich, C.M., Dach, H., Gattermayer, T., Engelbrecht, G., Benkner, S., Hofmann-Apitius, M.: @neuLink: a service-oriented application for biomedical knowledge discovery. Stud Health Technol Inform **138**, 165–172 (2008)
30. Geers, A., Larrabide, I., Radaelli, A.G., Bogunović, H., Gratama van Andel, H.A.F., Majoie, C.B., Frangi, A.F.: Reproducibility of image-based computational hemodynamics in intracranial aneurysms: comparison of CTA and 3DRA. In: IEEE Int. Symp. Biomed. Imag. pp. 610–613. IEEE Press, Piscataway, NJ, USA, Boston, MA, USA (2009)
31. Guglielmi, G., Viñuela, F., Dion, J., Duckwiler, G.: Electrothrombosis of saccular aneurysms via endovascular approach. Part 2: Preliminary clinical experience. J. Neurosurg. **75**(1), 8–14 (1991)
32. Hernandez, M., Frangi, A.F.: Non-parametric geodesic active regions: Method and evaluation for cerebral aneurysms segmentation in 3DRA and CTA. Med. Image Anal. **11**(3), 224–241 (2007)
33. Hoi, Y., Woodward, S., Kim, M., Taulbee, D., Meng, H.: Validation of CFD simulations of cerebral aneurysms with implication of geometric variations. J. Biomech. Eng. **128**(6), 844–851 (2006)
34. Iavindrasana, J., Lo Iacono, L., Müller, H., Periz, I., Summers, P., Wright, J., Friedrich, C., Dach, H., Gattermayer, T., Engelbrecht, G., Benkner, S., Hofmann-Apitius, M., Dunlop, R.,

Arbona, A., Rajasekaran, H., Fingberg, J., Chiarini, A., Moore, B., Bijlenga, P., Hose, R., Frangi, A.F.: The @neurIST project. Stud. Health Technol. Informat. **138**, 161–164 (2008)
35. Ishida, F., Ogawa, H., Simizu, T., Kojima, T., Taki, W.: Visualizing the dynamics of cerebral aneurysms with four-dimensional computed tomographic angiography. Neurosurgery **57**(3), 460–471 (2005)
36. Jou, L.D., Quick, C.M., Young, W.L., Lawton, M.T., Higashida, R.T., Martin, A., Saloner, D.: Computational approach to quantifying hemodynamic forces in giant cerebral aneurysms. Am. J. Neuroradiol. **24**(9), 1804–1810 (2003)
37. Jou, L.D., Saloner, D., Higashida, R.: Determining intra-aneurysmal flow for coiled cerebral aneurysm with digital fluoroscopy. Biomed. Eng. Appl. Basis Comm. **16**(2), 43–48 (2004)
38. Juvela, S.: Prehemorrhage risk factors for fatal intracranial aneurysm rupture. Stroke **34**(8), 1852–1858 (2003)
39. Kakalis, N.M., Mitsos, A.P., Byrne, J.V., Ventikos, Y.: The haemodynamics of endovascular aneurysm treatment: a computational modelling approach for estimating the influence of multiple coil deployment. IEEE Trans. Med. Imag. **27**(6), 814–824 (2008)
40. Kataoka, K., Taneda, M., Asai, T., Kinoshita, A., Ito, M., Kuroda, R.: Structural fragility and inflammatory response of ruptured cerebral aneurysms. A comparative study between ruptured and unruptured cerebral aneurysms. Stroke **30**(7), 1396–1401 (1999)
41. Kayembe, K., Sasahara, M., Hazama, F.: Cerebral aneurysms and variations in the circle of Willis. Stroke **15**(5), 846–850 (1984)
42. Kim, M., Larrabide, I., Villa-Uriol, M.C., Frangi, A.F.: Hemodynamic alterations of a patient-specific intracranial aneurysm induced by virtual deployment of stents in various axial orientation. In: IEEE International Symposium on Biomedical Imaging, pp. 1215–1218. IEEE Press, Piscataway, NJ, USA, Boston, MA, USA (2009)
43. Kim, M., Taulbee, D., Tremmel, M., Meng, H.: Comparison of two stents in modifying cerebral aneurysm hemodynamics. Ann. Biomed. Eng., **36**, 726–741 (2008)
44. Krings, T., Willems, P., Barfett, J., Ellis, M., Hinojosa, N., Blobel, J., Geibprasert, S.: Pulsatility of an intracavernous aneurysm demonstrated by dynamic 320-detector row CTA at high temporal resolution. Cent. Eur. Neurosurg. **70**, 214–218 (2009)
45. Kroon, M., Holzapfel, G.A.: Estimation of the distributions of anisotropic, elastic properties and wall stresses of saccular cerebral aneurysms by inverse analysis. Proc. R. Soc. A **464**(2092), 807–825 (2008)
46. Larrabide, I., Kim, M., Augsburger, L., Villa-Uriol, M., Rüfenacht, D., Frangi, A.: Fast virtual deployment of self-expandable stents: Method and in-vitro validation for intracranial aneurysmal stenting. Med. Image Anal. doi:10.1016/j.media.2010.04.009. http://www.sciencedirect.com/science?_ob=ArticleURL&_udi=B6W6Y-50297P9-1&_user=1517318&_coverDate=05%2F11%2F2010&_rdoc=1&_fmt=high&_orig=search&_origin=search&_sort=d&_docanchor=&view=c&_acct=C000053451&_version=1&_urlVersion=0&_userid=1517318&md5=5d3dad8469974f524b33d553ffa8aa13&searchtype=a (2010)
47. Larrabide, I., Radaelli, A.G., Frangi, A.F.: Fast virtual stenting with deformable meshes: Application to intracranial aneurysms. In: Medical Image Computing and Computer-Assisted Intervention – MICCAI, Lecture Notes in Computer Science, vol. 5242, pp. 790–797. Springer, Berlin, Heidelberg, New York, USA (2008)
48. Liou, T.M., Li, Y.C.: Effects of stent porosity on hemodynamics in a sidewall aneurysm model. J. Biomech. Eng. **41**(6), 1174–1183 (2008)
49. Lo, C., Don, H.: 3-D moments forms: Their construction and application to object identification and positioning. IEEE Trans. Pattern. Anal. Mach. Intell. **11**(10), 1053–1064 (1989)
50. Lylyk, P., Ferrario, A., Pasbon, B., Miranda, C., Doroszuk, G.: Buenos Aires experience with the Neuroform self-expanding stent for the treatment of intracranial aneurysms. J. Neurosurg. **102**(2), 235–241 (2005)
51. Ma, B., Harbaugh, R.E., Raghavan, M.L.: Three-dimensional geometrical characterization of cerebral aneurysms. Ann. Biomed. Eng. **32**(2), 264–273 (2004)
52. Millan, R., Dempere-Marco, L., Pozo, J.M., Cebral, J.R., Frangi, A.F.: Morphological characterization of intracranial aneurysms using 3-D moment invariants. IEEE Trans. Med. Imag. **26**(9), 1270–1282 (2007)

53. Morales, H., Kim, M., Villa-Uriol, M.C., Vivas, E., Frangi, A.F.: Influence of coil packing rate and configuration on intracranial aneurysm hemodynamics. In: Dössel, O., Schlegel, W.C. (eds.) 11th International Congress of the IUPESM, Medical Physics and Biomedical Engineering, World Congress 2009, IFMBE Proceedings, vol. 25/4, pp. 2291–2294. Springer, Berlin, Heidelberg, Munich, Germany (2009)
54. Narracott, A., Smith, S., Lawford, P., Liu, H., Himeno, R., Wilkinson, I., Griffiths, P., Hose, R.: Development and validation of models for the investigation of blood clotting in idealized stenoses and cerebral aneurysms. J. Artif. Organs **8**, 56–62 (2005)
55. @neurIST Consortium (2010) Integrated biomedical informatics for the management of cerebral aneurysms. http://www.aneurist.org
56. Novotni, M., Klein, R.: Shape retrieval using 3D Zernike descriptors. Comput. Aided Des. **36**, 1047–1062 (2004)
57. Olufsen, M.S., Nadim, A., Lipsitz, L.A.: Dynamics of cerebral blood flow regulation explained using a lumped parameter model. Am. J. Physiol., Reg. Int. Comp. Physiol. **282**, R611–R622 (2002)
58. Oubel, E., De Craene, M., Putman, C.M., Cebral, J.R., Frangi, A.F.: Analysis of intracranial aneurysm wall motion and its effects on hemodynamic patterns. In: SPIE Medical Imaging: Physics of Medical Imaging Image Reconstruction, vol. 6511, p. 65112A (2007)
59. Piotin, M., Mandai, S., Murphy, K.J., Sugiu, K., Gailloud, P., Martin, J.B., Rüfenacht, D.A.: Dense packing of cerebral aneurysms: an in vitro study with detachable platinum coils. Am. J. Neuroradiol. **21**, 757–760 (2000)
60. Pozo, J.M., Villa-Uriol, M., Frangi, A.F.: Efficient 3D Geometric and Zernike moments computation from unstructured surface meshes. IEEE Trans. Pattern. Anal. Mach. Intell. http://doi.ieeecomputersociety.org/10.1109/TPAMI.2010.139 April (2011)
61. Radaelli, A., Augsburger, L., Cebral, J., Ohta, M., Rüfenacht, D., Balossino, R., Benndorf, G., Hose, D., Marzo, A., Metcalfe, R., Mortier, P., Mut, F., Reymond, P., Socci, L., Verhegghe, B., Frangi, A.F.: Reproducibility of haemodynamical simulations in a subject-specific stented aneurysm model – A report on the Virtual Intracranial Stenting Challenge 2007. J. Biomech. **41**(10), 2069–2081 (2008)
62. Raghavan, M.L., Ma, B., Harbaugh, R.E.: Quantified aneurysm shape and aneurysm rupture. J. Neurosurg. **102**(2), 355–362 (2005)
63. Raymond, J., Guilbert, F., Weill, A., Georganos, S.A., Juravsky, L., Lambert, A., Lamoureux, J., Chagnon, M., Roy, D.: Long-term angiographic recurrences after selective endovascular treatment of aneurysms with detachable coils. Stroke **34**, 1398–1403 (2003)
64. Rohde, S., Lahmann, K., Beck, J., Nafe, R., Yan, B., Raabe, A., Berkefeld, J.: Fourier analysis of intracranial aneurysms: towards an objective and quantitative evaluation of the shape of aneurysms. Neuroradiology **47**, 121–126 (2005)
65. Satoh, T., Onoda, K., Tsuchimoto, S.: Visualization of intraaneurysmal flow patterns with transluminal flow images of 3D MR angiograms in conjunction with aneurysmal configurations. Am. J. Neuroradiol. **24**(7), 1436–1445 (2004)
66. Schievink, W.: Intracranial aneurysms. New Engl. J. Med. **336**, 28–41 (1997)
67. Singh, P., Marzo, A., Coley, S., Berti, G., Bijlenga, P., Lawford, P., Villa-Uriol M.C., Rüfenacht, D., McCormack, K., Frangi, A.F., Patel, U., Hose, D.R.: The role of computational fluid dynamics in the management of unruptured intracranial aneurysms: a clinicians' view. Comput. Intell. Neurosci. 2009(760364), 1–12 (2009)
68. Sluzewski, M., van Rooij, W.J., Slob, M.J., Bescós, J.O., Slump, C.H., Wijnalda, D.: Relation between aneurysm volume, packing, and compaction in 145 cerebral aneurysms treated with coils. Radiology **231**, 653–658 (2004)
69. Steinman, D., Milner, J., Norley, C., Lownie, S., Holdsworth, D.: Image-based computational simulation of flow dynamics in a giant intracranial aneurysm. Am. J. Neuroradiol. **24**, 559–566 (2003)
70. STEP Consortium (2007) Seeding the EuroPhysiome: A roadmap to the Virtual Physiological Human. http://www.europhysiome.org/roadmap
71. Stuhne, G.R., Steinman, D.A.: Finite-element modeling of the hemodynamics of stented aneurysms. J. Biomech. Eng. **126**(3), 382–387 (2004)

72. Taylor, C., Humphrey, J.: Open problems in computational vascular biomechanics: Hemodynamics and arterial wall mechanics. Comput. Meth. Appl. Mech. Eng. **198**, 3514–3523 (2009)
73. Ujiie, H., Tachibana, H., Hiramatsu, O., Hazel, A.L., Matsumoto, T., Ogasawara, Y., Nakajima, H., Hori, T., Takakura, K., Kajiya, F.: Effects of size and shape (aspect ratio) on the hemodynamics of saccular aneurysms: A possible index for surgical treatment of intracranial aneurysms. Neurosurgery **45**(1), 119–130 (1999)
74. Viceconti, M., Clapworthy, G., Van Sint Jan, S.: The Virtual Physiological Human – a European initiative for in silico human modelling –. J. Physiol. Sci. **58**(7), 441–447 (2008)
75. White, J.B., Ken, C.G., Cloft, H.J., Kallmes, D.F.: Coils in a nutshell: a review of coil physical properties. Am. J. Neuroradiol. **29**(7), 1242–1246 (2008)
76. Wiebers, D.: The international study of unruptured intracranial aneurysms investigators. Unruptured intracranial aneurysms: natural history, clinical outcome, and risks of surgical and endovascular treatment. Lancet **362**(9378), 103–110 (2003)
77. Zhang, C., De Craene, M., Villa-Uriol, M.C., Pozo, J.M., Bijnens, B.H., Frangi, A.F.: Estimating continuous 4D wall motion of cerebral aneurysms from 3D rotational angiography. In: Medical Image Computing and Computer-Assisted Intervention – MICCAI, Lecture Notes on Computer Science, vol. 5761, pp. 140–147. Springer, Berlin, Heidelberg, London, UK (2009)
78. Zhang, C., Villa-Uriol, M.C., De Craene, M., Pozo, J.M., Frangi, A.F.: Morphodynamic analysis of cerebral aneurysm pulsation from time-resolved rotational angiography. IEEE Trans. Med. Imag. **28**(7), 1105–1116 (2009)
79. Zhang, C., Villa-Uriol, M.C., Frangi, A.F.: Evaluation of an efficient GPU implementation of digitally reconstructed radiographs in 3D/2D image registration. In: SPIE Medical Imaging: Image Processing, p. 762333 (2010)

MIX
Papier aus verantwortungsvollen Quellen
Paper from responsible sources
FSC® C105338

If you have any concerns about our products,
you can contact us on
ProductSafety@springernature.com

In case Publisher is established outside the EU,
the EU authorized representative is:
Springer Nature Customer Service Center GmbH
Europaplatz 3, 69115 Heidelberg, Germany

Printed by Libri Plureos GmbH
in Hamburg, Germany